David Dary

FRONTIER MEDICINE

David Dary is the author of more than a dozen previous books including *The Buffalo Book, Cowboy Culture, Entrepreneurs of the Old West, Seeking Pleasure in the Old West, Red Blood and Black Ink, The Santa Fe Trail, The Oregon Trail,* and *True Tales of the Prairies and Plains.* He is the recipient of two Wrangler Awards from the National Cowboy and Western Heritage Museum, two Western Writers of America Spur Awards, the WWA's Owen Wister Award for lifetime achievement, the Westerners International Best Nonfiction Book Award, and the Oklahoma Center for the Book Arrell Gibson Award for lifetime achievement. *Frontier Medicine* won the Alvarez Award from the American Medical Writers Association. He lives in Norman, Oklahoma.

FRONTIER MEDICINE

FRONTIER
MEDICINE

FROM THE ATLANTIC TO
THE PACIFIC, 1492–1941

David Dary

Vintage Books
A Division of Random House, Inc.
New York

FIRST VINTAGE BOOKS EDITION, OCTOBER 2009

Copyright © 2008 by David Dary

All rights reserved. Published in the United States by Vintage Books,
a division of Random House, Inc., New York, and in Canada by Random House of
Canada Limited, Toronto. Originally published in hardcover in the United States by
Alfred A. Knopf, a division of Random House, Inc., New York, in 2008.

Vintage and colophon are registered trademarks of Random House, Inc.

The Library of Congress has cataloged the Knopf edition as follows:
Dary, David.
Frontier medicine : from the Atlantic to the Pacific, 1492–1941 / by David Dary.
—1st ed.
p. cm.
Includes bibliographical references and index.
1. Medicine—United States—History. I. Title.
[DNLM: 1. History of Medicine—United States.
2. History, Early Modern 1451–1600—United States.
3. History, Modern 1601—United States. WZ 70 AA1 D228F 2008]
R151.D37 2008
610.973—dc22 2008011407

Vintage ISBN: 978-0-307-45542-0

Author photograph © Ned Hockman
Book design by Robert C. Olsson

www.vintagebooks.com

Printed in the United States of America
10 9 8 7 6 5 4 3 2 1

CONTENTS

PREFACE

One day a cowboy in the Old West was asked how his workday had gone. He responded, "Well, I started up one canyon and came out another." The cowboy meant he'd started out in one direction but soon found he was going in another. So it was with this book.

When I embarked on the research, my focus was on medicine in the American West only during the nineteenth and early twentieth centuries. But it soon became evident that what can be considered the frontier period of American medicine began much earlier, with the arrival of the first Europeans during the sixteenth century, and did not really end until about 1941, just before U.S. entry into World War II. And a major part of this long story lies in the contribution of American Indians, whose herbal and psychological lore were combined by early European settlers with the medical theories and practices they brought with them. It is fair to say, in fact, that Indian medical knowledge is what gives early American medicine its particular character, and this rare combination becomes the true foundation for the growth and slow evolution of our practice of medicine, especially during the era of westward expansion following the American Revolution.

This book, then, is the story of that extended frontier period. It tells of the people involved and describes the contributions of Indians and of frontiersmen, explorers, and settlers of European origin, of mountain men, fur traders, immigrants bound for Oregon and California or the promised land of Utah, and soldiers from revolutionary times to beyond the Civil War and the Indian Wars that followed. Individual chapters tell the stories of each of these groups and discuss medicine on homesteads, on ranches, in towns, and in the picturesque and pris-

tine West that attracted health-seekers. Also included are stories about
midwives and other women who fought to break the barriers imposed
by male opposition to their entry into the field. There are also chapters
about patent medicines and quacks of every stripe. The book concludes with a chapter that sketches the significant changes that
occurred during the early twentieth century, when American medicine
moved steadily toward, and at last achieved, the status of a fully scientific enterprise.

In no way is this work definitive. It sketches in broad outline the
story of how medicine struggled, evolved, and ultimately emerged
from its frontier period. Certainly, the forces that have shaped it since
the Revolution still exist. But they have largely taken on different
forms in an atmosphere where scientific methods are now of greater
influence than the botanical medicine and the often primitive beliefs
and superstitions that once dominated the profession. Today's medicine, more subject to scientific practices, along with better education,
scholarship, and the development of standards, is responsible for
Americans living longer than their ancestors.

The history of frontier medicine in America between 1492 and
1941, as sketched between this book's covers, is important to the
understanding of the medicine of today and the changes that undoubtedly will continue to occur in the future. Medicine will change, and
perhaps it will someday bring good health to all American citizens.

David Dary
Along Imhoff Creek
Norman, Oklahoma

FRONTIER MEDICINE

INDIAN MEDICINE

Wisdom begins in wonder.

—Socrates

M AY IS A DELIGHTFUL TIME to visit the Wichita Mountains in southwestern Oklahoma. The little bluestem, the big bluestem, switch, Indian, and grama grasses are green after their winter sleep, and the wildflowers display a variety of colors. Groves of post oak, black-jack, and eastern red cedar dot the landscape. Countless birds, including rare black-capped vireos, search for nourishment. Everywhere there is a promise of nurture and it warms the soul, as do the warm and gentle breezes from the south. The Wichita Mountains are about 300 million years old, and among the oldest mountain ranges on earth. They consist of two rugged ranges of red granite reaching nearly 2,500 feet at the highest point. They run several miles east and west and enclose a natural prairie where buffalo, elk, prairie dogs, and other wildlife still roam in what is today the Wichita Mountains Wildlife Refuge administered by the U.S. Fish and Wildlife Service. While the Wichitas may lack the majesty of the Rocky Mountains, they are impressive islands projecting upward from a sea of rolling prairie.[1]

The Wichitas are rich in lore which includes legends of Indian battles and Spanish treasure. The Spanish penetrated the area in the 1600s, and French traders first traversed the region during the 1770s. Long before the first Europeans arrived, Indians found protection from their enemies in the Wichitas. They also found solace at what is called Medicine Bluff, located near the eastern edge of the mountains. The bluff rises three hundred feet above a creek whose waters were thought by Indians to have special qualities. Indians—Wichitas, Comanches, and Kiowas—most likely named the bluff in their native languages, designing it as a place of mystery with great spiritual pow-

ers. The first white men in the area named it Medicine Bluff after
learning of this Indian belief. The word *medicine* probably derived
from *médecin*, the French word for physician, which early French fur
traders would have introduced into North America. The term was
widely applied by whites. In time, Indians used the word to identify
their own healing methods and spiritual mysteries.

Medicine Bluff is just one of countless natural places with distinc-
tive features that Indians believed had special spiritual power because
they could not rationally explain why they existed. Such natural places
conveyed to them the essence of a religious experience but were not
actually worshipped. Not all things with spiritual power, to be sure,
were natural. Indians created smoking pipes, bundles, and other
objects that became sacred and powerful once the makers performed
special rituals to imbue them with qualities of sacredness or good medicine. For the American Indian, almost anything could attain such a
therapeutic or mystical quality, emphasizing how great a role spiritual
power plays in Indian medicine.

In "Letter Six" of his *Letters and Notes on the Manners, Customs, and
Conditions of North American Indians* (1844), the artist George Catlin
noted that "Indian country is full of doctors, and as they are all magi-

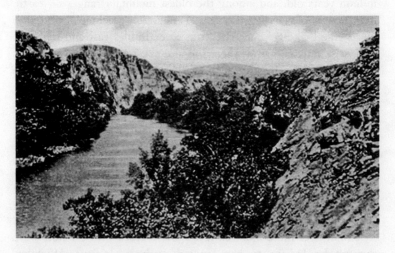

*This view of Medicine Bluff in the Wichita Mountains of southwestern Oklahoma was
copied from a mid-twentieth-century postcard. The bluff rises three hundred feet above
Medicine Creek. (Author's collection)*

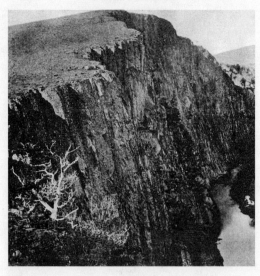

This close-up view of Medicine Bluff, with its three-hundred-foot drop to Medicine Creek (visible at lower right), was taken in the 1870s. (Courtesy Western History Collections, University of Oklahoma Libraries)

cians, and skilled, or profess to be skilled in many mysteries, the word 'medicine' has become habitually applied to every thing mysterious or unaccountable and the English and Americans . . . have easily and familiarly adopted the same word, with a slight alteration, conveying the same meaning; and to be a little more explicit, they have denominated these personages 'medicine-men,' which means something more than merely a doctor or physician."

Catlin related that every Plains Indian male has a medicine bag. When a boy is fourteen or fifteen, he leaves his father's lodge, locates a secluded spot, cries out to the Great Spirit, and fasts. At night, he sleeps on the ground. He may stay there from two to five days, or until he dreams of an animal, bird, or reptile in his sleep. He believes the first such creature to appear to him in a dream is his protector for life, so designated by the Great Spirit. The young Indian then returns to the lodge of his father, tells of his dream, breaks his fast, and leaves again to find and kill the animal, bird, or reptile in question. After killing it, he skins it and uses the full skin to fashion his medicine bag, which he stuffs with grass, or moss, or something of the kind. He then

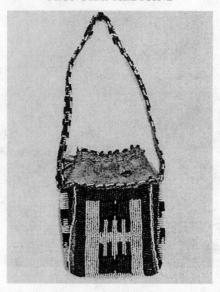

A Sioux Indian medicine bag, circa 1880. Constructed with a beaded sinew strap, the bag is made of tanned leather that has been braided. It measures ten inches high and three inches wide. (Author's collection)

closes it and will rarely open it again. He will carry the bag throughout his life, frequently paying homage to it and looking to it for safety and protection. Catlin saw medicine bags made from a variety of creatures, including otter, beaver, muskrat, weasel, raccoon, skunk, frog, toad, bat, mouse, mole, hawk, eagle, magpie, sparrow, and even a wolf. The size of the skin determines the size of the bag. When its owner dies, the medicine bag is placed with his remains.

Indians practiced their medicine long before Christopher Columbus arrived in 1492. Believing he had reached the Indies, Columbus called the natives Indians, a name that stuck. Since most native cultures in North America were exclusively oral, the recorded history of Indian medicine begins with the arrival of the Europeans and their written observations. One exception was the Aztecs in what is now Mexico, who did have written records. After the Spanish arrived in 1519, however, most of these records were destroyed with great zeal. The Spanish did express their amazement at the Aztecs' vast knowledge of

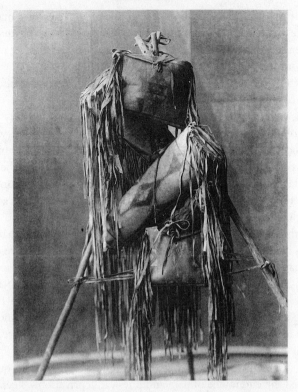

Edward S. Curtis (1868–1952) took this photo in 1910. It shows four Piegan fringed medicine bags hanging on a tripod. (Courtesy Library of Congress)

medicinal plants, and noted that their practice of medicine was an intrinsic part of their spiritual life.

At the time, Europeans used the word *medicine* to describe any substance, regimen, or physical procedure that had a beneficial effect on the human body and restored health, and they viewed medicine as separate from religion. Among Indians, however, their medicine encompassed much more. "While they used herbal remedies to treat simple physical conditions such as burns, broken bones, sore eyes, and dislocations, the majority of Indian medicine was used to cure conditions which had no obvious physical cause," writes one authority, Clara Sue Kidwell. "Symptoms included not only overt aches and pains, but could include what modern medicine might term neuroses, any behavior that was excessive or out of the ordinary. . . . Illness is a matter of balance and harmony with one's physical surroundings, spiritual environment, and social group. Thus, it goes far beyond mere physical symptoms. If one's balance is disturbed (witchcraft is a good example of how fear of an individual as a witch can have a disruptive effect in a group of people), illness results."[2]

Eric Stone, a Rhode Island physician, wrote in 1932 that Indian "mythology and theology are peculiarly rich and endowed with an unexpected symbolism and beauty, bespeaking an unusual ability to express their emotional and esthetic appreciation of their all-important physical environment. Their métier was not pictorial, but lay, on the one hand, in decorative design and, on the other, in a wealth of folklore and poetry."[3]

Anthropologists, ethnologists, and historians tell us that early Indian medicine was closely tied to their reverence for nature and its supernatural powers. Indians lived most of their lives out of doors, and nature charmed them, but, as Clara Sue Kidwell points out, "Nature is threatening as often as it is benevolent. Ceremonies were held to restore balance that had been disrupted, or to assure that balance continued and nature produced the results that the people desired. The natural environment of the Great Plains was a source of spiritual power for individuals through vision quests, but vision questing required the endurance of pain and physical deprivation—sleep, food, water. Going alone into special places where spirits were thought to make their presence known was a way of acquiring access to that power. Going alone into the environment could also be a source of illness if one encountered a spiritual being without proper preparation."[4]

In most tribes, the principal person overseeing such matters was a medicine man or sometimes a medicine woman. After the arrival of the Spanish in the Southwest, this person was often called a *curandero* (or *curandera*), but ethnologists have sometimes used the Asian term *shaman*, defined by Merriam-Webster as a priest or priestess who uses magic for curing the sick. Kidwell, however, points out that a shaman or medicine man's role is not just in healing, nor is it necessarily one of high prestige. The shaman or medicine man/woman supposedly had learned to control and use the spiritual power of nature. At the same time it followed for the people who believed in his or her powers that those powers might be used to do harm as well as to help. Moreover, Kidwell added that "being a shaman is also a dangerous position for the individual who must confront the power that is causing the illness and uses his or her power to exorcise it or bring it under control. If the curer's power weakens, the illness may affect him or her."[5]

Whatever their title, such individuals received what others believed was a vision or a deep spiritual insight into their patients. They never lost sight of the spiritual side of health and disease, realizing the power of the mind. Most were viewed as wise, as knowing the secrets of healing, and as visionaries who mastered death. They were thought to be able to go into a trance, leave their bodies, and visit unearthly kingdoms. Some were also poets and singers who danced and created works of art. Their medicine simply denoted a spiritual power used for many purposes including healing with natural herbs and plants.

The role of the shaman varied from tribe to tribe. The Harvard anthropologist Roland B. Dixon wrote in 1908 that in numerous instances the position of shaman descended by inheritance in either the male or the female line, depending upon the prevailing tribal system of descent. In most cases, it was mandatory that the person in line for the position accept it and the duties and responsibilities that went

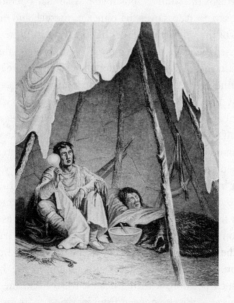

Artist Seth Eastman (1808–1875) depicts a Sioux medicine man (left) ministering to a patient. (Courtesy Library of Medicine)

with it. If the person refused to do so, Dixon said, tradition had it that spirits would punish him or her in the form of sickness or death.

In some tribes, young Indians wishing to possess medicine were severely tested. In 1858, Thomas Kennard described such a test as carried out among various tribes:

> At a certain period of each year, all young braves, who are ambitious to become great or medicine men, assemble and go through the horrible ordeal which is to render them immortal. . . . After three or four days of fasting, praying and privation, and after having witnessed all the mysterious movements of those advanced in the science, the ambitious young men present themselves for the last and most trying test of greatness. They enter the great medicine lodge, where the ceremonies have been celebrated for four days, and place themselves in a reclining position, when immediately the executioners commence their work, by pinching up an inch or two of the integument and pectoralis major muscle on each side, and thrusting a ragged knife through the flesh beneath the fingers; after which skewers are passed through the wounds thus made. A similar operation is performed in several places over the trapezius muscle, and often on the front part of the thigh, the leg or the forearm. To these skewers or sticks, passed beneath the integument and through the muscles, cords are attached, by means of which the candidates are raised clear of the ground, and left dangling until apparently dead, having fainted repeatedly. They are then lowered down and left without the slightest aid or comfort until reaction takes place, when heavy weights, such as buffalo heads, are attached to the skewers and kept dragging on the ground or suspended in the air as the poor sufferers are hurried from place to place, until they are torn loose by their own weight, or by being caught in some way as they madly rush over the plains around the encampment. The Sioux have even a more refined process of testing or torturing the ambitious than that just described as common to most North American Indians. They pass skewers through the pectoral muscles as above mentioned, and then fasten their victims to a strong sapling just stiff enough to raise them on tiptoe, in which position, with the head thrown back, they are compelled to gaze at the shining sun from its rising to its setting; and if one faints or falls whilst undergoing the trial before the sun has disappeared, he is forever disgraced as a man without medicine.[6]

Among the Apaches, the shamans or medicine men usually acted as individuals, but among the Pawnees, Zuñis, and a few other tribes, they were organized in one or more societies and kept their secrets concealed from people at large. An herbalist was consulted for less serious health problems. If the herbalist failed to relieve symptoms, a "hand trembler," or diviner, was called in. If the patient still did not show signs of improvement, a medicine man would finally be summoned. Healers in all tribes, however, did have one thing in common: they had complete and sincere faith in their practice and took great pride in their work as healers.

Unlike native peoples elsewhere in the world, most early American Indians did not stress ancestor worship; but many Indian peoples believed that if the dead were not properly buried, their spirits would haunt those responsible and bring illness and other misfortunes upon the living. Some believed that if a person entered an area haunted by such spirits, he would soon die, and if a dead relative called to you in a dream, you would soon die. In some tribes, it was the custom to wear small medicine bags of herbs and roots next to the body to ward off bad spirits—which might take the form of owls or wolves—and the illnesses they could cause.

Many Indians saw enemies or bad spirits as the cause of illness, but the healing methods used by medicine men varied from tribe to tribe. The medicine man would usually conduct a ceremony that supposedly created magical power to effect a cure, or that called upon spirits to aid a sufferer. From his medicine bundle, usually made of animal skin, he might produce a charm or fetish such as a deer tail, bird feather, or bone, and sometimes the stomach of a buffalo or other animal. He might use a medicine stick to serve as an offering, a warning, or an invitation.

Nearly all Indians subscribed to a particular notion of how human or spirit enemies did their work, specifically, that "disease was due to the presence in the body of some tangible, albeit mysterious, object placed there magically by a sorcerer or inimical spirit."[7]

It was then the medicine man's responsibility to extract this harmful object from the body of the patient, and this was usually accomplished by sleight of hand. The object might be a bone fragment, stone, thorn, hair, or even a tiny worm or small animal. Before removing it, the medicine man might blow on the person's body, make a small incision, or use a feather, the tip of which was placed on the body while holding the other end in his mouth. Once removed, the object might be shown to the patient and others as proof the medicine had worked. The medicine man would then destroy the object by burning it, swallowing it, tossing it into running water, or burying it in the ground.

In some tribes, instead of seeking to remove an object from a patient's body, medicine men sought to cure the patient by repeating a traditional prayer successfully used earlier on someone else with the same illness. Some medicine men might also use certain plants ceremonially to relieve the patient's pain. Such treatments varied among tribes. The Navahos and Apaches in the Southwest had complicated ceremonials lasting several days that included numerous songs and dances, and the creation of elaborate sand paintings. The Apaches used drumming, singing, the application of amulets, the laying on of hands, and incantations to placate or expel the evil spirits. The whole tribe would participate in these ceremonies, under the medicine man's leadership and guidance, making his role much more like that of a priest. But according to one account, an Apache medicine man was permitted to lose only six patients before he himself would be done away with. In one instance, the *Arizona Sentinel* reported on February 16, 1878, that an Apache medicine man, with the permission of his tribal chief, placed two babies dying of smallpox back-to-back and with a single bullet killed both of them. In this way the medicine man protected his own future.

A medicine man might also be called to resuscitate someone who had fainted or fallen into a coma. In such cases, most Indians believed, the person's soul had left the body. The medicine man would usually go into a trance, and either send his spirit to search for the missing soul or ask his guardian spirits to make the search. This practice was widespread among Indian medicine men, especially in the Pacific Northwest. In most tribes there was little separation between diagnosing an illness and curing it, but there were some in which a medicine man would stop after determining the nature or cause of a problem, and call upon another medicine man to effect the cure.

On the upper Missouri River, George Catlin in the early 1840s observed that when a medicine man was called, he first prescribed roots and herbs. If they failed, he turned to the treatment of last resort, which included putting on "a strange and unaccountable dress, conjured up and constructed during a life-time of practice, in the wildest fancy imaginable, in which he arrays himself, and makes his last visit to his dying patient, dancing over him, shaking his frightful rattles, and singing songs of incantation, in hope to cure him by a charm." If the patient did not recover and died, the medicine man changed his dress and joined in doleful lamentations with the mourners. The medicine man, Catlin added, sought to maintain his influence over his people by assuring them that the patient had died because it was the will of the Great Spirit.

In many tribes the medicine man also functioned as a teacher and historian, preserving the tribe's history, myths, and traditions, and it was his responsibility to teach them to the younger generation. Together, this responsibility and his role as a healer gave the medicine man a great deal of prestige among his people in times of peace, when most tribes had a peace chief. When a tribe turned to defensive wars or wars of conquest, however, a war chief would be appointed and the responsibilities of the medicine man/woman were greater, as he or she was expected to make medicine to help the tribe gain victory in battles. If the outcome was favorable, the medicine man gained still greater standing and honor.

Indian healing practices evolved slowly over the centuries before the arrival of Europeans, and once they arrived the Europeans gradually learned more and more of Indian medical lore. Likewise, in time, as contact between the two peoples increased, the Indians absorbed ideas from European medicine. One of the earliest instances of this occurred in the 1530s, when a Spanish physician, Álvar Núñez Cabeza de Vaca, and three other men, including a black African named Esteban, made their way across modern-day Texas to modern-day Mexico after being shipwrecked on the Gulf coast. Cabeza de Vaca and the others in his party treated sick Indians along the way using medicial knowledge brought with them from Spain and by saying blessings and making the sign of the cross over people, water, food, and other objects while adding suitable prayers. In one instance, a supposedly dead Indian got up and walked after Cabeza de Vaca made the sign of the cross and prayed over the man. Another time, Indians brought him a man who had been wounded by an arrow. The Indian was in pain because the arrow point was embedded in his right shoulder. Cabeza de Vaca cut the arrow point out and then made two stitches in the incision using a deer-bone needle. By the next day, the wound was healing and the Indians danced and celebrated. The Indians asked for the arrow point and sent it with runners ahead to show it to other Indians as Cabeza de Vaca and his party resumed their journey. He later wrote: "We all came to be physicians, although in daring and in readiness to attempt any cures whatever I was most distinguished among them. And we never cured anyone who did not tell us that he got well . . . they believed that as long as we were there none of them would die."[8]

When the Spanish explorer Francisco Vásquez de Coronado set out to find the legendary Seven Cities of Cibola in 1540, he had at least one doctor to care for his three hundred soldiers and the thousands of Indians who followed his party. When the Spanish later extended their sway and influence into modern California, Arizona, Texas, and New Mexico, Spanish doctors were there fighting the plagues that ravaged Spaniards and Indians alike. These physicians were trained in Spain, or at what is now the University of Mexico in Mexico City, which had a medical school as early as 1578. Some were Jesuits who carried not only the cross but a medicine kit. In 1570, Francisco Bravo published apparently what was the first medical book produced in the New World. A second such book was written by a Jesuit, Alonso López de Hinojosis, and dealt with surgery, while Friar Agustín Farfán wrote a third work in 1579, which concerned anatomy, surgery, and medicine, and included sixty cures credited to the Aztecs. The Spanish effort to study native medicine in New Spain soon stagnated, however, because of Spanish orthodoxy across the Atlantic: the church authorities in Spain regarded it as dangerous and smacking of heresy to accept any knowledge or understanding from "heathens." The Spanish study of Indian medicine was not revived until about 1711, when a Jesuit lay brother named Steinheofor—his Spanish name was Juan de Esteyneffer—arrived at the order's college in Chihuahua, Mexico, to care for old and ailing missionaries. Steinheofor compiled a 522-page book titled *Florilegio Medicinal* (a metaphor for the gatherings of the bee). He first listed eighty-six internal diseases, their symptoms, and their treatments. He next wrote about tumors, wounds, ulcers, fractures, and dislocations and how to treat them. His last section was a catalog of herbal lore including where to find plants and how to prepare them as medicines. The book was published in 1712 and by 1719, two years after Steinheofor died, reprinted in New Spain as well as in Madrid and Amsterdam. The work standardized herbal therapy in the Southwest, and its influence is still felt today.[9]

In 1767, Franciscans took over the missions in Baja California. Two years later Father Junípero Serra led the Franciscans north to found missions at San Diego and Monterey, to convert Indians to Christianity, and establish the Spanish right to California. Serra would eventually direct the construction of twenty-one missions along El Camino Real, from San Diego to Sonoma. In terms of health and medicine, Father Serra is personally credited with getting people to eat citrus fruits to control scurvy. His fellow Franciscans provided the Indians with regular medical treatment, and in so doing often sought to make use of local flora or indigenous drugs. But it must also be noted that many Indians died because of the mission system, which congregated Indians in large settlements against their will and so made them more vulnerable to European diseases.

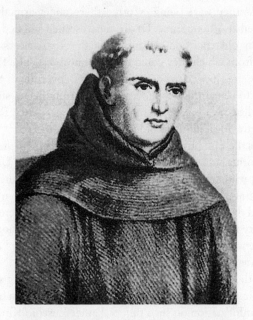

Father Junípero Serra (1713–1784), the leading founder of Roman Catholic missions in California. He noted in his diary that Indians used the oil crushed from beans of the jojoba shrub (Simmondsia chinensis) to treat cuts, sores, bruises, and burns, including sunburn and windburn. They also roasted jojoba seeds to produce a coffee-like drink and used the beans as an appetite suppressant when food was not available. (Courtesy San Diego Historical Society)

While Cabeza de Vaca probably was the first *curandero* in the Spanish Southwest, a Spanish doctor arrived in what is now New Mexico in 1693. He was Francisco Javier Romero, a native of Mexico City. Two years later, he moved north to the Española Valley. To make a living he worked as a shoemaker and farmer when not practicing medicine. According to the well-known historian Marc Simons, records indicate that Romero was a *cirujano*, or surgeon, suggesting he probably received his formal medical training in Mexico City. Dr. Romero apparently served as a battlefield physician, looking after both Spanish and Indians who had been wounded. One day he and some friends went hunting but found no game. They did find an ox belonging to the governor of a nearby pueblo, killed the animal, and butchered it. For this, they were tried, found guilty, and sentenced to two years' exile at El Paso. As they were being escorted there under armed guard, the party paused at Albuquerque. Dr. Romero escaped and fled to a nearby church. An old tradition permitted fugitives to take sanctuary in churches, from which they could not be removed. While Romero was holed up there, local citizens petitioned the governor in Santa Fe to allow him to remain in Albuquerque as their physician, since the village then had no doctor. The governor did, and later Romero was appointed the local minister of justice. He died in 1745.[10]

Perhaps the first physician of record to practice medicine in what is now California was Don Pedro Prat, a graduate of the University of Barcelona, who arrived in 1769 aboard the *San Carlos*, one of the two ships bringing Father Serra and his mission-builders to San Diego Bay. Scurvy and dysentery nearly wiped out the *San Carlos*'s crew. When a rescue party from the other ship helped the survivors ashore, Dr. Prat treated them in a makeshift hut constructed of driftwood and canvas. This hut was probably California's first hospital.

Before the Spanish arrived, Indians were already using some plants and herbs in treating illness and injury, but letters written by Prat provide little information on such things. Father Eusebio Kino, however, described a medicinal plant found in what is now southern Arizona called jojoba, a member of the boxwood family (*Buxaceae*). Indians ate its fruit, which contains a liquid chemically identical to the oil of the sperm whale. Indians used the liquid to treat cancer and kidney disorders. Apaches were already mashing poison ivy leaves to prepare a remedy for ringworm, and Karankawas, who lived along the Gulf coast, relied on various plants to control diarrhea.

Most authorities believe that nearly all Indian tribes in North America had long experimented by trial and error with natural plants and herbs to determine their properties and effects. In time, they learned their benefits and the best times to gather plants and herbs, the times when they contained the highest concentration of the desired active ingredients. For instance, Indians gathered inner bark in the spring, and they picked the leaves of plants, and dug the roots of annuals just before blooming. They dug roots of perennials in the autumn, when the plants were storing nutrients for winter. Many roots and leaves were dried for later use—although the Indians appeared generally unaware that in many cases the active ingredient would be lost over time.

The Indians discovered two ways to obtain the needed ingredients. One was to boil leaves or roots in water to concentrate the solution in liquid form, a process called decoction, and the other was to extract the solid form of the desired ingredients in boiling water and remove it after cooling. This process, called infusion, produced a crude drug.

Many Indian healers developed a system whereby each ingredient or drug from a plant or a root was assigned to one of the four directions of the compass—north, south, east, and west—reflecting the universal circle of life, energy, influence, and relationship. This is sometimes referred to as the medicine wheel, though it is more properly called the medicine circle. Medicines assigned to the east represented illumination, freshness, peace, understanding, spring, and the light of wisdom. Those belonging to the south enhanced the power of life, fertility, warmth, and growth. Those representing maturity, autumn rain, thunder, or the quality of things coming to an end were assigned to the west, while those medicines that promoted the cleansing of austerity, cold purifying winds, the strength of endurance, or the white snows and hair of old age belonged to the north. Many tribes also assigned importance to two other directions, up and down. The direction up represented the Grandfather—the Great Spirit—while down represented the Grandmother—the Earth.

Medicine circles date back about 4,000 years, to the time of the Egyptian pyramids and English megaliths like Stonehenge. Some circles functioned as calendars, but their symbolism and meaning have widely varied, making it nearly impossible to provide one description that fits all. The English who arrived along the east coast of North America could not understand Indian medicine because it included spiritual aspects and was much broader in scope than their own. In England, and Europe generally, medicine and the spiritual world—religion—were separate. Therefore in matters of healing and medicine, the only common ground for understanding between the early English settlers and the Indians was their use of plants, herbs, extracts, minerals, and trees that had medicinal value. To begin with, of course, the Indians knew vastly more about North American cures than the English, having learned by trial and error over the centuries. Gradually, however, the English absorbed much of the Indians' knowledge and discoveries.

At Jamestown, Virginia, the first permanent English colony, established in 1607, Captain John Smith struggled to hold his small band of about two hundred colonists together. Because of hardships and illness during a drought, many died from typhoid, dysentery, and influenza. In 1610, the colonizing company sent Lawrence Bohun, a physician, from England to save lives at Jamestown. When not treating the ill, Bohun experimented with native flora, seeking remedies to treat his patients with and to take home to England.

Bohun found sassafras (*Sassafras albidum*)* growing in the Jamestown area, and it was one of the first exports that John Smith sent to England. Sassafras was already known in Europe, and thought to have medicinal qualities. Spaniards first found it in the New World and took plantings to Spain and cultivated it in the middle 1500s. The Spanish and later the English thought its root useful in the treatment of venereal disease and the plague. In time the Spanish and English concluded that sassafras had little medicinal value, but when boiled, its roots and leaves produce a palatable tea, and the oil extracted from the root bark can be used in some soap. The English also used its wood as fuel and in the construction of barrels and canoes. Some people in England believed bugs would never infest bedsteads constructed of sassafras wood. By 1601, it was highly valued in England, selling for £322 per ton.[11]

Captain Bartholomew Gosnold, an English explorer, also found sassafras in New England early in the seventeenth century, after he

---

*About 1736, Swedish naturalist Carolus Linnaeus developed the binomial system (two words in Latin) for classification purposes. Since plants also have more than one common name in any given language, the scientific Latin name is the only dependable and universal one.

arrived off the coast of Maine aboard the ship *Concord*. He then sailed south to what is now Massachusetts, where he named Cape Cod. Gosnold spent three weeks in the area, during which time Indians helped his men dig sassafras roots that were taken back to England. But by the time Gosnold returned home with his cargo, the London price of sassafras had dropped.[12]

As more English arrived in the colonies, they learned more about the Indians' use of plants and herbs for healing. John Josselyn, an English gentleman, arrived in Boston in July 1638 to tour New England. Boston was then a town of not more than thirty houses. Josselyn's brother Henry, who lived in Maine, came down to Boston to meet him, and together they toured New England. Josselyn stayed for fifteen months, then visited again twenty-four years later, in 1663. On his visits, Josselyn made notes on the birds, animals, reptiles, fishes, and plants he found. After he returned to England the second time, he published a book in 1671 titled *New England's Rarities Discovered: In Birds, Beasts, Fishes, Serpents, and Plants of That Country*. In this small book, Josselyn gives the impression that everything he found possessed marvelous medicinal properties. He described the plant green hellebore (*Veratrum viride*). He called it white hellebore, as something the Indians used to heal wounds. Josselyn wrote that Indians would anoint the wound first with raccoon grease or wildcat grease, and then sprinkle on it powdered hellebore root. He observed that Indians also used the plant for toothaches, by putting the powdered root into a hollow tooth. Josselyn also praised the merits of the bearberry (*Arctostaphylus uva-vrsi L Spreng*), especially against scurvy and fever, and he wrote that sassafras could produce an ointment for bruises.

Josselyn's book became popular in England, but it was not widely distributed in the colonies, where many settlers were slow to accept anything of Indian origin. From their arrival, most English looked down on the native peoples and considered them savages, and rejected anything associated with them. This contempt appears to have been rooted in a widespread English interpretation of the Old Testament, whereby they were the chosen people destined to exterminate the Philistines (i.e., Indians) who occupied the Promised Land (America). Instead of turning to Indian remedies that were readily available, most early settlers relied on English medicines exported to the colonies. However, in the early eighteenth century, as the cost of English medicines became greater in America, this gradually changed.

In 1670, when German physician John Lederer explored the Appalachian Mountains in modern Virginia with an Indian guide, he was stung on his finger in his sleep by a "Mountain-spider." His guide treated Lederer by sucking out the poison and then putting on the wound a small dose of powder from the root of snakeroot (*Aristolochia serpentaria*) that had been made into a plaster. Lederer recovered, and a few days later became the first recorded European to see the Shenandoah Valley. Looking down from a peak in the Blue Ridge Mountains in August 1670, he mistook the haze in the valley for an ocean's surface, and became convinced that an arm or bay of the Indian Ocean was located just west of the Appalachian Mountains.[13]

During the 1680s in Pennsylvania, Indians showed the colony's founder, William Penn, many plants, including sassafras and wild myrtle (*Myrtus communis L.*), that they said were used to reduce swellings and to treat burns and cuts. A few years later another Englishman, Gabriel Thomas, compared Indian medicine in Pennsylvania favorably to medicine in Europe, and he described the Indians as being "as able doctors and surgeons as any in Europe." Thomas was particularly impressed with the roots of a plant (*Phytolacca decandra L.*) called in England by various names, including black snakeroot, rattlesnake root, pokeroot, and jalap. When it was added in powdered form to wine, brandy, or rum, it was believed to be a cure for the plague. Indians used the roots as an emetic and to treat skin diseases. Colonists used the plants as a heart stimulant and a strong purgative, and to treat venereal disease. When chewed, its seeds and berries supposedly relieved the pain of arthritis.[14]

In Virginia, Robert Beverley, a planter and colonial official, was also favorably impressed with Indian medicine. In his *History and Present State of Virginia* published in London in 1705, Beverley observed that medicine men knew much about "the hidden qualities of Plants, and other Natural things." The Indians, he wrote, also "take great delight in Sweating, and therefore in every Town they have a Sweating House, and a Doctor is paid by the Publick to attend it." Beverley, however, found the Indians reluctant to disclose their medical secrets for fear of offending the spirits. They told him only about snakeroot, he said, and a few other antidotes for snakebites, which had to be applied immediately after a person was bitten. Beverley also observed the Indians making an ointment by crushing the roots of red puccoon or bloodroot (*Sanguinaria canadensis L.*) and wild angelica (*Aralia spinose L.*) and mix-

THE

DISCOVERIES

OF

JOHN LEDERER,

In three several Marches from

VIRGINIA,

To the West of

Carolina,

And other parts of the Continent :

Begun in *March* 1669, and ended in *September* 1670.

Together with

A General MAP of the whole Territory
which he traversed.

Collected and Translated out of Latine from his Discourse
and Writings,

By Sir *William Talbot* Baronet.

Sed nos immensum spatiis confecimus æquor,
Et jam tempus equum fumantia solvere colla. Virg.Georg.

London, Printed by *J. C.* for *Samuel Heyrick,* at Grays-
Inne-gate in Holborn. 1672.

In 1669–70, John Lederer, a German physician, became the first European to explore the lands west of the Blue Ridge Mountains. He wrote an account of his journeys in Latin. It was translated into English by Sir William Talbot and published in London in 1671. This is the title page of the translation. The English were embarrassed that it was a non-Englishman who was brave enough to venture first into this unknown region. (Courtesy University of North Carolina Libraries)

ing the powder with bear's oil. The ointment was then rubbed on the skin to "conserve the substance of the Body." The ointment, added Beverley, kept away lice, fleas, and other troublesome vermin.[15]

French missionaries also gained much knowledge from the Iroquois' use of herbs and plants in the Mohawk Valley between modern Albany and Niagara, New York. The missionaries were particularly impressed with the Indians' use of herbs in treating illness. Two centuries later, Iroquois' medical knowledge was still being praised by Eric

Stone, M.D., who wrote in 1934 that the Iroquois recognized the syndrome of a dry, hot skin, chills, thirst, prostration, and muscular pains.

Their treatment, he noted, seems quite modern, as it included rest, sweating purgation, and a diet restricted to liquids. "Copious infusions of elderberries (*Sambucus candensis*), the fruit or the inner bark, caused sweating and diuresis or an increased excretion of urine. When the thirst had subsided and the skin had become moist, elimination was further promoted by sweat baths. The plant boneset (*Eupatorium perfoliatum L.*), a perennial with opposite perfoliate leaves and white-rayed flower heads, was used in a hot decoction or the bush beam [*Phaseolus vulgaris L.*] was chewed in this or in other conditions where purgation was desirable. They also practiced phlebotomy [bloodletting] for fever."[16]

John Lawson, an English explorer, naturalist, and writer, collected natural history specimens in the Carolina colony for James Petiver, a London apothecary. Lawson later wrote *The History of North Carolina*, published in London in 1714, in which he describes how Indians beat the bark of the sassafras tree and then spread it on painful parts of the body, reducing the pain. Lawson also observed Indians making tea from the leaves of the yaupon; on drinking the tea, they vomited, purging the body. Lawson tells of one drunken Indian who was seriously burned when he fell into a fire, but was cured with the bark of the sassafras tree in ten days. "I never," Lawson wrote, "saw an Indian have an Ulcer, or foul Wound in my life; neither is there any such thing to be found among them."[17]

Twenty-three years after Lawson's book was published, John Brickell, a native of Ireland, accompanied the future provincial governor, George Burrington, to what is now North Carolina. Brickell went inland from the coast as far west as modern Tennessee, and was fascinated with the flora and fauna he observed. When he returned to Ireland about six years later, he wrote *The Natural History of North-Carolina*, published in Dublin in 1737. Brickell borrowed much of Lawson's material but added new information on Indian remedies. Brickell, like Lawson, thought highly of the Indians' medical skills.

As there are in this Country many poisonous Herbs and Creatures, so the Indian people have excellent Skill in applying effectual Antidotes to them; for Medicinal Herbs are here found in great Plenty, the Woods and Savannas being their Apothecary's Shops, from whence they fetch Herbs, Leaves, Barks of Trees, with which they make all their Medicines, and perform notable Cures; of which it may not be amiss to give some Instances, because they seem strange, if compared with our Method of curing Distempers [illnesses].[18]

Brickell described how the Indians cultivated herb gardens to guarantee a ready supply of plant remedies. He cited scarlet root (possibly

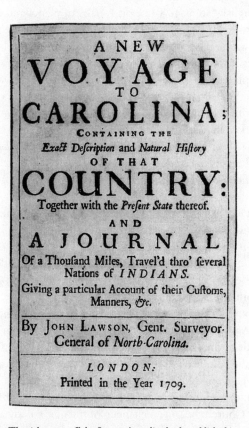

The title page to John Lawson's earlier book, published in London in 1709. Lawson wrote of Indian life in North Carolina and the Indians' use of herbs and plants as medicines. (Courtesy University of North Carolina Libraries)

Ceanothus americanus), a plant found at the foot of the mountains, which the Indians mixed with bear's oil to anoint their bodies to kill lice. He added that its leaves were like spearmint and could cure women's sore nipples and sore mouths.

Mark Catesby, a thirty-year-old English naturalist and artist, arrived in Virginia in 1712 and spent ten years touring the colonies observing, researching, and painting native plants and animals. Catesby, who is often called the "Father of American Ornithology," devoted another ten years to writing and illustrating the first comprehensive English-language work on American plants and animals, his two-volume *Natural History of Carolina, Florida, and the Bahama Islands.* Volume 1 was published in 1731, Volume 2 in 1743. On Indian medicine, Catesby observed that the Indians could identify "vulnerary [curative] plants of virtue, which they apply with good success." He noted that they cured ulcers and dangerous wounds by a regimen of severe abstinence, which they endured with resolution and patience, and he marked in passing that they had not suffered from venereal disease until it was introduced by Europeans. Catesby also, however, found the Indians to be wholly ignorant of anatomy and to have only a very superficial knowledge of surgery, knowing nothing of amputation or bloodletting.

Catesby, as had other English observers of Indian medicine, described how they used yaupon tea. Catesby called it "emetick Broth" and wrote that it "restores the Appetite and strengthens the Stomach."[19]

Still another frequently mentioned Indian remedy adopted by at least some colonists was the dried root bark of wahoo (*E. atropurpureus*), both a mild purgative and a mild heart stimulant. Wahoo is a shrubby spindle tree sometimes called the "burning bush" because of its purple capsules with scarlet-ariled seeds. Indians had used the bark for its cardiac stimulant properties for many years by the time William Withering, an English physician, discovered digitalis, an active ingredient derived from the foxglove plant, late in the 1700s.

In 1735, the English evangelist John Wesley, who later founded the Methodist Church, became a chaplain of the new colony at Savannah, Georgia, arriving about two years after the colony was founded. As an agent for the Society for the Propagation of the Gospel, he was to oversee the colonists' spiritual lives and to convert the Indians. Not long after he arrived, however, he wrote in his journal, "I came to convert the Indians, but, oh, who will convert me?" Wesley failed to convert the Indians, but was impressed with their rugged health and their medical practices. After he returned to England in 1737, Wesley wrote a book called *Primitive Physic*, in which he suggests that knowledge of the art or discipline of healing disease, which he called "physic," was very similar to religion. He observed that it was traditional among the Indians, and that the medicines they used to cure diseases of each season and climate were handed down from generation to generation. "It is certain that this is the method wherein the art of healing is preserved among the Americans [Indians] to this day. Their diseases, indeed, are exceedingly few; nor do they often occur, by reason of their continual exercise, and (till of late) universal temperance. But if any are sick, or bit by a serpent, or torn by a wild beast, the fathers immediately tell their children what remedy to apply. And it is rare that the patient suffers long; those medicines being quick, as well as generally infallible."[20]

By the middle 1700s, it was obvious to many colonists that Indians were skilled in identifying flora that could be used in treating externally caused injuries such as fractures, dislocations, wounds including snake and insect bites, skin irritations, and bruises. Otherwise, the colonists found the Indians' understanding of medicine limited. This was especially evident in the light of the new diseases brought from Europe to America by the colonists—chiefly contagious ones such as measles, yellow fever, and smallpox, diseases that the Indians had never experienced. Their immune systems lacked the genetic resistance passed along from generation to generation among Europeans who had recovered from such diseases, against which the Indians' traditional herb, plant, and other remedies were of little use. When the Indians sought to cure these imported plagues by applying traditional methods such as bringing people together in sweathouses and then having them jump into cold streams, these treatments only spread disease more effectively and usually made those already ill even sicker.

European diseases carried to the New World took a deadly toll among the Indians. Between 1616 and 1619, what was probably smallpox swept through the Massachusetts and other Algonquin tribes along the northeastern coast, reducing their population by 1620 from about 30,000 to 300. Some Indians may have been affected when measles broke out in Boston in 1657 and again in 1687, when a yellow fever epidemic struck New York in 1690, and when smallpox attacked Boston in 1702. Authorities burned the bodies of the dead without funerals to prevent the spread of disease.

When another smallpox epidemic occurred in Boston in 1721, Rev. Cotton Mather urged Dr. Zabdiel Boylston to try inoculations. Mather said a slave, Onesimum, had told him how he had been inoculated as a child in Africa, and that the practice was ancient. Dr. Boylston inoculated his son and two slaves by making in each case a small wound and infecting it with pus taken from a smallpox sore. The resulting illness was mild and the doctor's patients recovered within days. Many Boston residents objected to the practice on religious grounds, but with the support of the Puritan clergy, Boylston inoculated a total of 244 residents. Only 6 died. When smallpox hit Charleston, South Carolina, in 1738, physicians inoculated 683 residents using Boylston's method, and only 16 died, whereas of 1,600 people who did not receive inoculations, 295 died. Nonetheless, Boylston's technique was also vigorously opposed by the medical establishment of the day. It would be another seventy-five years before Dr. Edward Jenner in England would come up with a generally acceptable form of inoculation using matter taken from lesions on cows with cowpox instead of pus from an infected person's smallpox lesions.

As smallpox spread among the Cherokee Indians in the Carolinas, authorities feared a loss of revenues from the Indian trade, and Thomas Dale, a Charleston physician, was sent to inoculate the Indians, but many Cherokees suspicious of any offer of help from whites refused inoculations. As a result, perhaps half of the Cherokee population in the Carolinas died from smallpox.

In 1763, near the end of the French and Indian War when France allied with the Indians to drive the British out of North America, Lord Jeffrey Amherst, commander of British forces in America, suggested that smallpox be used to reduce the number of hostile Indians. Amherst wrote to one of his officers, Colonel Henry Bouquet, who commanded the British forces in Pennsylvania, suggesting that he come up with a way to infect with smallpox the Indians who were then threatening Fort Pitt, where the disease had broken out. From Fort Pitt, Captain Simeon Ecuyer replied on June 24, 1763, that two blankets and a handkerchief from the fort's hospital had been given to the Indians outside the post, and that he hoped these would have the desired effect. It is unclear whether they did, but by the following spring a smallpox epidemic was raging among Indians in the Ohio River Valley.[21]

While the English and French, usually though not always unwittingly, spread new diseases to the region east of the Mississippi, the Spanish conquest of New Spain similarly brought smallpox and other diseases unknown to Indians in modern California and the American Southwest. The Spanish probably spread disease as they traversed the prominent trade routes. Spanish Franciscans reported in 1638 that 20,000 Pueblo Indians had died from smallpox, and by 1640 another 30,000 Indians had died; that was only the beginning of the decline of the Indian population in the West, due in large degree to diseases brought to America by Europeans.[22]

CHAPTER TWO

EARLY AMERICAN MEDICINE

The remedy is worse than the disease.

—Francis Bacon

THE THEORY OF MEDICINE brought to the colonies by the English goes back to the first medical school in Europe, established in southern Italy at Salerno around AD 1000. It was there that Arab, Greek, and Jewish medical thought merged from earlier beliefs, especially those of the Greek physician Hippocrates, widely hailed as the "Father of Medicine." Scholars at Salerno posited that everything in the universe is made up of four basic elements—fire, air, water, and earth. They believed that the human body contains four corresponding "humors," as Hippocrates called them: blood is fire, yellow bile is air, black bile is water, and phlegm is earth. Good health depended upon the maintenance of a proper balance and harmony among the humors, and illness and disease arose from any imbalance among them. The Salerno scholars regarded medicine as a philosophy that could neither be proved nor tested; in fact, the head of the medical department at Salerno was also head of the philosophy department. Slowly these beliefs spread across Europe and to England, where in time physicians saw it was their job to maintain a balance among the four humors and to treat each human's dominant humor, which determined the treatment to be used. The therapies prescribed were bleeding, purging either by emetic or by enema, blistering, and medicines.

While the Romans had used surgery much earlier to treat the injuries of gladiators and warriors, the evolving Catholic Church forbade physicians to perform surgery because it believed the human body was, as proclaimed in the Book of Genesis, made in God's own image and should not be violated. The clergy were ordered not to practice medicine, on the grounds that it would distract them from

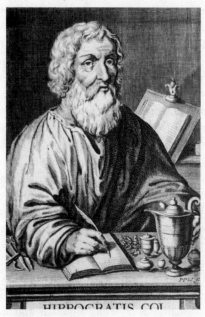

HIPPOCRATIS COL

The Greek physician Hippocrates (460–370 BC) is often called "the Father of Medicine." He founded a medical school on the island of Cos, wrote more than fifty books, and developed a system of medical methodology and ethics that is still with us today. Hippocrates once wrote, "Walking is man's best medicine." He also observed, "Everyone has a doctor in him or her; we just have to help it in its work. The natural healing force within each one of us is the greatest force in getting well. Our food should be our medicine. Our medicine should be our food. But to eat when you are sick, is to feed your sickness." (Courtesy National Library of Medicine)

their holy duties. Thus the practice of medicine fell into the hands of laymen. The job of bleeding and otherwise cutting people went to barbers, who had evolved from ancient medicine men who believed the hairs on the head allowed both good and bad spirits to enter the body. Therefore, the medicine men cut hair to drive out bad spirits. In time, medicine men became barber-surgeons who also pulled teeth and even removed gallstones without anesthesia. Barber-surgeons were seen as mere craftsmen until 1686, when one of them, Charles François Félix, was commanded by the French king Louis XIV to examine his bottom. Félix did so and six months later, after practicing the surgery on several peasants, he operated on the king's anal fistula. Whether the king's problem was caused by his great fondness for enemas is not known, but the operation was a success and he showered Félix with money, titles, and other honors. The king's operation significantly raised the stature of surgery in Europe. (Many of Louis's courtiers thereupon insisted on being examined to see if they, too, had anal fistula, *la maladie du roi*. And the delight of those who did knew no bounds.)

In those days people located barber-surgeons by the red-and-white-striped pole outside of their establishment. Atop the pole was a brass bowl or basin symbolizing the vessel used to catch blood from blood-letting, which was then a common cure for all illness. The red-and-white pole, representing bloody rags hung out to dry, identified members of the Barber-Surgeon Guild until 1745, when barbers and surgeons began to split into separate groups. The barbers kept the pole and still use it to mark their places of business. Afterward barbers were limited to shaving, haircutting, removing teeth, and bloodletting. Surgeons became one of three distinct groups in the English practice of medicine—physicians, surgeons, and apothecaries. Physicians usually held university degrees and were part of the upper class. In contrast, surgeons learned their craft as apprentices or were trained in a hospital. Apothecaries, the ancestors of modern-day pharmacists, also learned to compound, prescribe, and sell medicines through apprenticeships.

By 1750, more and more medications were used to heal. If a patient was lethargic, weak, and had a fever, the body was given counterirritants and a restricted diet. Such treatment gave rise to the old adage "Feed a cold and starve a fever." By 1780, however, what later was labeled by the pejorative term "heroic medicine" was aggressively practiced. Heroic medicine meant the patient had to be more heroic than the physician whose treatments included bloodletting, intestinal purging, vomiting, profuse sweating, and blistering. For instance, physicians originally treated a disease like syphilis with salves containing mercury. While heroic medicine treatments were well intentioned, they were actually harmful to the patient. By the mid-nineteenth century, heroic medicine treatments were superseded by scientific advances.

But while the division of medicine—physician, surgeon, and apothecary—worked in England, it was impractical in America. In the colonies, each physician had to engage in all three branches to survive financially. Most American doctors had little if any medical training, and even those with some training knew relatively little about what made a person sick or well. Medicine in the colonies, as in England, was very rudimentary. The practice had not changed greatly for centuries, except in obstetrics. In the early 1700s William Smellie, a Scottish doctor, invented the steel-lock, curved, and double-curved forceps to rotate the fetus's head in birthing. Aside from Smellie's invention, the English trial-and-error process of adopting remedies from flora was very similar to that used by Indians for centuries. Internal surgery was unknown. Operations were limited to the amputation of limbs or the drilling of a hole in a person's skull (trepanning) to relieve pressure on the brain. Most practicing physicians in the colonies had little time to seek better treatments and remedies. They were too busy trying to make a living.

Physicians were scarce in the colonies because there were few incentives to attract more doctors from England. A few colonizing companies in England did contract with physicians and barber-surgeons to practice in America, but many of them did not like life there and soon returned to England. Perhaps it was natural, then, that midwives came to expand their practice from attending women in childbirth, their traditional function, to dealing with injuries and routine illnesses and medical problems. Doctors would be sought out for surgery or serious medical conditions that eluded the skills of midwives. Because most Americans were poor and could not afford to pay doctors, most physicians held other positions that provided income. Villages and towns were widely scattered, and most were sparsely populated and somewhat isolated. Life in the colonies was hazardous for everyone, and disease and sudden death were commonplace. To compound the problems, anyone in the colonies who wanted to practice medicine could do so without credentials or certification. There were many quacks* who passed themselves off as physicians. The numerous lay practitioners ranged from midwives, as noted above, to bonesetters to charlatans peddling a wide range of remedies to cure all ills. Even the rare qualified doctors had only a limited store of medical knowledge and skills at

---

*The word *quack* is a shortened form of *Quacksalver*, the old Dutch word for mercury, and originated as an insult to physicians in Europe who used mercury salves in their treatments.

best; they knew something about easing pain and healing with herbal mixtures but little else. It is not surprising that poor colonists turned to home remedies or what historian Albert Deutsch called "kitchen physic," which he described as astrological lore, time-tested grand-mother remedies, and a plenitude of superstitious ingredients.[1]

Such homemade remedies were also sold to the public, as witness one remedy advertised in Ben Franklin's *Pennsylvania Gazette* on August 19, 1731: "The Widow READ, removed from the upper end of Highstreet to the New Printing-Office near the Market, continues to make and sell her well-known Ointment for the ITCH. . . . It is always effectual for that purpose, and never fails to perform the Cure speedily. It also kills or drives away all Sorts of Lice. . . . It has no offensive Smell, but rather a pleasant one; and may be used without the least Apprehension of Danger, even to a sucking Infant. . . . Price 2 s. a Gallypot containing an Ounce." It is doubtful that Widow Read had to pay anything for the advertisement. She was Ben Franklin's mother-in-law.

From their earliest arrival, English physicians brought patent medicines to America, and it was not long before they were being commercially marketed. Produced by enterprising Englishmen who combined medical lore with promotional skills, such products as "Anderson's Pills," "Elixir Salutis: The Choise [*sic*] Drink of Health or, Health-bringing Drink, Being a Famous Cordial Drink," "Steer's Opodeldoc," "British Oil," and others found their way to America beginning in the seventeenth century. Anderson's Pills first appeared in the 1630s and supposedly were prepared from a formula learned in Venice by a Scot who claimed to be physician to King Charles I. The pills were a cathartic and emmenagogue that included aloes. Daffy's Elixir claimed to prolong life but apparently consisted mostly of alcohol with a few other ingredients. British Oil and Steer's Opodeldoc were liniments. Later came Turlington's Balsam, an oily and resinous substance extracted from various plants containing benzoic or cinnamic acid. These early over-the-counter preparations, however, chiefly offered ingredients that were already widely employed in medicines. Later patent medicines, some described as "new inventions," really were nothing more than variations of early potions containing either new combinations or new proportions.*

Many if not most colonists did not understand that the body's own

---

*There is more information on patent medicines in Chapter Twelve.

natural capacity for healing might restore them to health without the aid of medicines or physicians. When they recovered from an illness, they sought to credit something they had taken or done as the reason for their cure, and they would pass it along by word of mouth. For instance, some colonists believed warts could be cured by placing a hand with a wart in "spunk water," water that had collected in a rotting stump. Others insisted that warts would disappear when treated with milk made from the milkweed plant, or by rubbing raw potato slices or raw meat on them. Still others apparently believed warts could be cured by holding their hands in the air during a waxing moon. If any of these cures actually did work, it was probably due to the placebo effect so familiar to us today. They worked because patients believed they would work.

There is no truth to the legend, dating back to colonial times in New England, that to stretch scanty winter food supplies, old people were given herbs and moonshine until they passed out and were then taken outside, frozen, and packed in wood and straw until spring when they were thawed out. But many strange-sounding remedies supposedly were effective. Gunpowder was used to treat wounds; whiskey to treat sore throats, snakebites, and burns; and tobacco mixed with an onion and held to the ear could cure earaches.

Nightmares, sometimes called *incubi*, were a different matter. Many people believed nightmares were caused by intense thought, and could be cured by purifying the blood. One remedy consisted in putting five quarters of water in a large copper kettle and adding one handful each of the bark of yellow sarsaparilla (*Aralia nudicaulis L.*), and wild cherry (*Prunus virginiana L.*), boiling the mixture until only two quarts of liquid remained, and then adding one pint of whiskey. The patient took one tablespoon of the liquid twice each day until the nightmares stopped.

The colonies had no hospitals in the modern sense until 1751, when one was established in Philadelphia. After Dr. Thomas Bond told Benjamin Franklin the town needed a hospital, Franklin conducted a public campaign through leaflets and pamphlets to raise the funds to build one. Fourteen years later, in 1765, the first medical college in the colonies was established, also in Philadelphia. Until then, nearly all physicians began their practice of medicine after a short apprenticeship with a doctor who taught them the then current theory of medicine; disease was caused by an imbalance in body fluids, and purging, starving, vomiting, or bloodletting could restore health. Physicians either added fluids or drained them away by diet, therapy, medications, or physicial procedures. Emetics, diuretics, and scalpels were used in treatments when blood would be drained from patients.

There were three methods of bloodletting. Using a lancet was most common. The physician would select a vein, usually at the elbow, apply a tight bandage, and when the vein swelled, he marked it with his thumb; with his other hand, he used a lancet to make a slit obliquely across the blood vessel. The common practice was to bleed the patient until he became faint. When a physician was not available to perform bloodletting, barbers performed the task. Many physicians believed there was far more blood in the human body than there really is. At times, they took too much blood and killed their patients.

The second form of bloodletting was by the use of leeches. The

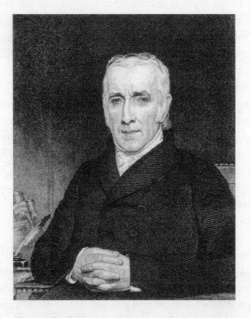

Thomas Bond (1712–1784) was a physician in colonial Philadelphia. Benjamin Franklin helped Bond raise money to establish Pennsylvania Hospital in Philadelphia, the first hospital in America designed to treat the sick, injured, and mentally ill. (Courtesy National Library of Medicine)

word *leech* comes from the Angle-Saxton *laece*, which means "reliever of pain." Leeches were removed from the box in which they were kept and dried on a linen cloth. Then the part of the patient's body on which they were to be used was cleansed. The leeches were placed in an open pillbox or a wineglass and applied to the spot on the body at which the physician desired they draw blood. If they did not attach themselves quickly, they were induced to bite by moistening the desired portion of the body with milk or blood. Most leeches could draw slightly more than an eighth of an ounce of blood. When full, the leech would detach itself from the body. Leeches could be applied to almost any part of the body and were sometimes applied to the inside of the mouth or nose. Occasionally a patient might swallow one. If that happened, the patient was given a glass of wine every fifteen minutes to destroy the leech.

The third method of bloodletting was called "cupping." A physician made a small incision with a lancet and placed a cup made of tin, brass, horn, or glass over it to catch the blood. Another technique was to use a scarificator, a device that made in one moment many shallow cuts with a dozen blades. A cup would then catch the blood. Still another form was called "dry cupping," in which the skin was not punctured. A cup was heated over a candle flame. The physician then created suction in the cup by placing it on the body so that the skin under the cup became engorged. The purple skin supposedly indicated that evil humors had been drawn to the surface. When the cup was removed and the skin returned to its normal color, physicians and patients believed the bad humors had been removed. By the early nineteenth century, cupping gave way to the lancet method, which dominated until that practice declined during the second half of the nineteenth century. The use of leeches began to decline in the 1830s.

During the early nineteenth century physicians performed amputations without anesthetic, often giving the patient a swig of whiskey for the pain. Because internal surgery was unknown, stomach ailments were usually treated by "blistering," the practice of placing a harsh substance on a selected portion of the patient's skin to induce a second-degree burn. Steaming hot poultices would create infections on scalded portions of the skin. Physicians thought the resulting pus flowing from the wound was beneficial.

Eighteenth-century theories of medicine ignored cleanliness; doctors did not wash their hands before treating patients or performing surgery. But then, washing and bathing were uncommon everywhere. Although most colonists chose to live near creeks and rivers, people only occasionally bathed in them. In many homes, the only facilities for washing were a basin and a towel. Most colonists could not afford soap, which was considered a luxury. Colonists who could not afford to build an outhouse or buy a chamber pot defecated outside, often in the same stream from which they obtained their drinking water. Colonists with chamber pots or commodes thought nothing of tossing excrement and garbage out the front door, just as was done in England. The lack of personal cleanliness among the early colonists, including physicians, no doubt contributed to the spread of illness and disease.

During the mid-seventeenth century, the existing American colonies, with a combined population then slightly more than one million, could claim no more than about 3,500 physicians. Few colonists ventured very far from their homes. Roads were poor. Most settlements were only villages. If a trusted physician lived in one, he was a person of high social standing, like the schoolmaster. Only ministers had a higher ranking. The physician was usually present at every birth and every funeral, and often put his name with that of a lawyer to wills. The principal role of a colonial doctor was to provide patients with support and comfort, to set broken bones, and occasionally to prescribe herbal remedies. Opium, an extract from the seedpods of the opium poppy (*Papaver somniferum*) was administered freely by physicians to relieve pain. Many colonists cultivated opium poppies in their gardens and used their resin in whiskey to relieve coughs, aches, and pains. Opium had been around for centuries. Physicians viewed it as a medicine and not a drug and there was no concept of any addiction from medicines. The same was true of laudanum, a derivative of opium. Early in the sixteenth century, a German wanting to cure disease by medicine discovered that the alkaloids found in opium were less soluble in water than in alcohol. Philippus Aureolus Theophrastus Bombast von Hohenheim, better known as Paracelsus, concocted laudanum by extracting opium into brandy. Thomas Sydenham, an Englishman, later standardized the recipe for laudanum: two ounces of opium, one ounce of saffron, and a dram of cinnamon and cloves, all dissolved in a pint of Canary wine.

If someone had a medical emergency, he usually had three choices: find a doctor or perhaps an apothecary, treat himself, or die. If a trusted doctor lived nearby, the average house-call charge was the equivalent of 50 cents. If the patient had no money, which was usually the case, payment could be made in food, goods, or promised services. Like teachers, doctors generally did not receive money for their services. If a physician set a broken leg, he might receive two chickens. If he delivered a baby, his payment might be some household object or tool. When patients could not locate or afford a doctor whom they trusted, they might turn to an apothecary, if there was one in their town. If no doctor or apothecary was available, the patient turned to either home or Indian remedies.

John Tennent, who arrived from England about 1725 and settled in Spotsylvania County, Virginia, compiled a book to help colonists treat themselves. It is not known whether Tennent was a physician, but his little book of less than a hundred pages titled *Every Man His Own Doctor; Or, The Poor Planter's Physician* was the first popular manual of American medicine. First printed in Williamsburg in 1734, it became avidly sought after and was reprinted by others, including Benjamin Franklin in Philadelphia. Tennent told readers, with a distinct note of irony, that his book was designed for those who could not afford to die by the hand of a doctor. He said it was his aim to create an aid for the poor so they could have good health, and to show them the cheapest and easiest ways of getting well again.

The first remedy that Tennent offered in his book is a cure for a *cough*:

Begin with riding moderately on horseback every day, and taking only a little Ground Ivy Tea sweetened with Syrup of Horehound at night when you go to bed. In case the cough is violent, bleed eight ounces, and be constant in the use of the other remedies. Meanwhile, use a spare and cooling diet without either flesh or strong drink. Do not stove yourself up in a warm room, but breathe as much as possible in the open air. Do not make yourself tender, but wash every day in cold water, and very often your feet.

Tennent's remedy for *pleurisy*:

For *pleurisy*, noted by a brisk fever and a sharp pain pretty low in one of the sides, shooting now and then into the breast, and sometimes back into the shoulder-blades each time, one draws his breath. One must take away 10 ounces of blood, and repeat the same three or four

days successively unless the pain stops. On the third day he may
vomit with 80 grains of Indian Physick [*Virginia ipecoacanna*] and
every night drink seven spoonfuls of *Pennyroyal Water* [a tea of fresh
or dried *Hedeoma pulegioides*] or the decoction of it, moderately
sweetened. In the meantime, every three hours, take half a spoonful
of *Honey* and *Linseed Oyl* mixed together. Also stew *Indian Pepper*,
upon *Pennyroyal Plaister*, and apply it very hot to the place where the
pain lies, and be sure to keep warm, and abstain from cold water. If
the pain does not leave, you must apply a *Blister* to the neck, and one
to each arm on the fleshy part of the elbow. The patient's diet should
be light and cooling, and his constant drink should be either *Linseed*
or *Balm Tea* with a little sweetener.

Toward the end of his book Tennent points out that almost all of
the remedies he has prescribed come from more than eighty plants
that his readers could grow in their gardens, that no more than five or
six foreign medicines are included, and even these are cheap. As clearly
shown in these two examples, Tennent, like many other physicians of
the day, believed in bloodletting. Most doctors thought the human
body held twenty quarts of blood, not the five quarts it actually contains.[2]

Some of the remedies prescribed by Tennent probably originated
with Indians, who believed, for instance, that a bad headache would go
away if they chewed the bark of the willow tree. They also learned that
witch hazel (*Hamamelis virginiana*) helped sore muscles, that pennyroyal (*Hedeoma pulegioides*) would repel insects, and raspberries could
treat diarrhea. Willow, poplar, and wintergreen were used as remedies.
Neither the Indians nor the colonists, of course, knew that these flora
all contain salicylate, which is chemically related to acetylsalicylic acid,
better known today as aspirin, though chemically modified so that
humans can more easily tolerate it. The bark of the cherry tree contains hydrocyanic (prussic) acid, which was utilized as a cough suppressant. Coniferous trees such as balsam, fir, pine, and cedar contain
volatile oils used to reduce nasal and pulmonary congestion. The resin
from coniferous trees was applied as an antiseptic on wounds, and the
inner bark was mashed and used as a poultice. Oak, raspberry, sumac,
dogwood, alumroot, and many other plants contain astringent ingredients such as tannin, which helps to reduce the flow of blood and other
fluids.[3]

Numerous Indian remedies relying on the use of plants were eventually adopted by the colonists, and became a mainstay of early American medicine because English medicines were costly and often scarce, especially during the American Revolution. The use of herbal remedies was passed from physician to physician, and from one generation to another in families, to treat injuries and to keep minor ailments from becoming chronic. A partnership developed between physicians and home folk medicine.

One herb thought to strengthen the body and remove stress was American ginseng (*Panax quinquefolium*), identified in southern Canada by a French Jesuit priest in the 1700s. He took a sample to Paris, where his fellow Jesuits sensed it could produce a profit and sent more missionaries to Canada to find ginseng. Soon they were shipping tons of American ginseng to China, where it was thought to have more cooling properties than its Asian counterparts, provided its roots were at least four years old. As news of the herb's commercial value spread along the Eastern Seaboard, Americans learned that Indians had long recognized ginseng's health value. Americans including Daniel Boone soon found ginseng in the Appalachians and elsewhere and reportedly made money in the ginseng trade.

One physician who began studying Indian herbal medicine in the 1770s was Benjamin Rush of Philadelphia, who became the most prominent of four doctors who signed the Declaration of Independence and the most famous American physician and medical teacher of his generation. Born near Philadelphia in 1745, Rush thought of becoming a lawyer or minister, but after his schooling at Princeton, he changed his mind and returned to Philadelphia to study medicine. He completed his studies in London and Edinburgh, where he received his medical degree in 1768. He then toured Europe and in Paris became friends with Benjamin Franklin, then the American minister to France. In August 1769, Rush returned to Philadelphia, established his medical practice, and soon was the leading proponent of heroic medicine. He participated in pre-Revolutionary movements, and renewed his friendship with Franklin when he also returned home. The two men had much in common, and Franklin, as a printer, published eighteen books on medicine between 1732 and 1765.

Rush made a point of talking with Indians who visited Philadelphia in order to gather information about their medicine. He was intent on learning how their lifestyle influenced their health and survival. In

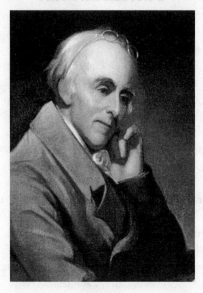

Benjamin Rush (1746–1813) as painted by
Charles Wilson Peale about 1818. Dr. Rush
was a signer of the Declaration of Indepen-
dence. He attended the Continental Congress
and treated soldiers during the American
Revolution. He practiced heroic medicine and
had an interest in Indian medicine. Rush has
been described as "the American Hippocrates"
and "the Father of American Psychiatry."
(Courtesy Carpenters' Hall, Philadelphia)

1774, he presented a paper titled "An Inquiry into the Natural History
of Medicine Among the Indians" to the American Philosophical Society in Philadelphia, and concluded that Indians generally maintained
good health because they anointed their bodies with oil, which supposedly promoted longevity in warm climates because it checked perspiration; they took one cold bath each day to fortify the body, rendering it
less subject to those diseases that arise from the extremes and vicissi-
tudes of heat and cold; and they refrained from drinking before dinner,
work, or travel, which made their systems less receptive to overheating.

Rush concluded that Indian children were healthy because as babies
they were breast-fed by their mothers for two years, giving them extraordinary vigor. The children, he added, gained strength against heat

and cold by being plunged into cold water every day, and he pointed out that babies were strapped to a board for six to eighteen months in order to facilitate their being moved from place to place and to preserve their shape. Rush also believed that the Indians' mixed diet of wild game, roots, and fruits was one of the most efficient ways of warding off disease. He also theorized that because Indians avoided drinking water during long marches, they were able to stay alert, resist fatigue, and accomplish their daily goals.

Rush believed that Indian women generally had strong immune systems because of their heavy, constant domestic labor, which was why their bodies maintained an intimidating firmness. He concluded that this firmness delayed the onset of menstruation until they were eighteen to twenty. And because their menstrual cycles started so late, when they did marry their reproductive systems had a greater vigor that enabled them to better support the convulsions of childbirth. He added that because there is hardly a period in the interval between the eruption and ceasing of the menses in which the women are not pregnant or breast-feeding, this is the most natural state for Indian women and is similar to the best state of health of women in the "civilized" world.

From the information he gathered, Rush concluded that fevers were the only diseases among Indians before the arrival of Europeans, and that their fevers were caused by the "insensible" qualities of air breathed because they lived primarily out of doors. He believed inflammatory fevers were produced by cold and heat, while intermitting, remitting, malignant fevers, and dysentery were caused by insensible qualities of air or putrid exhalations. In his opinion, Indians relied on the powers of nature for their primary cures, especially the drinking of cold water for fevers. He noted that sweating was another natural remedy, along with the Indian custom of confining a patient to a closed tent or wigwam with red-hot stones in the middle. Water poured over the stones created a thick, warm cloud of moist air that caused sweating.

To cure fractures, breaks, and other wounds, Rush believed that Indians usually relied on nature to be the surgeon. He said natural remedies were also used for purging and vomiting, but Rush did not pay much attention to Indian herb and plant remedies in his paper; he considered their use to be only secondary cures. They sometimes bled their patients, restricting the bleeding to that part of the body affected, and using sharp stones and thorns to draw the blood. They also employed caustics, usually a piece of rotten wood placed on the affected area. The wood would be set afire and the hot ashes would burn a hole in the flesh. Astringent vegetables were applied in cases of intermittent fever. Rush summed up his view on Indian medicine with these words: "We have no discoveries in the materia medica to hope for from the Indians in North America. It would be a reproach to our school of physic, if modern physicians were not more successful than the Indians, even in the treatment of their own diseases."[4]

Rush's failure to examine in depth the use of herbs, plants, and trees in Indian medicine was one major flaw in his presentation; a second was that he studied Indians only in the vicinity of Philadelphia. In no way did his conclusions represent all Indians in North America, and certainly not those to the southwest and west, in regions unexplored by colonial Americans. Rush assumed the lifestyle of Indians everywhere was the same. He did not realize there were significant differences from tribe to tribe westward to the Pacific.

In 1790, after practicing medicine for twenty years, Rush began to publish his own medical theories and conclusions. He stressed the use of bloodletting and purgative medicines to cure consumption (tuberculosis), dropsy (swelling of the body), hydrocephalus (the buildup of excessive spinal fluid), apoplexy (uncontrolled bleeding that caused strokes), gout (a painful type of arthritis), and other diseases of the body. But when a yellow fever epidemic struck Philadelphia in 1793 and he attempted to apply his theories, he, as well as other doctors, was unsuccessful in treating the disease. Frustrated, Rush turned to his library and read everything he had acquired that concerned yellow fever. He found a paper written by a Dr. Mitchell of Virginia, who earlier had succeeded in curing yellow fever by using powerful evacuates. Rush immediately began administering calomel and jalap, and cured four of the first five patients to whom he applied this method. He quickly passed along this form of treatment to the two other physicians remaining in Philadelphia who had survived the disease and not deserted their patients and left town. All told, the three doctors treated about 6,000 patients. For several days Rush treated as many as 120 patients each day, and along with his two colleagues saved many lives.

Much of Benjamin Rush's fame as a physician came from his Philadelphia practice, but he is also remembered for his unparalleled intellectual curiosity about Indians and their health. Rush never convinced his friend Thomas Jefferson that the doctors of their time did more good than ill; Jefferson favored herbal over heroic medicine. Even so, he still had great respect for Rush.

Early in 1803, President Jefferson sent Congress a secret communication seeking authorization to send an expedition into the West beyond the Mississippi River. Jefferson chose his personal secretary, Meriwether Lewis, to lead the expedition and sent Lewis with letters of introduction to Philadelphia to meet with selected members of the American Philosophical Society, including Rush. There Lewis reportedly discussed paleontology and botany with Caspar Wistar, a prominent physician, and met Andrew Ellicott, America's foremost surveyor and an accomplished astronomer and mathematician. Lewis also met Robert Patterson, professor of medicine at the University of Pennsylvania. While Lewis spent much of his time in Philadelphia buying camp equipment and supplies, he also talked with Benjamin Rush, who not only gave his advice freely but also provided him with a carefully prepared list of questions to answer about the history, medicine, morals, and religion of the Indians he would meet:

> What are the acute diseases of the Indians? Is the bilious fever attended with a black vomit?
>
> Is Goiture [*sic*], apoplexy, palsy, Epilepsy, madness . . . ven. [venereal] Disease known among them?
>
> What is their state of life as to longevity?
>
> At what age do the women begin and cease to menstruate?
>
> At what age do they marry? How long do they suckle the Children?
>
> What is the provision of their Childr[e]n after being weaned? The state of the pulse as to frequency in the morning, at noon & at night— before & after eating? What is its state in childhood. Adult life, & old age? The number of strokes counted by the quarter of a minute by glass, and multiplied by four will give its frequency in a minute. What are their Rem[e]dies?
>
> Are artificial discharges of blood ever used among them?
>
> In what manner do they induce sweating?
>
> Do they ever use voluntary fasting?
>
> At what time do they rise—their Baths?
>
> What is the diet—manner of cooking & times of eating among the Indians?
>
> How do they preserve their food?[5]

Rush undoubtedly lectured Lewis on his principles of medicine, including the bloodletting Thomas Jefferson opposed. On June 11, 1803, after Lewis left Philadelphia, Rush sent the president a letter in which he wrote that "[Lewis's] mission is truly interesting. I shall wait with great solicitude for its issue. Mr. Lewis appears admirably qualified for it. May its advantages prove no less honorable to your administration than to the interest of science."[6]

Meriwether Lewis was certainly qualified to lead Thomas Jefferson's Corps of Discovery and to gather information about the land and the inhabitants of the newly acquired Louisiana Territory. Before becoming Jefferson's personal secretary, Lewis, as an Army officer, had acquired some medical knowledge and the skills needed to set broken bones and tend to boils, tumors, cuts, and gunshot wounds. Lewis also knew herbal medicine—which Jefferson, as noted above, favored. Jefferson knew Lewis's family well; they were his neighbors in Charlottesville, Virginia, and he had much respect for Lucy Marks, Lewis's mother, who was well known for her herbal cures. It was she, Jefferson knew, who had taught her son herbal medicine.

After returning to Washington from Philadelphia, Lewis met with Jefferson to finalize plans for the expedition. On June 1, 1803, Lewis had sent a long letter to William Clark, asking him to be co-leader of the expedition. Clark accepted. On July 3, official word was received that James Monroe and Robert Livingston had arranged the purchase of the Louisiana Territory from France for the United States. By then Lewis was ready to head west. On July 4, 1803, Jefferson, Lewis, and others celebrated not only the purchase but also the nation's twenty-seventh birthday. Jefferson wished Lewis well and told him to "bring back your party safe." The following day Lewis left the capital and traveled west to Harper's Ferry to pick up equipment he had previously ordered and to arrange for its delivery by wagon to Pittsburgh, where a keelboat was being constructed. The boat builder, a heavy drinker, was behind schedule. It was seven weeks before the keelboat was finished, on August 31, and supplies were immediately loaded aboard. Lewis and a crew of ten men started down the Ohio River the same day.

Their journey was slow because of low water caused by a drought. When they reached Wheeling on September 7, they loaded on additional equipment and rested. While they were there, William Patterson, a physician, approached Lewis and volunteered to join the expedition. Patterson probably was the son of Robert Patterson, professor of medicine at the University of Pennsylvania, whom Lewis had visited in Philadelphia. Lewis agreed to take him on the expedition, but told Patterson he had to be ready to travel by three o'clock the next afternoon. When Patterson failed to show, Lewis and his party left without him and set off again down the river.

William Clark joined Lewis and the others at Clarksville, Indiana, and the keelboat continued down the Ohio toward Wood River, Illinois. Since agreeing to join the expedition, Clark had spent time studying astronomy and learning to make maps. When he joined Lewis, the medical capabilities of the expedition were also doubled, because Clark, like Lewis, had the usual military training required for treating common injuries but had learned other medical skills as well, such as how to prepare poultices and calculate proper dosages of medicine. Even though Jefferson favored herbal medicine for curing illness, Lewis took a good supply of the medicine and implements recommended by Dr. Rush in Philadelphia.

Lewis purchased a hardwood chest in Philadelphia, and by the time the expedition started up the Missouri River it was stocked with medical supplies, costing $90.60, that included a mortar and pestle for preparing remedies, a scale for weighing ingredients, a measuring beaker, syringes, lancets, and one tourniquet for use, if needed, with amputation. The chest also contained fifteen pounds of powdered Peruvian bark containing quinine to treat fevers, one-half pound of powdered jalap derived from the Mexican morning glory, and one-half pound of powdered rhubarb, both used as laxatives. Lewis included four ounces of powdered ipecacuan, a Brazilian root used as an emetic, purgative, or diaphoretic for the treatment of fevers. He also included in the chest two pounds of powdered cream of tartar (potassium bitartrate) used as a purgative or diuretic, two ounces of gum camphor, used as a stimulant and as a diaphoretic, one-half pound of common poppy for producing opium to be used as a painkiller, and four ounces of tragacanth, an inert gum for making pills. There also was a supply of benzoin, a disinfectant, plus six pounds of Glauber's salt (sodium sulfate), used as a purgative, plus two pounds of saltpeter (potassium nitrate), employed in the treatment of fevers and gonorrhea. Other medicines in the chest included six ounces of Sacchar or sugar of lead (lead acetate) used in the treatment of eye problems, and a penile syringe for the treatment of gonorrhea. There also were fifty dozen "Bilious Pills" (six hundred) ordered by Benjamin Rush, containing a combination of calomel (mercurous chloride) and jalap.[7]

Lewis also carried with him a list of eleven commandments "for preserving your health" that had been prepared by Dr. Rush:

1. When you feel the least indisposition, do not attempt to overcome it by labor or marching. Rest in a horizontal position. Also, fasting and diluting drinks for a day or two will generally overcome an attack of fever. To those preventatives of disease may be added a gentle sweat obtained by warm drinks, or gently opening the bowels by means of one, two or more of the purging pills.
2. Unusual costiveness is often a sign of an approaching disease. When you feel it, take one or more of the purging pills.
3. Want of appetite is otherwise a sign of approaching indisposition. It should be banished by the same method.
4. In difficult and laborious enterprises or marches, eating sparingly will enable you to bear them with less fatigue and more safety to your health.
5. Flannel should be worn constantly next to the skin, especially in wet weather.
6. The less spirits you use, the better.
7. Molasses or sugar victuals with a few drops of the acid of vitriol will make a pleasant and wholesome drink with your meals.
8. After having your feet much chilled, it will be useful to wash them with a little spirit.
9. Washing your feet every morning in cold water will fortify them against the notion of cold.
10. After long marches or much fatigue from any work, you will be more refreshed from lying down in a horizontal position for two hours than by resting a much longer time in any other position of the body.
11. Shoes made without heels by affording equal action to all the muscles of the legs will enable you to march with less fatigue than shoes made in the ordinary way.[8]

As the expedition pushed up the Missouri River from St. Louis, the men began to be plagued with gastrointestinal problems caused by their mostly meat diet and the drinking of muddy river water. Lewis began handing out Dr. Rush's Bilious Pills, which the men soon nick-named "Thunderclappers." They were not a cure but a quick-acting laxative that provided almost immediate relief.[9]

The account of their more-than-two-year round-trip expedition (1803–6) across the continent is well known, so here we will highlight only the medical aspects. This journey of 8,000 miles in twenty-eight months is itself remarkable, considering that only one member of their party, Sergeant Charles Floyd, lost his life. Two weeks before his death on August 20, 1804, near modern-day Sioux City, Iowa, Floyd apparently came down with a respiratory infection, then seemingly recovered. But suddenly he again became ill with severe, colicky abdominal pain, vomiting, and diarrhea and died within a single day. Many people have speculated that he died from a ruptured appendix, but as Bruce C. Paton, M.D., more recently concluded, "the evidence and clinical course do not fully fit with this diagnosis." Paton believes Floyd may have died from an overwhelming gastrointestinal infection, a ruptured organ (other than the appendix), or a burst aneurysm. But early-nineteenth-century physicians, including Benjamin Rush, knew little of these things.[10]

While the evidence suggests that Lewis conscientiously sought to follow Dr. Rush's medical advice, he was not always able to do so because some of the doctor's recommendations were impractical in the unsettled western country. Lewis and Clark had to adapt to the conditions they found, using their own training and skills to resolve a variety of medical ailments. Probably the most common problems were boils and swellings on their men's feet and lower legs. These were treated with poultices. Several men contracted venereal disease (it was then called the pox) from Indian women, which was treated by applying a mercury ointment to the infected areas until the sores healed. Lewis himself may have used the ointment. There were many cases of dysentery, which were treated with Glauber salts, a purgative first produced in 1668 from sulfate of sodium, and laudanum (Tinctura Opii), a pain reliever containing opium. When a member of the expedition was bitten on his ankle by a prairie rattlesnake, causing pain, bruising, and swelling, he was treated with a poultice of Peruvian bark. The poultice did not work, but because there was not much venom in the bite, the man nonetheless recovered.

On January 10, 1805, at Fort Mandan, the winter quarters they constructed in modern North Dakota, Lewis wrote that an Indian boy about thirteen arrived with his feet frostbitten after he'd spent a night in the frigid cold under a buffalo robe but without a fire. The boy's feet were put in cold water, and he appeared to be recovering. However, seventeen days later Lewis had to amputate the toes on one of the boy's feet. That day, January 27, 1805, Clark wrote that he bled a man "with the Plurisy . . . & Swet him."

It was at Fort Mandan that forty-five-year-old Toussaint Charbonneau, a French-Canadian fur trader who lived among the Hidatsa and Mandan Indians, was hired as an interpreter. On the evening of February 11, 1805, Sacagawea, one of Charbonneau's two wives, delivered her first child, a fine boy who was named Jean-Baptiste. Lewis wrote that in such cases labor was often tedious and the pain was intense. He was told that if one administered a small portion of the rattle of the rattlesnake, the birth would be quick. Lewis noted that two rings of a rattle were broken in small pieces and added to a small quantity of water: "Whether this medicine was truly the cause or not I shall not undertake to determine, but I was informed that she had not taken it more than ten minutes before she brought forth . . . perhaps this remedy may be worthy of future experiments, but I must confess that I want faith as to its efficacy."[11]

Six months later Sacagawea almost died when the expedition reached the Great Falls of the Missouri. Clark wrote in his journal that "if she dies, it will be the fault of her husband as I am now convinced." Lewis noted that Sacagawea suffered from "an obstruction of the mensis [menses] in consequence of taking could [sic]," suggesting, as Washington University historians Peter Kastor and Conevery Bolton Valenčius reported in 2004, that her illness may have been the result of a miscarriage.[12] She survived after Lewis and Clark ignored heroic medicine and turned to herbs and the use of mineral water.

While Lewis and four other men were traveling overland from the mouth of the Marias River to the Great Falls of the Missouri, Lewis got very sick from dysentery. Having no heroic medicines with him, he turned to a herbal remedy: he had chokecherry twigs cut and boiled to produce a liquid, which he drank. By the next day, he had recovered. On another occasion when a member of the expedition, Peter M. Weiser, became ill from a stomach disorder, Lewis administered peppermint, a resin derived from the *Pistacia lentiscue* tree, and laudanum for relief.

When the expedition reached the Pacific and built Fort Clatsop, William Bratton could not walk because of the pain in his lower back, probably due to lumbago or rheumatism. Heroic medicine did not cure him either. He was only able to walk again after an Indian technique of putting Bratton in a sweat lodge and alternating that with immersion in a cold stream. Only then did Bratton's back loosen up, enabling him to walk. While George Gibson and a few other men were making salt on the coast some miles from Fort Clatsop, Gibson cut his knee badly with his tomahawk. The wound was washed, poultices applied, and then wrapped in bandages. He got well. On their return journey, William Clark became so ill at Three Forks in present-day Montana that the expedition had to stop and let him rest for several days until he recovered from what may have been tick fever. Near the end of their two-year journey, Lewis was accidentally shot in the thigh. Clark washed and treated the wound with poultices and bandages.

We know a great deal about the practice of medicine on Lewis and Clark's journey because the expedition was carefully planned and everything recorded in journals and diaries. Meriwether Lewis was meticulous in his attention to detail in solving medical problems because he had the ability to differentiate symptoms, which is the basis for diagnosis, a knack sorely lacking in many early-nineteenth-century physicians. It is doubtful that Lewis realized it at the time, but diagnosis would form the foundation for the revolutionary change in American medicine that would occur a few decades later.

The co-leaders' preparations for the journey and the advice Lewis received from Dr. Benjamin Rush were important, but Lewis's understanding and use of herbal medicine was certainly a vital factor as well. Another plus was that the explorers and their men were in excellent physical condition and had army discipline ingrained in them. Lewis and Clark's leadership and their persistent concern for the health and well-being of their men made the Corps of Discovery function like a well-oiled machine adjusting to change. Their journals reflect this, as do the known diaries kept by men on the expedition. For instance, Private Joseph Whitehouse wrote in his diary of his "utmost gratitude . . . for the humanity shown at all times" by Captains Lewis and Clark.[13]

While the expedition came into contact with nearly fifty Indian tribes and witnessed their way of life in varying degrees, more pressing concerns regarding diplomacy and trade apparently gave Lewis little time to seek all of the answers Benjamin Rush had asked him to obtain about the history, medicine, morals, and religions of the Indians he met. Lewis and Clark's journals contain at least bits and pieces of information relating to Rush's questions, but no comprehensive or extended accounts such as the Philadelphia doctor would have wished to receive. After the expedition returned east, Meriwether Lewis spent more than two months in Philadelphia, but there is no evidence that he or William Clark ever met with Rush to discuss what they had learned about Indians on their expedition.

CHAPTER THREE

OVER THE APPALACHIANS

Nothing is more fatal to health than over-care of it.

—Benjamin Franklin

BEFORE THE AMERICAN REVOLUTION, colonists along the Atlantic coast were hemmed in on the west by the rugged Appalachian Mountains, which stretch south from Canada through New England, Pennsylvania, West Virginia, Virginia, and the Carolinas to northern Georgia and Alabama. Some adventurous hunters and trappers began penetrating the mountains by the early 1700s, but most colonists gave little thought to moving west of the Appalachians because the British government, wishing to avoid antagonizing or provoking the Indians living there, forbade settlement in that area. By the late 1760s, however, as tensions mounted between the colonies and their mother country, Richard Henderson, a former merchant in Virginia, moved to North Carolina to study law. He soon became a judge and land speculator, and he hired the frontiersman Daniel Boone to explore beyond the mountains, with an eye to establishing new settlements. Boone made several forays into present-day Tennessee and Kentucky. Encouraged by what he reported, Henderson successfully negotiated for Cherokee Indian land west of the Appalachians. In 1769, Boone led a group of families out of North Carolina through the Cumberland Gap over an old Indian trail that soon became known as the Wilderness Road. Boone established a settlement on the Kentucky River and named it Boonesborough. It still exists, but today it is an unincorporated community in Madison County in central Kentucky.

James Robertson, a frontiersman from what is now Wake County, North Carolina, had accompanied Boone on one of his explorations over the mountains. Roberts liked the country and about 1770, as the leader of twelve families from North Carolina, blazed a trail that became known as the Yellow Mountain Road across the mountains to the present site of Elizabethton, Tennessee. There Robertson helped to establish the Watauga colony. In 1778, three years into the American Revolution, he led a group of 250 frontiersmen and their families, including the author's great-great-great-great-grandfather, James Russell, to establish Fort Nashborough, now Nashville, Tennessee, on the Cumberland River. By then more English, German, and Scottish immigrants were moving south into the Shenandoah Valley and into western Pennsylvania and along the headwaters of the Ohio River. The nation's great westward migration was under way, and it led to the creation of a new pioneer society. From this society evolved characteristics that are today regarded as typically American, including individual freedom, rugged individualism, self-reliance, equality of opportunity, hard work, material wealth, and competition.[1]

As settlers moved into what is now Virginia, Kentucky, Tennessee, western Pennsylvania, and southern Ohio, Indiana, and Illinois, most were looking for land on which to settle, grow crops and livestock, and raise their families. In 1800, when the nation's population had grown to more than five million, only 10 percent of all Americans lived west of the Appalachians, primarily in Tennessee, Kentucky, and Virginia, including what is now West Virginia; but by 1824, 30 percent of all Americans were settled between the Appalachians and the Mississippi River. The westward migration was gradual and did not occur in an orderly fashion. Once a family or group decided to move west, they simply packed up and started out. Some followed the wagon road that ran west from Philadelphia and south through the Shenandoah Valley and through North Carolina into South Carolina. Boone's Wilderness Road was a particularly popular route for those going to Kentucky and Tennessee. Still others favored river transportation, and by 1810 flatboats floating down the Ohio River— bringing settlers and goods westward toward the Mississippi, then the nation's western boundary—were a commonplace sight. Settlements sprang up along the rivers.

Gradually doctors arrived. Dr. Patrick Vance was the first white physician in Tennessee following the American Revolution, while an army doctor named Skinner, a native of Maryland, probably became the first physician in Kentucky when he was assigned to the military post founded in 1778 by George Rogers Clark on the site of modern

Louisville. Most people, being farmers, settled in the countryside. Unlike Indians who had long farmed the region and cultivated several crops on a single plot of land, the newcomers farmed on several pieces of land, dedicating each to a single crop, usually corn, and later wheat or some other grain. These pioneers tried to produce more than they needed for their own use so they would have a surplus to sell. But this approach to crop cultivation exhausted the soil more quickly than the Indian method of farming, and soon people were moving westward again seeking uncultivated land, much of which had to be cleared of trees.

Settlers learned quickly that courage and hard work overcame most natural obstacles, but a major and unrelenting concern was sickness. They measured happiness by their health and came to realize that when they settled on rich farmland in the river bottoms, their health became poor. Unfortunately, they did not understand that the mosquitoes, fleas, lice, ticks, rats, and snakes which abounded in areas with stagnant water, swamps, and muddy river bottoms carried disease and infection. The settlers viewed them as nothing more than unavoidable nuisances, especially on the river bottomland made rich by the silt deposited by frequent floods. High ground was healthier, but few settlers built their houses there because the land was poorer and often rocky or forested.

Since few people associated disease with where they built their houses, the land they farmed, or where they established settlements, they continued to locate along rivers for the convenience of boat transportation and trade. The oldest river town between the Appalachians and the Mississippi was New Orleans, founded as a French colony in 1718. Residents, however, found its location unhealthy. In 1803, the year the United States purchased Louisiana Territory, including New Orleans, from France, Pierre du Lac, a French visitor, wrote that "nothing equals the filthiness of New Orleans unless it be the unhealthfulness, which has for some years appeared to have resulted from it. The city, the filth of which cannot be drained off, is not paved. . . . Its markets, which are unventilated, are reeking with rottenness. . . . Its squares are covered with the filth of animals, which no one takes the trouble to remove. Consequently there is seldom a year that the yellow fever or some other contagious malady does not carry off many strangers."[2]

Another unhealthy settlement was Louisville, Kentucky, near the falls of the Ohio River and what was then the western end of the Wilderness Road. By 1820, Louisville had a population of about 4,000 people, but it was becoming known as the "Graveyard of the West." The town was built over ponds that in the summer were breeding places for mosquitoes. The ponds extended south and west to the mouth of the Salt River, some twenty miles away, along a strip of land about twenty miles wide. Residents did not associate the mosquitoes with malaria or other diseases. Many level streets in the town drained poorly and held moisture, creating more breeding places for mosquitoes. When an epidemic of "bilious fever" struck Louisville in 1823, aroused citizens appointed a board of health. The legislature approved a lottery to raise funds to fill in the ponds, but the project faltered.

The English writer Charles Dickens recognized the unhealthy conditions in various areas when he visited America a few years later and traveled on the Mississippi and Ohio rivers. In his *American Notes* (1842) he observed that at the junction of the two rivers where the town of Cairo, Illinois, was founded in 1817, the ground was "so flat and low and marshy, that at certain seasons of the year it is inundated to the house-tops." Dickens described Cairo as a "breeding-place of fever, ague, and death" and labeled the Mississippi River as "an enormous ditch, sometimes two or three miles wide, running liquid mud, six miles an hour." He described the residents of Cairo as being "more wan and wretched than any we had encountered."

During the hot summers, dysentery and malaria were common in most low-lying areas. When settlers became sick they were soon debilitated, making them susceptible to dropsy, jaundice, and consumption. Their weakened condition also made them candidates for measles, mumps, smallpox, scarlet fever, pneumonia, and typhoid fever, some of which were carried west by new settlers and travelers. Because of the scarcity of physicians, medicine, like cookery, was mostly home-grown. Settlers treated themselves as best they could with home remedies such as mustard plasters, sulfur, sassafras, rhubarb, molasses, and herbs. These expedients often relieved symptoms, but they did not cure disease. The existence of germs was unknown, and the universal ignorance of proper sanitation made the spread of disease commonplace. Most people believed that bathing removed protective oils from their skin. As for cookery, food was prepared in dirty and pest-ridden conditions, and what people ate often did not help their health. James Fenimore Cooper wrote in his book *The American Democrat* (1838) that "Americans are the grossest feeders of any civilized nation known . . . food is heavy, coarse, ill-prepared and indigestible. . . . The predominance of grease in the American kitchen, coupled with the habits of hasty eating and of constant expectoration, are the cause of the diseases of the stomach so common in America."

American medicine was still primitive. In 1810, not one in fifty physicians along the Atlantic coast, and not one in a hundred west of the Appalachians, had a diploma from a school of medicine. There were only seven medical schools in the United States, serving a grand total of no more than 650 students. However, an American system of medical education did begin to develop in the early 1800s, and twenty-six additional medical schools opened between 1810 and 1840. A pattern developed whereby the medical education for new doctors consisted of three years of apprenticeship with a practicing physician, and attendance at two short annual sessions in a medical school at which the same lectures would often be given in the second year as in the first. These became the accepted requirements for a medical degree. New medical schools sprang up not only in large cities but in country towns. They were launched whenever a handful of doctors wanting to teach could form a faculty and attract students. Many of these schools established some loose attachment with an established college, either locally or at some distance. Since no licensing exams were required, the quality of the education provided largely depended upon the ability, sincerity, honesty, and energy of the doctors teaching.

Many physicians who moved west over the Appalachians early in the nineteenth century practiced the heroic medicine of Philadelphia's Benjamin Rush. They treated patients with powerful drugs and blood-letting that often did more harm than good. There were, however, other doctors disposed to let nature have its way. One old doctor who practiced "nature's way" from the late eighteenth into the early nineteenth century recalled that he had great difficulty with the new names of diseases and was frank enough to admit it. He also was plagued when physicians east of the Appalachians changed the names of medicines. This unidentified doctor admitted that he had never used drugs much and had never seen the inside of a cadaver. It appears that many old-time physicians rebelled against the new and what they did not understand as the scientific inquiry into medicine, which was just beginning.[3]

UNTIL THE UNITED STATES purchased Louisiana Territory in 1803, the Mississippi River was the nation's western boundary. Some Virginians had pushed westward by 1800, settling along the river's eastern bank on the strip of land called "The American Bottom," which extended from modern-day Chester to Alton, Illinois, and from the river east to the bluffs. It was rich bottomland, and rather picturesque. To the west, in the middle of the Mississippi River, was Blood Island, so named because it was the scene of several duels, a rendezvous point for gamblers, and a place where cockfights were held.

In 1801, a group of Pennsylvania Dutch arrived and founded Belleville, Illinois, located about ten miles southeast of present-day St. Louis, Missouri. Around 1815 a physician named Estes became Belleville's first doctor. Little is known about his medical training, but from all accounts he was of strong mind and an experienced frontiersman. He built a house south of the public square and soon became captain of a band of "regulators" who dealt out justice to the horse thieves and other crooks who plagued the area. It wasn't long, however, before Dr. Estes sought greener pastures. By then another physician, identified only as Dr. Schogg, had set up practice in Belleville, but he, too, did not stay long. An unidentified writer in *St. Clair County History* (1881) described Schogg as "a noxious vapor, shedding light and darkness so close to each other, that he put the whole town in an uproar. He had two shooting matches, using pistols, and their targets were their own bodies."

Probably neither of these doctors had much formal medical education. They may have, like many other physicians on the frontier, served apprenticeships with practicing doctors and perhaps read medical textbooks from the physicians' libraries. If so, those books most likely lacked illustrations. The apprentice had to memorize the names of muscles without seeing a diagram or illustration, and the names of the bones in the human body without ever seeing a human skeleton. Conditions were slightly better when the physician taught the apprentice how to compound medicines. Each physician mixed his own medicines, so the student could learn by watching the physician and then making his own. Since most apprentices paid to study with physicians, the arrangement provided a mentoring doctor with needed extra income and cheap labor.

One young man who started his medical career as an apprentice was Ephraim McDowell. Born in Rockbridge County, Virginia, in 1771, McDowell was twelve when his parents moved to Danville, Kentucky, about thirty-five miles southwest of Lexington. When he was about twenty, he apprenticed himself to Dr. Alexander Humphreys in Staunton, Virginia, who had received his medical degree from the University of Edinburgh in Scotland. Humphreys came to the United States just after the American Revolution, and settled in Augusta County, Virginia, where his brother lived. In 1787, Humphreys moved to Staunton, a frontier town of about eight hundred people located on the north–south wagon road running between Philadelphia and South Carolina. Dr. Humphreys was soon impressed with young McDowell, a serious student, and urged him to study at the University of Edinburgh.

Although McDowell's father, Samuel, was not wealthy, he wanted his son to get the best possible medical education. And so, about six years later, in 1793, McDowell, now a tall and broad-shouldered young man of twenty-two, crossed the Atlantic and enrolled as a first-year medical student at Edinburgh. He attended as many lectures as he could and learned anatomy and the basics of surgery, which included amputations, how to treat wounds, and the removal of tumors. McDowell had hoped to remain in Scotland three years to earn his medical degree; at the end of his second year, financial conditions forced him to return home to Danville, where he opened a medical practice. The fact that he lacked a formal degree did not matter to the people of Danville. They were sufficiently impressed that he had studied at a great university, and were soon even more impressed with his ability to treat hernias, do amputations, and perform other medical procedures.

In December 1809, Dr. McDowell was asked to visit the log cabin home of Mrs. Jane Crawford in Green County, Kentucky. The request came from two physicians already caring for her who believed that she was struggling to deliver overdue twins. After a vaginal examination, McDowell concluded that she was not pregnant and that her distended belly was caused by an enlarged ovarian tumor. He realized that the only thing that could save her life was to remove the tumor, but he knew no such operation had even been successful. In fact, abdominal surgery in general was positively taboo. Medical school professors were emphatic in warning students never to operate on the abdomen, pointing out that attempts at cesarean section had always been fatal. McDowell, however, had heard Dr. Humphreys describe a successful cesarean operation. Fifteen years earlier, Dr. Jesse Bennett, a graduate of the University of Pennsylvania, had performed a successful cesarean section on his own wife at Edom, in what is now West Virginia, in 1794. A few physicians in the area knew about the operation, but Bennett never reported it, because as a rule doctors did not operate on their own family members.[4]

Dr. McDowell confronted Mrs. Crawford and frankly explained that she could stay home and die, or there was a chance she could live if she was willing to come to his home in Danville and let him operate. Her husband opposed the operation. McDowell again explained her chances. Finally, the Crawfords agreed. McDowell left for Danville to make preparations. A few days later Mrs. Crawford dressed warmly and mounted her horse, resting her distended stomach on the pommel of her saddle. With a neighbor's wife, she rode sixty miles in the winter cold to Danville. Once she was in the doctor's home, McDowell had her rest to regain her strength while he made plans for the operation. He decided to operate on Christmas Day 1809, saying, "God's beneficence will be at its highest." As was his custom before every operation, he wrote out a prayer: "Direct me, Oh! God in performing this operation for I am but an instrument in Thy hands. . . . Oh! Spare this afflicted woman." With the assistance of his nephew James McDowell, who had studied medicine, and another physician, Dr. Alban Smith, McDowell began the operation.

Without sedating Mrs. Crawford, Dr. McDowell used a pen to mark the path of his incision. He then made a nine-inch cut into the abdominal cavity, exposing the large tumor. Mrs. Crawford endured the pain by reciting psalms and singing hymns even as her intestines rolled onto the wooden table beside her. The tumor was so large that McDowell could not remove it in one piece. So he cut it open and took out 15 pounds of a dirty, gelatinous-looking substance. He next removed the sack, which weighed 7½ pounds. He then rinsed Mrs. Crawford's intestines with warm water and replaced them. He then turned his patient on her side to allow the blood to drain from the abdominal cavity before he carefully sutured the edges of his incision

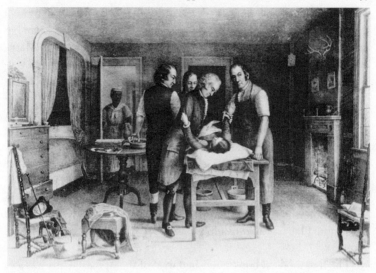

Dr. Ephraim McDowell's operation on Mrs. Jane Crawford, the world's first abdominal surgery, as portrayed by an unidentified artist. (Courtesy National Library of Medicine)

together and apposed the edges with adhesives. The operation had taken twenty-five minutes.

Twenty-five days later Mrs. Crawford returned home in good health and lived to age seventy-eight. This was the world's first ovariotomy. McDowell waited seven years before submitting his report for publication, but it took many more years before the medical profession would admit that a small-town physician in Kentucky had the ability to make medical history.[5]

Exactly how many medical practitioners were scattered between the Appalachians and the Mississippi during the early 1800s is not known. A reasonable guess is about 10,000, with the majority lacking formal medical schooling. Dr. Samuel McAdow, the first physician in the new settlement of Chillicothe, Ohio, in 1796, was unlike most. He was a native of Maryland, where he received a classical education before studying medicine in Philadelphia with Dr. Benjamin Rush. In 1793, McAdow crossed the Appalachians and practiced medicine for a time in Bourbon County, Kentucky. When he learned about a new settlement at Chillicothe in south-central Ohio, he joined a party from

Kentucky and moved north with his wife and family. Living in a small
town, McAdow had to obtain the drugs he needed in his practice in big
cities in the east. In 1802, he rode on horseback to Baltimore, Maryland, and purchased a new stock of drugs. Dr. McAdow was one of several doctors in Ohio who played a healing role in treating patients in
1807 when an influenza and fever epidemic occurred. They tried all
sorts of remedies to treat the fever, including calomel and borax. A
favorite remedy of Dr. Walter Buell of Chillicothe, an educated friend
of McAdow, was bicarbonate of soda. Buell theorized that it neutral-
ized "septic acid in the stomach and bowels . . . rendering the fever
mild and more manageable." Bicarbonate of soda worked well when
given internally, but a few doctors actually wrapped their patients in
sheets made wet with a mixture of bicarbonate of soda, alcohol, and
capsicum. This treatment supposedly cooled the patient and broke the
fever.[6]

The first medical book published west of the Appalachians was *The
Indian Doctor's Dispensatory, Being Father Smith's Advice Respecting Dis-
eases and Their Cure* . . . printed in Cincinnati in 1813 for the author,
Peter Smith, who was born in Wales in 1753 but raised in New Jersey.
After moving successively with his family to Virginia, the Carolinas,
Georgia, and Kentucky, Smith settled near Cincinnati about 1794.
There he farmed and practiced medicine, using remedies he had
learned from Indians or drawn from his own experiences. The book,
now rare, contains nearly two hundred prescriptions for botanical
remedies and descriptions of curative roots, leaves, barks, and barriers
found in eastern North America.[7]

Two years after Smith's book appeared, Dr. Richard Carter published a book of cures in 1815 at Frankfort, Kentucky, titled *Valuable
Vegetable Medical Prescriptions, for the Cure of All Nervous and Putrid Disorders*. In this 187-page work, Carter lists the following remedy for
gout and rheumatism: "Take a young fat dog and kill him, scald and
clean him as you would a pig, then extract his guts through a hole previously made in his side, and substitute in the place thereof, two handfuls of nettles, two ounces of brimstone, one dozen hen eggs, four
ounces of turpentine, a handful of tansy, a pint of red fishing worms,
and about three-fourths of a pound of tobacco, cut up fine; mix all
those ingredients well together before [they are] deposited in the dog's
belly, and then sew up the whole, then roast him well before a hot fire
as hot as you can bear it, being careful not to get wet or expose yourself

to damp or night air, or even heating yourself, or in fact you should not expose yourself in any way." The patient with rheumatism was supposedly made to feel better by the fumes from the oily substance seeping from the belly of the roasted dog and the heat of the fire.

Most practicing physicians reached their own individual conclusions concerning health and freely expounded them. At least some probably agreed with William Buchan, an English physician, when they learned his theory that men would improve their health by bathing frequently, avoiding strong drink, and regulating their diet. In 1769, Buchan published a book in Edinburgh called *Domestic Medicine, or, the Family Physician*. The work was reprinted in America in 1772. It was the first book in English to combine instructions for home treatment with general advice about diet, lifestyle, and how to live longer. During the century that followed, the book was reprinted more than 140 times, until Buchan became almost a brand name. Most doctors west of the Appalachians knew well that men on the frontier might go for months without taking a bath, and that they consumed a great deal

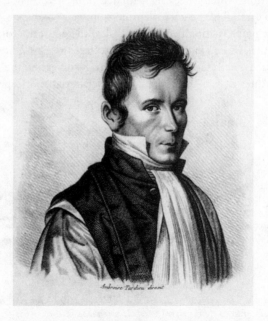

French physician Théophile Hyacinthe Laënnec (1781– 1826) invented the first stethoscope in 1816. (Courtesy National Library of Medicine)

of whiskey, brandy, and rum. Some accounts suggest that each man annually consumed about five gallons of distilled liquor.

Something else invented in Europe would help American doctors. In 1816, Théophile Hyacinthe Laënnec, a physician in France, found himself embarrassed to place his ear on the chest of a female patient to listen to her heart. He then remembered learning as a child that sound travels through solids. Laënnec rolled up twenty-four sheets of paper, placing one open end on the woman's chest and the other to his ear. He could hear her heartbeat loud and clear. When he went home, he used his woodworking equipment to turn a piece of walnut wood, hollow in the center, on his lathe. He then hollowed out a cone at one end of the piece of wood. By placing the cone end on his ear and the open end on the chest of a patient, he could easily listen to heart sounds and breathing. The *stethoscope*, as it was called, was slow to catch on, but as word of its development spread, the tool was refined by others, one of whom about 1829 produced a binaural stethoscope with two earpieces. It became popular because physicians did not have to assume uncomfortable positions when checking patients. The stethoscope has since become a symbol of the doctor's profession.

Anatomy instruction became central to the education of new doctors by the 1820s, but a serious difficulty arose. Medical schools needed cadavers to teach anatomy, but laws—reflecting the deep concern, in America and elsewhere, for proper burial and respect for the

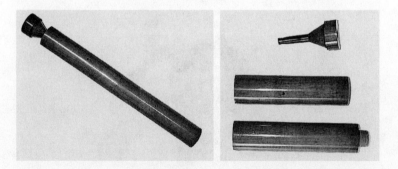

These photos show the original version of Laënnec's monaural stethoscope, constructed of turned, finely grained, light-colored wood. It was made in three parts (right) that fit together by means of a wood screw thread and brass tube fitting. Broken down, it was easy to carry in the doctor's bag. The photo on the left shows the stethoscope assembled. The overall length is 12.6 inches, the diameter 1.5 inches. (Courtesy Wood Library Museum)

dead—prohibited doctors from obtaining specimens for the classroom. Many if not most medical schools therefore resorted to robbing
graves. But when local residents heard that a grave was robbed, it usually brought a public outcry, and did little to improve popular perceptions of the medical profession. For instance, Yale University's medical
school in New Haven, Connecticut, felt the public's wrath in 1824
when someone removed a body from a fresh grave in nearby West
Haven. A constable, suspecting who had taken it, went to the school
and found the body in the cellar. When the news reached the townspeople, who were steeped in a Puritan tradition that fostered strong
religious feelings, they became furious. That evening a mob of perhaps
six hundred armed men stormed the school, pelting the building with
stones and shouting "Tear down the college!" and "Death to the students!" The mob dispersed about midnight, but only after the governor's foot guards were called out and marched toward the crowd to the
music of the fife and drum.[8]

One disease apparently unknown east of the Appalachians during
the early 1800s but widespread in the West was milk sickness or "milk
sick," also called puking stomach, sick stomach, the slows, and the
trembles. Milk sickness entailed a loss of appetite, weakness, vague
pains, muscle stiffness, vomiting, abdominal discomfort, severe constipation, bad breath, and finally coma. It was often fatal because milk
contained the toxin tremetol found in white snakeroot (*Aristolochia serpentaria*), a plant the cows ate. The amount in each plant varied with
local conditions, but this fact was not known in the early 1800s. The
plant is not usually found in pastures but grows well in or near woods.
When other forage was not available or when pastures were scarce or
in times of drought, cattle grazed on its leaves in the woods. One of the
earliest known deaths from milk sickness occurred on Little Pigeon
Creek in southern Indiana in the fall of 1818: Thirty-four-year-old
Nancy Hanks Lincoln, mother of Abraham Lincoln, died from drinking poisoned milk. The future president later remembered helping to
carve pegs for his mother's coffin.

About 1828, in Hardin County in southeastern Illinois, a midwife
named Anna Bixby or Bigsby was puzzled by the deaths of several people, including relatives of hers, as well as many cattle, from milk sickness. She may have saved some people by using a folk remedy of hot
sugar, whiskey, and plenty of rest. People in the area believed the disease was caused by poison sprinkled on the ground by witches, but not

Anna, an intelligent woman who realized that milk sickness occurred only during the summer and early fall. She warned her neighbors not to drink milk until after the first frost. One day she described the sickness to an elderly Shawnee woman well versed in herbal medicine. The woman took Anna into the woods and pointed out the plant—white snakeroot—and explained how her people used its roots—in small doses—to treat fevers, stomach problems, sore throat, and snakebites. Anna experimented and fed some of the plant's leaves to a calf. The animal was soon sick. Convinced that the white snakeroot was the cause, she warned settlers in southern Illinois about it, and through her efforts white snakeroot was eradicated and milk sickness virtually eliminated in the area during the three years that followed.

Anna's discovery, however, went unnoticed outside of her home area because she was a midwife and not a physician. Milk sickness persisted widely elsewhere until the 1920s, when the U.S. Department of Agriculture officially discovered the cause to be white snakeroot. Unlike many other medical practitioners of the early nineteenth century, Anna Bixby had the ability to diagnose the problem and find a solution.[9]

One of the best-known pioneer physicians in the Ohio Valley was Daniel Drake, who was born on a farm near Plainfield, New Jersey, in October 1785. When he was two years old, his parents, Isaac and Elizabeth Shotwell Drake, moved to Mayslick, Kentucky, about sixty miles southeast of Cincinnati. There Daniel was educated and learned to read by age seven. He grew up in a log cabin across the road from a tavern and store owned by his father's brother, Abraham Drake, who sent his son John to study medicine with Dr. William G. Goforth at Washington, Kentucky. Two years later, John Drake entered the University of Pennsylvania to continue studying medicine. Both families planned for John to return to Mayslick and teach his cousin Daniel medicine. John, however, died soon after graduation in Philadelphia. But Daniel's father was determined his son have a medical education, and when he learned that Dr. Goforth had moved to the new settlement of Cincinnati, population about 750, Isaac Drake traveled there and arranged for Daniel to study medicine with Goforth, a tall man with a long and slender neck, who had the reputation of being the homeliest person anyone had ever seen. Goforth agreed to take the fifteen-year-old Daniel as an apprentice for $400 for four years. Daniel began his apprenticeship in December 1800.

Daniel did well. He learned all he could about medicine and not only helped Dr. Goforth with patients but was soon handling the doctor's business affairs and serving as well as a pharmacist, compounding medicine and making pills. Daniel was also expected to feed, water, curry, and saddle the doctor's horse. By 1804, Drake became a partner in Goforth's practice. The next year Goforth granted Drake a diploma to practice medicine on his own. It was the first medical diploma granted west of the Appalachians. After practicing medicine in Cincinnati for several years, Drake went to the University of Pennsylvania to study and received his medical degree in six months. He returned to Mayslick, where he practiced medicine for about a year. When Dr. Goforth moved to Louisiana in 1807, Drake returned to Cincinnati, took over Goforth's practice, and became active in community affairs, helping to establish Cincinnati's first circulating library and its first medical society, which he served as secretary.

In 1810, Drake published a small book called *Notices Concerning Cincinnati*, and in 1813 *Statistical View or Picture of Cincinnati and Its Environs*, both works describing the city and written to encourage people to settle there. That same year he was elected to what is now the Cincinnati city council and proposed sanitation legislation. In 1817, Drake accepted the position of Professor of Materia Medica and Medical Botany in the Medical Department at Transylvania University in Lexington, Kentucky. It was the sixteenth college in the United States and the first college west of the Allegheny Mountains.

Drake, however, was not prepared for the academic polemics he found at Transylvania. When the medical faculty met to organize at the start of the school year, Benjamin Dudley, a professor of anatomy and surgery, objected to the presence of William Richardson, a professor of obstetrics, who held no medical degree but had considerable experience. After one year at Transylvania, Drake resigned from the faculty in March 1818. Dudley openly accused Drake of breaking a promise to remain on the faculty for two years, and of seeking to destroy the Transylvania Medical College. Dudley made insulting references about Richardson. When Richardson learned this, he challenged Dudley to a duel. Although duels were illegal in Kentucky, Dudley accepted and chose pistols as the weapons. When summer arrived, the duel took place in secrecy. Dudley's shot struck Richardson in the groin, lacerating a major artery. Richardson probably would have bled to death from the wound had Dudley not rushed to his side

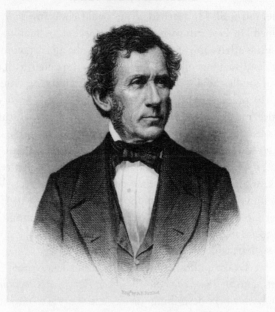

Daniel Drake (1785–1852) as he appeared about 1825. He was one of the founders of a medical school in Cincinnati, Ohio, crusaded against quack doctors, supported social reform movements, and recorded valuable data on the geology, botany, and meteorology of the Ohio River region. This illustration appears in Memoirs of the Life and Services of Daniel Drake, M.D., *written by Edward Mansfield and published in 1835. (Courtesy National Library of Medicine.)*

and pressed his thumb on the artery until Richardson's surgeon tied the vessel without the benefit of anesthesia.

In the meantime, Drake refuted Dudley's accusations against himself by publishing two pamphlets addressed to the citizens of Lexington that destroyed Dudley's arguments. Drake also asked the College of Physicians and Surgeons in New York to grant Richardson an honorary degree, which they did. With no intention of returning to Transylvania, Drake, back in Cincinnati, founded the Medical College of Ohio in 1819 and a year later established a teaching hospital staffed by physicians from the medical college. In 1827, Drake founded Cincinnati's first eye infirmary and created and edited *The Western Medical and Physical Journal.* He believed passionately in high professional standards in medical practice and in medical education, and in diagnostics over the shotgun approach of heroic medicine, even though he considered bloodletting to be of value under some circumstances. In 1822, Drake published a series of essays advocating hospital-based medical training for new physicians and recommending a requirement of four years of training for new doctors. A forceful and eloquent public speaker, Drake spoke during Cincinnati's forty-fifth-anniversary celebration and extolled the virtues of the buckeye tree, suggesting it as the state's emblem. Ever since, Ohio has been called "the Buckeye State."

Drake taught at a new medical school in Louisville from 1839 to 1849. While there he received a letter from an Illinois lawyer, Abraham Lincoln, who described various symptoms he was experiencing and asked Drake to suggest treatment. The doctor replied that he could not do so without a personal interview and physical examination. Lincoln probably contacted Drake because by the late 1840s the doctor was known widely as a scientific doctor. His reputation would grow even more after he published two volumes titled *Treatise on the Principal Diseases of the Interior Valley of North America* (1850 and 1854), totaling more than a thousand pages. Among other things, Drake wrote on the relationship between the environment and disease and included descriptions of cities, villages, mountains, and rivers and the diseases found in and around them. Drake's work was the most important contribution to medical geography since the days of Hippocrates. Drake hoped to produce a third volume, but in late October 1852 he became ill. He bled himself, but his condition did not improve. He died a few days after his sixty-seventh birthday on November 5, 1852.[10]

AT THE TIME OF Andrew Jackson's inauguration as president in 1829, the medical profession was suffering from a wave of Jacksonian democracy that was sweeping the country, glorifying the equality of all adult white males collectively labeled as "the common man." It rejected the elitist view that only the proven "best" men should be chosen to manage public affairs. In medicine, patients correspondingly rejected elitist doctors, and countless Americans came to believe that anyone could cure the sick by just applying common sense. By then the number of state and local medical societies had increased. They had established regulations, standards of practice, and certification of their members after they qualified. Fifteen states had already instituted the practice of licensing physicians. But during the 1830s, the nation's new attitude toward the profession resulted in the abolishment of state licensing in most of the fifteen. By the early 1840s, anyone was free to practice medicine without the certification of a professional society, or any formal credentials at all. Scientific medicine took a backseat to medical quackery, which became inextricably linked to the religious revivalism and social reform movements that were sweeping the country.

Organized religion in this period saw a change from authority resting chiefly in the hands of individual religious leaders to a participant-run activity, and revivals and competition among denominations replaced established religious orthodoxies. Evangelical Protestants, including the Baptist, Methodist, and Presbyterian denominations, became the wealthiest, biggest, and most influential group. Their rivals included non-evangelical Protestants, Roman Catholics, and Jews, among others. Soon there arose small communitarian religious sects that sought fundamental social reform, including utopian groups that preached withdrawal from the larger society as their response to urban growth and industrialization, and the radical Shakers, who abolished families, practiced celibacy, and established full equality between the sexes. Not least, there were also the Mormons, organized in 1830 by Joseph Smith.

The social reforms of this period included compulsory elementary education in every state. This movement was led by Horace Mann, who secularized the curriculum. There were still other movements for women's rights, abolitionism emphasizing racial equality, and temperance groups led by women who first called for moderation, then abstinence, and, finally, the outright prohibition of alcohol.

While many Americans were confused by these new movements of religious and social reform, they were even more confused by the medical profession, where there was now no clearly defined standard, no real sense that medicine was a developing science, and no acknowledged authority. There was a serious time lag between new discoveries and their assimilation into medical practice. There were perhaps two dozen competing medical systems in use by the 1840s and no single system dominated. One group of physicians, known as heroics, used bloodletting and toxic metals such as mercury compounds to treat disease. There were the allopaths (now called homeopaths) inspired by Christian Friedrich Samuel Hahnemann, a German doctor who put forth his ideas in *The Organon of Homeopathic Medicine* (1810), advocating the use of minute quantities of drugs that in larger doses produced effects similar to those of the disease being treated, thus theoretically restoring the body to harmony and balance. There also were the botanists (sometimes called herbalists or rootists) who evolved into eclectics, treating diseases by the application of single herbal remedies to effect specific cures of certain signs and symptoms. There also were, among others, the hydropaths, who used water as their chief mode of treatment; Thomsonians, named for Samuel Thomson, who favored distillates of native American vegetables and baths; mesmerists, who used hypnotism; phrenologists, who studied the shape and size of the skull to determine a person's mental faculties and character; and Indian healers who relied on traditional native methods. Every practitioner, whether trained or untrained, was called *doctor*. The term *quack* came to identify anyone medically unqualified and untrained who pretended to be a medical doctor. It is little wonder that countless people living west of the Appalachians distrusted all doctors and turned to using home remedies passed down in their families from generation to generation.

When Dr. John C. Gunn of Knoxville, Tennessee, published *Gunn's Domestic Medicine, or Poor Man's Friend in the Hours of Affliction, Pain, and Sickness* in 1830, his apparent aim was to fill the medical needs of Americans in the age of Jacksonian democracy. Gunn complained to his readers that more learned persons used highfalutin language to conceal the naked poverty and emptiness of the sciences. He added that if the masses knew to what pains scientific men go to throw dust into their eyes by using ridiculous and high-sounding terms, they would realize there is little difference between the very learned and themselves.

In his book, Gunn indicates that he wrote it for families living west of the Appalachians and in the South. The 440-page book repeats age-old hygienic wisdom, but its central theme is individual self-reliance. Gunn argues that good health is largely within the control of each man and woman, and knowledge based on experience could make each American head of household the primary physician and provider of medications for his or her own family. Gunn places emphasis on moderation and restraint in every aspect of life, warning his readers that excesses in eating and drinking can lead to sickness. He stresses the role of women, calling for women to be educated, and emphasizes their primary role in child-rearing. Gunn inveighs against the emotionally and physically destructive consequences of a loveless marriage, and he stresses the need to treat the sick in their homes rather than in a hospital or clinic. He describes disease as a shifting, holistic phenomenon and stresses the connection between body and mind, with the brain being the "father" and the stomach the "mother." He warns that disease, insanity, and even death can be caused by moral or psychological factors. Gunn views disease as the sum of an individual's symptoms at a particular moment in time, and sees the physician's task as one of eliminating those symptoms.

Gunn's book describes more than fifty-six diseases and their treatments, provides a section on diseases of women and children, discusses the value of specific plants and herbs and how to use them, and offers an illustrated guide on how to bleed a person. The drugs he freely recommended include mercury, opium, South American ipecac (*Cephaelis ipecacuanha*), and the African plant senna (*Cassia acutifolia*), items that had to be purchased, unlike the plants and herbs that grew wild or in people's gardens west of the Appalachians. But Gunn assures his readers the drugs and even instruments needed for home medical treatment could be obtained from physicians.

Gunn presents himself as a simple frontier doctor writing unpretentiously for "country folks." But in fact he had studied in New York and practiced in Virginia before moving to Knoxville. The medical authorities cited in his book include Benjamin Rush and Rush's successor, Nathaniel Chapman, and other physicians from what was then America's preeminent medical school at the University of Pennsylvania. Gunn also refers to leading New York medical teachers, including Samuel Latham Mitchill, Valentine Mott, and David Hosack. His book's subtitle—*Poor Man's Friend*—implies that he wrote it for the poor who could not afford doctors, but one wonders how many of them could have afforded to buy the book, which probably sold for $2 or $3, not a small sum in those days. Nonetheless, the book was more successful than Gunn could have imagined and went through nearly seventy printings between 1830 and 1920. Its importance would even be noted in two distinguished literary works, Mark Twain's *Huckleberry Finn* (1884) and John Steinbeck's *East of Eden* (1952).

Physicians often had to confront frontier superstitions. In southeast Arkansas Dr. Charles Martin was asked to treat an elderly woman who thought she had a frog in her stomach because of a dispute with a neighbor. The woman was in bed ready to die when Dr. Martin arrived to examine her. He soon realized he could not change her mind and left, promising to return. On his next visit he carried a small toad in his pocket. He first gave the woman a dose of ipecac and waited for the results. When she began reacting to the medicine, the doctor secretly took the toad from his pocket and placed it in an empty jar. When she recovered from the medicine, Martin showed her the toad. Within minutes the woman was out of bed and praising the doctor for curing her.[11]

Biographies of early-nineteenth-century doctors west of the Appalachians convey the many difficulties and hardships they encountered in frontier communities. Hiram Rutherford was born and grew up in Millersburg, Pennsylvania, and went to Philadelphia to study medicine during the 1830s. After receiving his degree he returned to Millersburg and practiced there for a time. Rutherford, however, was soon convinced that he would have a brighter future moving west. In 1840 he settled in sparsely populated Cole County in east-central Illinois. There was already one doctor in the area, but he lacked formal medical education.

Rutherford lost no time in making certain that everyone in the area knew of his medical diploma, written in Latin and listing his prominent professors. Rutherford ordered his medicine from a Harrisburg, Pennsylvania, drug company. The bill for one order, of calomel, opium, quinine, and catheters, was more than $66. Rutherford learned quickly that patients came to see him after their home remedies had failed. He developed a good practice and when he visited patients by horseback, he carried previously prepared doses of drugs in his saddlebags, along with bandages, splints, and the equipment he might need to deliver a baby, remove kidney stones, lance boils, or extract teeth.

In a letter to a friend, Dr. Rutherford provides one of the better descriptions of a typical day in the life of an Illinois doctor in 1841:

My first care of a summer morning is to feed my horses. After breakfast I mount & take the road; having escaped the timber, I strike into the prairie & steer for a distant arm of the river well wooded for miles, into this forest I plunge & after doing my business on its near side, I take across to the other, & again emerge on an endless expanse of green: here the tools of the art are again employed, & again I mount for some distant point. In the afternoon a different direction is pursued and as night sees me again at home, & claims repose after the fatigues of the day; I draw bridle for a new day and the exertions

under another sun is contemplated for future hours. But ere my foot
is out of the stirrup, here comes a man at full gallop with his coat of
Jean fluttering in the evening breeze. Some one is bad. I must go with
all haste, and soon the forest echoes with the rapid footfalls of our
high mottled horses.[12]

By the early 1840s another physician in the West was seeking to
duplicate the success of Gunn's self-help medical book. John W. Bright
of Louisville, Kentucky, published *The Mother's Medical Guide: A Plain,
Practical Treatise of Midwifery, and the Diseases of Women and Children*
(1844). Bright noted that his 792-page work was designed especially
for the use of "mothers and nurses." Nine other doctors then practicing medicine in Louisville endorsed the work. Bright, a native of Virginia, came to Kentucky with his parents when he was two years old.
He grew up at Eminence, about thirty-five miles northeast of
Louisville, and attended Transylvania University at Lexington, where
he studied medicine and also mastered Greek, Latin, and French. After
graduation in 1820, he practiced medicine at New Castle. Fifteen years
later, he moved to Louisville, where, according to most accounts, he
became one of the ablest physicians in Kentucky.

Bright's book, illustrated with several lithographic plates, examines
a variety of children's diseases, pregnancy, delivery, taking care of a
baby, raising a female child, menstruation, and countless other topics.
His appendix includes recipes for antimonial wines, ointments, pills,
tonics, plasters, and even a diet drink made up from half a pound of
Chany briar root (*Similax balbisiana*), half a pound of Saint-John's-wort
(*Hypericum perforatum*), and half a pound of Life Everlasting (*Helichry-
sum scorpioides*). Bright calls for this mixture to be boiled in five gallons
of water until only one gallon remains, at which time the liquid is
strained and one quarter of spirits added. Bright writes that a person
should drink a full wineglass two or three times a day, and adds, "This,
in common language, is a good purifier of the blood. If it should fer-
ment, it will operate on the bowels." Dr. Bright's book apparently
never enjoyed the sales Dr. Gunn's book did, but it did go through at
least one reprinting with revisions, under the title *Bright's Family Practice*. Bright was the oldest practicing physician in Kentucky when he
died at Lexington in July 1879.[13]

A year after Bright's book was published, Nathan Davis, a young
New York doctor, introduced a resolution at a meeting of the New

York Medical Society endorsing the establishment of a national medical association. By then many physicians were looking for some way to bring order to the nation's medical profession and to protect the interests of the more orthodox physicians. Some doctors at the meeting called Davis's proposal impractical or utopian. But others realized that something needed to be done to bring order to the medical profession, establish standards for medical education, establish a code of ethics, find ways to inform the public about the increase in quack remedies, and generally warn the public about the dangerous direction in which American medicine was headed. Davis's idea caught on and on May 5, 1847, nearly two hundred delegates, representing forty medical societies and twenty-eight colleges within twenty-two states and the District of Columbia, convened in Philadelphia and organized the American Medical Association.

A strong supporter of the new association was a Kentucky physician, William Loftus Sutton, a large man of medium height with dark hair and blue eyes. He attended the 1850 meeting of the AMA in Cincinnati and many others that followed. His story is typical of educated physicians who wanted to see order in the profession. Sutton was born in 1797 in Scott County, Kentucky. His parents had moved to Kentucky from Virginia, where his father had been a prominent planter in Albermarle County, not far from Thomas Jefferson's Monticello. Young William walked to school in nearby Georgetown and then studied at Bourbon Academy in Paris, Kentucky. He was an avid reader and a very good student, and in 1814 he became a teacher. The following year he began studying with Dr. Richard Ferguson in Louisville, where he assisted the doctor in his apothecary shop. He soon found time to read the doctor's medical books.

As already noted, Louisville was a very unhealthy place in 1815 because of the many marshes and swamps in and around the town. When William Sutton was about nineteen, he contracted some form of fever, probably malaria, but he continued his medical studies until the spring of 1817. By then his health was so poor that he left Louisville and returned to his parents' home in Lexington, a town that had grown. It was now the home of Transylvania University, which had a new medical department. Sutton became one of twenty students of the department's faculty, whose members included doctors Benjamin Dudley, William H. Richardson, and Daniel Drake. Sutton studied hard and received his medical degree. Soon after his twenty-first birthday, he began practicing medicine in the small village of Catlettsburg in Greenup County, Kentucky. His experiences in his practice, however, convinced him that he needed more advanced training, preferably at one of the five leading medical schools in the East—the University of Pennsylvania, Harvard, Dartmouth, the College of Physicians and Surgeons in New York, and the Maryland Medical College, in Baltimore. Sutton chose Baltimore, and there earned his second medical degree. He then returned to Catlettsburg, where in the spring of 1819 he rented an office from Horatio Catlett, for whom the town was named. Instead of paying rent, Sutton agreed to provide medical care for the Catlett family. Sutton fell in love with Mary Belle Catlett, daughter of George and Lactita Buck Catlett. But this branch of the family soon suffered financial reverses and moved to Morganfield, Kentucky. Sutton followed, moving his medical practice to Morganfield, where he married Mary Belle.

For Sutton the practice of medicine in the undeveloped region of western Kentucky was often difficult. He traveled by horseback and sometimes had to leave his horse and walk to his patients' cabins over rugged trails. Distances between patients were great in the sparsely populated area. When making calls in the winter, Sutton wore a fur cap and used leggings over his high-top boots. After he obtained a buggy, a lantern underneath became standard equipment on night calls. His wife would heat bricks and wrap them for him to take in the buggy to keep his feet and hands warm.

Because currency was scarce, Sutton, like other doctors, often took his fees in whatever medium of exchange was available, including tobacco, hay, cows, clover seed, pork, soap, fish, and butter. For instance, two steers were equal to $20, one cow equaled $9, and a set of dessert spoons equaled $14. Sutton's account books list many other items he accepted in exchange for his services. When one patient died without making any effort to pay, Sutton simply wrote in his account book "Gone Hellward."

Through experience, Dr. Sutton established standard fees for his services:

For visiting	$1.00
For more than 18 miles	.50
For cathartics	.25 to .50

Emetics	.25 to .50
Tinctures per ounce	.50
Blisters to ankles & wrists	.50
Blisters to chest	.50
For administering	$2.00
For bleeding	.50
For extracting teeth	$1.00
For delivery	$5.00 to $20.00
For curing gonorrhea	$10.00
For curing Lues Venera [venereal disease]	$20.00
For pacacenteis	$20.00
For amputation	$50.00
For trepanning [skull-boring]	$50.00
For reducing fractures	$10.00–$20.00
For reducing Luxation [kneecap dislocation]	$10.00–$20.00

Sutton remained in Morganfield until 1833, when a recurrence of fever forced him to relocate to Georgetown, Kentucky. There his health improved. He rented, and later purchased, a four-story brick house on the north side of East Main Street as his family home. Nearby he established an office in a small frame building but later erected a brick building next to his home for his office. Sutton bought one of the first kerosene lamps in Georgetown, but it was used only for special occasions. He and his family continued to mold and use home-made candles because they were more economical. They were used until the introduction of coal-oil lamps.

Sutton's practice of medicine was conservative. He did not bleed patients often, or in large quantities. His case histories mention the use of an onion poultice for hoarseness along with a gargle of nitrate of potash and honey and a flannel compress wrung out of the hot ooze of oak bark. He used a mustard poultice to treat an ulcer and an oak bark poultice for an injured knee. Dogwood and spruce tea were frequently prescribed, along with chamomile tea made from the chamomile plant (*Matricaria chamomilla*) grown in most gardens. Early in his practice, Sutton used blistering on painful areas of the body. In one case, after removing the burnt skin of a patient, he applied fresh cabbage leaves. In time, Sutton concluded that blistering was an unnecessarily harsh or severe treatment, and he substituted mustard plasters. In treating typhoid fever during the 1840s, Sutton favored frequent sponging of a patient, including the lips and nose, with cool water. His case studies suggest his methods of treatment were never as drastic as the ones used by his contemporaries who favored heroic medicine. He did not believe in purging or inducing vomiting, and he consistently prescribed arrowroot (*Maranta arundinacea L.*) as a convalescent nutrient to eat and mucilage to drink. Mucilage was made by combining flaxseed or quince seed with boiling water, which produced a sticky, gelatinous concoction for patients to imbibe. He was ahead of most other doctors of his time by insisting that drinking water be boiled. If the patient objected to downing it warm, he told them not to drink until it had cooled. He believed that if a typhoid patient's symptoms were mild, no medicines should be given but diet should be relied on exclusively as a cure.

Sutton did not solely use local plants and herbs for medicines. He often prescribed drugs from overseas, especially from the tropics. These included gamboge, a strong laxative obtained from a tree (*Garcinia hamburyi*) in East Asia; copaiba (*Capaifera officinalis*), a diuretic from South America; kino juice from a tree (*Marsupium Roxburgh*) in Madras and the East Indies that was used to treat diarrhea; and jalap, the dried juice from a Mexican morning glory (*Ipomoea purpurea*) named for the town of Jalap, used to treat chills and fevers. Sutton's records indicate he imported large quantities of *Zingiber*, commonly known as ginger, from the tropics, and aloes, a bitter herb, from Africa and the East Indies. One part of aloes was combined with three parts of calomel and two parts rhubarb to form the well-known and widely used 3.2.1. pill to treat chills and fever.

Sutton's case history files indicate he also used Dower's Powder, an opium-based medicine to induce vomiting; Hooper's pills, supposedly a sure cure in all hypochondriacal, hysteric, or vaporish disorders in women after childbirth; pills of asafetida to treat chronic bronchitis; pulmonary balsam to treat closed airways and improve expectoration; tincture of Valerian to reduce anxiety and improve sleeping; and blue mass pills containing mercury to treat depression. Abraham Lincoln reportedly took blue mass pills during the Civil War to fight his depression caused by the war. Sutton also used lactucarium, a milky fluid secreted from the base of several species of lettuce, that had sedative and analgesic properties. Sutton often used it as a substitute for opium.

Sutton was also a pioneer in the use of anesthesia.* Chloroform was discovered in 1831, but its anesthetic properties were not known until 1847, when Dr. Jacob Bell of London and Dr. James Simpson of Edinburgh used it in an operation. Barely two years later, on June 24, 1849, Dr. Sutton was called to see the brother of a Georgetown physician. The patient was having convulsions. Sutton suggested trying chloroform, and the patient's brother approved. "In about five seconds from its application to his nostrils the convulsions ceased. . . . As soon as they recommenced the chloroform was reapplied with the same result. . . . After the third application there was no return, but he remained insensible for twelve or fifteen hours."[14]

*The word *anesthesia* was coined by Oliver Wendell Holmes, M.D. (the father of the Supreme Court justice) in 1846. Although ether was discovered in 1275 by the Spanish chemist Raymundus Lullius and called "sweet vitriol," its first use as a surgical anesthetic occurred in 1842 when Dr. Crawford Williamson Long employed it in removing two tumors from the neck of James Venable in Jefferson, Georgia. Chloroform was widely used for a time, but was later dropped as an anesthetic because it is quite toxic to the kidney and the liver.

CHAPTER FOUR

BEYOND THE MISSISSIPPI

*The art of medicine consists in amusing the
patient while nature cures the disease.*

—Voltaire

I N 1763, the year France transferred Louisiana Territory to Spain
and forty-five years after the French colony of New Orleans was
founded, Pierre Laclède Liguest and a group of traders traveled seven
hundred miles up the Mississippi River from New Orleans and established a fur-trading post on the site of modern St. Louis, Missouri.
The settlement grew slowly and had more than a hundred buildings by
1797, the year a Spanish official invited Dr. Antoine Saugrain to move
to St. Louis from Ohio. The Spanish authorities offered him land
grants near St. Charles to make the move attractive. Dr. Saugrain
accepted and became the first physician in St. Louis.

Born near Paris, France, in 1763, Saugrain came from a family of
prominent booksellers. His three sisters married well, one of them to
Joseph Ignace Guillotin, the inventor of that highly efficient means of
execution named for him, the guillotine. Saugrain, who stood less than
five feet tall, was educated in Paris as a physician and chemist and
moved to New Orleans in 1783, where he was soon admitted to the
practice of surgery. Four years later, he journeyed to the United States
with a letter of introduction to Benjamin Franklin, who arranged for
Dr. Saugrain to join a scientific expedition on the Ohio River in 1788.
Indians killed most members of the expedition, including the leader,
and Saugrain was wounded, but he recovered and returned to France.
When, however, the French Revolution broke out in 1789, Dr.
Saugrain fled France and returned to the United States, where he
helped to establish a community of French exiles at Gallipolis, Ohio. It
was there he met and married Geneviève Rosalie Michau in 1793.
When not practicing medicine, Saugrain experimented with phospho-

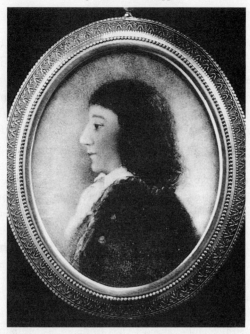

Dr. Antoine François Saugrain (1763–1820), the first and only physician in St. Louis from 1800 to 1807. He treated residents during the smallpox outbreak of 1801. From 1805 to 1811, he was also an assistant surgeon stationed at Fort Bellefontaine, north of St. Louis. (Courtesy Missouri Historical Society)

rus matches and manufactured barometers and thermometers, interests he maintained after moving to St. Louis in 1799. During the smallpox epidemic that struck St. Louis in 1801, the doctor worked long hours trying to save lives. Eight years later, he became the first physician west of the Mississippi to use Edward Jenner's cowpox vaccine to vaccinate residents of St. Louis against smallpox.[1]

In May 1804, the doctor was a member of a small group of men who escorted Meriwether Lewis overland from St. Louis to St. Charles as the Corps of Discovery was preparing to head west. When Lewis and Clark and the Corps returned to St. Louis in September 1806, Lewis remained there for five weeks instead of hurrying back to Washington. There is evidence to suggest that Lewis delayed his trip east to receive monthlong mercury treatments for syphilis from Dr. Saugrain, who from 1805 to 1811 was assistant surgeon at Fort Bellefontaine, north of St. Louis.

Reimert T. Ravenholt, M.D., a modern-day physician, well-known epidemiologist, and serious student of history, cites the journals kept by Lewis and his own medical knowledge of the disease as evidence that Meriwether Lewis suffered from neurosyphilis, and that he probably caught it in August 1805 from Shoshone women when he was negotiating with Chief Cameahwaite for horses needed for crossing the mountains. Lewis could ill afford to be rude to the chief by refusing his hospitable offer of a tepee and pleasing female company. Dr. Ravenholt notes that five weeks after his meeting with the Shoshones the explorer wrote in his journal of "breaking out or eruptions of the skin have been common with us for some time." This, writes the doctor, would be the usual interval for secondary-phase skin eruptions of syphilis to appear. At the time Dr. Saugrain was, in Ravenholt's words, "surely one of the most capable syphilologists in America." He also points out that after reaching Washington and staying at the White House with President Thomas Jefferson, Lewis was ill on several occasions, and he often failed to demonstrate good judgment. The effects of the disease probably caused Lewis to delay his preparation of the expedition's report for publication. He withdrew from public circles for several months, staying with his mother in Albemarle County, Virginia, where he was probably treated by her and his physician brother Reuben. By March 1808, Lewis was well enough to assume his responsibilities as governor of Louisiana Territory in St. Louis, but by September of that year, his condition had worsened as the disease attacked his mind. He attempted suicide twice while traveling on a steamboat from St. Louis to Memphis and spent two weeks in the care of a friend at nearby Fort Pickering before setting out on horseback to return to Washington. On October 10, at Grinder's Stand on the Natchez Trace, Lewis again became deeply disturbed. During the night, he shot himself twice; he lived until dawn, then died.

Lewis's behavior, according to Dr. Ravenholt, clearly corresponds to "the ultimate agony of advancing neurosyphilis—losing his mind and verging on utter madness." Ravenholt acknowledges that some Americans "dislike the thought that Meriwether Lewis died of neurosyphilis; but others will mourn anew, with greater understanding, admiration, and compassion, this truly heroic leader who, I believe, died an agonizing death from an infection acquired in the line of duty while on a dangerous mission for his President and country."[2]

Antoine Saugrain, who treated Lewis and other members of the Corps, died on March 5, 1820, in St. Louis, about a year before Missouri became a state. By then Missouri was the nation's farthest western frontier. It was generally unhealthy for settlement, especially in poorly drained areas. St. Louis had become the gateway to Missouri primarily because the Missouri River provided the easiest route west from the city. Settlers from Ohio, Indiana, Illinois, Kentucky, Tennessee, and elsewhere came through St. Louis traveling up the river or following trails and roads along it to seek land and new opportunities. One new settlement that grew up on the banks of the Missouri was Franklin, about 150 miles west of St. Louis. Nearby was Arrow Rock, where a ferry had been established in 1811 to take people and animals across the river and where, in 1812, Factor George Sibley established a post for fur trading with the Osage Indians.

It was in the area around Franklin that Dr. John Sappington arrived in 1817, settling on land west of the river crossing at Arrow Rock. Sappington had studied with his physician father in Maryland and then headed west, becoming the first physician in Nashville, Tennessee, in 1785. After three years there, he moved farther west, settling in the area of modern Franklin, Tennessee, a town he helped to lay out in 1799. By then he had become known as a physician who compounded pills covered with a coating of sugar. Dr. Sappington remained in Tennessee until 1817, when he joined a westbound caravan heading for Missouri.

Locating in west-central Missouri, Dr. Sappington found his practice growing and soon extending to Jefferson City and west to Lexington. Pneumonia, rheumatism, and colds were common ailments because of damp cabins, hard winters, and frontier hardships; malaria, called the "Missouri chills" by local residents, was a particular problem, producing more sickness than any other disease in the region. In those days, people considered themselves fortunate if at least one family member did not suffer chills and fever at the same time as the others during late summer and fall. Malaria attacks came every second day or, in some cases, every third. They were so regular that many settlers knew the exact hour to finish the morning's work and sit down to await the chill or "lague fit," as some called it. The typical attack lasted six to twelve hours and began with stretching and yawning followed by chills until the whole body shivered, teeth chattered, fingers turned dead-white, and fingernails turned blue. Once the attack ended, a dry fever developed, with the skull feeling very hot and flushed, after which the sufferer was drenched with sweat and finally left weak and exhausted. The next day the person felt better, but as the attacks continued, the person's health grew worse.

Late in 1820, Sappington learned that two French pharmacists had succeeded in purifying an extract called quinine from Peruvian cinchona bark, which had been discovered in South America during the 1600s. By the early nineteenth century it was being used in England to treat fevers. Sappington acquired a supply of quinine from France by 1823 and developed a tonic that contained one grain of quinine, one-half grain of licorice, one-half grain of myrrh, and oil of sassafras. By this time he believed that fever was a symptom of the disease rather than the cause. He soon learned that his tonic prevented malaria if given in small daily doses, and he would carry a good supply of the tonic in his saddlebags when he rode to treat patients. At some point, he used his formula to produce pills that were easier to carry and distribute. The demand for his pills increased as Missourians learned of the treatment.

Dr. Sappington made money. He acquired several thousand acres of land, engaged in agriculture, and became a moneylender. By the early 1830s he had tired of his strenuous medical practice and decided to focus on manufacturing his quinine pills and selling them to the public. He knew he was breaking the code of medical ethics by doing so, but he realized his pills would save hundreds if not thousands of people from malaria. The doctor hired nearly twenty men to sell "Dr. John Sappington's Anti Fever & Ague Pills." Each box contained twenty-four pills and sold for $1.50. He told his salesmen to take the pills themselves, three each day, knowing that their good health would be the best advertisement. Dr. Sappington made a great deal of money from his pills. By the early 1840s his sense of public duty induced him to sit down, write, and publish a 216-page book called *The Theory and Treatment of Fevers* (1844). He included details of his treatments of malaria and ague, including the formula for his anti-fever pills, which was worth a fortune. This was probably the first medical book in English published west of the Mississippi River.[3]

When the doctor first settled near Arrow Rock, he became ac-

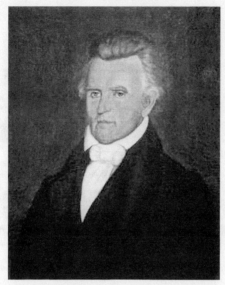

John Sappington (1776–1856) was born in Maryland, received his medical degree in Philadelphia, went west to Missouri in 1817, and settled on a farm near Arrow Rock. He concocted a remedy for fever containing quinine. It proved so effective against malarial fevers that he manufactured and sold it as "Doctor John Sappington's Anti Fever & Ague Pills" and became wealthy. He also wrote the first medical book published west of the Mississippi River. Artist George Caleb Bingham painted this portrait of Sappington about 1854. (Courtesy University of Missouri)

quainted with William Becknell, a Virginian who operated the nearby ferry. Becknell probably took Dr. Sappington's tonic to avoid malaria. Suffering from financial problems, Becknell organized a party ostensibly to trade horses and mules and to catch wild animals far to the west of Missouri. In truth, Becknell had his eyes on Santa Fe in Spanish New Mexico, where he hoped to make sufficient profit trading to solve his money problems. Becknell and his party left Franklin in 1821 and before reaching Santa Fe learned that the Mexican Revolution had occurred. Unlike other Americans who had earlier sought to trade in Santa Fe, only to be arrested or sent packing by the Spanish, Becknell and his party were welcomed, and they traded, made a profit,

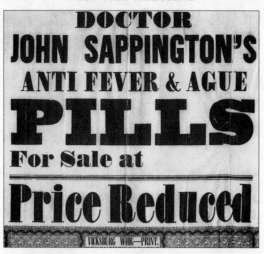

A poster used by Dr. John Sappington to advertise his anti-fever pills. (Courtesy University of Missouri)

and returned to Franklin. When news of the Becknell party's success spread in Missouri, the Santa Fe Trail was born and more Americans ventured westward onto the prairie and plains to make a profit in Santa Fe.[4]

During the 1820s and 1830s, the traders heading for Santa Fe left only bits and pieces of information relating to medical problems. Some of the traders probably were vaccinated against smallpox, and some probably carried bottles of Sappington's tonic and later boxes of his "Anti Fever & Ague Pills" to protect against malaria. Contaminated water produced typhoid fever and contributed to dysentery and diarrhea. An epidemic of Asiatic cholera in the vicinity of Arrow Rock in 1833 caused problems, but scurvy was a more common health hazard because of the lack of fruits and vegetables. On the plus side, at least in the view of some of the early travelers, the dry air on the plains and in the mountains improved health. For the early traders traversing the Santa Fe Trail, most medical problems seem to have been injuries sustained in accidents, occasional fistfights, and wounds received in Indian attacks. But once the trading caravans reached Santa Fe, there were other health problems to contend with, including lice, venereal disease, poor sanitation, and occasional outbreaks of smallpox.

When William Becknell opened up the Santa Fe trade in 1821, the southern plains across which the trail ran were still unexplored by the government in Washington. Lewis and Clark and the Corps of Discovery had crossed the northern prairies and plains, but it was not until 1806 that explorer Zebulon M. Pike led the first major government-sponsored exploration across the southern plains. Pike's reports, unlike those of Lewis and Clark, make no mention of medicines carried and contain little information about any medical problems. In fact, Pike's reports suggest that he made few if any provisions to take care of his men. Pike had been in St. Louis only two months after returning from a trip up the Mississippi River when he received orders to lead a government expedition to explore the Southwest. Pike escorted fifty Osage Indians to their homes after they were freed by the Army from the Potawatomis. He negotiated a peace treaty between the Kansas and Pawnee Indians, sought to make contact with the Comanches, explored the headwaters of the Arkansas River, and tried to locate the source of the Red River before returning east. Pike undoubtedly realized that he should learn what he could about the Spanish along the poorly defined southwestern border of Louisiana, and should move as close as possible to Santa Fe.

On his 1806 expedition Pike took along a physician, Dr. John Hamilton Robinson, twenty-four, a native of Augusta County, Virginia, who was then an acting surgeon's mate at Cantonment Belle Fontaine near St. Louis. Dr. Robinson, a nephew of Alexander Hamilton, was probably the first physician to accompany a major government expedition in the West. The exact nature of his medical education is hazy, but, like most other physicians of the day, he may have studied under an established doctor. Robinson married Sophie Marie Michau, Dr. Antoine Saugrain's sister-in-law, in St. Louis on December 24, 1805, before August Chouteau, a justice of the peace. The Robinsons' second child, a son, was born in St. Louis in October 1806, nearly four months after he left on Pike's expedition.

Pike thought highly of Robinson. On February 7, 1807, he wrote of the doctor's "good qualities," noting that he

> has had the benefit of a liberal education, without having spent his time as too many of our gentlemen do in colleges, viz. in skimming on the surfaces of sciences, without ever endeavoring to make themselves masters of the solid foundations, but Robinson studied and reasoned; with these qualifications, he possessed a liberality of mind

too great ever to reject an hypothesis, because it was not agreeable to the dogmas of the schools; or adopt it, because it had all the éclat of novelty—his soul could conceive great actions, and his hand was ready to achieve them; in short, it may truly be said that nothing was above his genius, nor any thing so minute that he conceived it entirely unworthy of consideration. As a gentleman and companion in dangers, difficulties and hardships, I in particular, and the expedition, generally, owe much to his exertions.[5]

Pike's logistical planning, however, was poor. He believed his men would not encounter cold weather, so he had them take only their summer uniforms. He failed to bring along a sufficient number of horses, or sufficient scientific equipment and other supplies. The government furnished Dr. Robinson with medicines, but what they were is not known. Pike, however, did carry a telescope and a copy of a map drawn by Baron Alexander von Humboldt, who had visited New Spain. Humboldt had given President Jefferson a copy of his map when he visited Washington in 1804, and it was the only map Pike used to guide him once the expedition reached the Arkansas River.

As planned from the beginning, part of the expedition split off, led by Lieutenant James B. Wilkinson, whose father was General James Wilkinson, a senior officer of the U.S. Army. He took five men and returned east to explore the Arkansas River to its mouth, going back up the Mississippi River to St. Louis. In late November, Pike, Dr. Robinson, and two other men set out to reach the top of a high mountain, but because they lacked food and winter clothing, they were forced to abandon their ascent of what is known today as Pikes Peak. In the course of their trek, fourteen men, including Pike's best hunters, suffered frostbitten feet. Pike does not indicate how they were treated in his report. Three of the men could not travel and were left behind. Even Dr. Robinson suffered vertigo for two days after eating some berries he found in the mountains.

Cold, hungry, and exhausted, Pike led his men over the Sangre de Cristo Mountains and found another stream, which he believed was the Red River. It was actually the Rio Grande, near what is today Alamosa, Colorado. While some of his men constructed a small stockade, Pike sent two relief parties to bring up horses and the three soldiers left behind who were suffering from frostbite. Only one of the three returned; the other two were too sick to move, but sent Pike pieces of their gangrenous toe bones in a desperate appeal not to be abandoned. The two men later were able to rejoin the party. Otherwise, Pike's reports convey much color and emotion but are of little value in learning about other medical problems that he and his men experienced. If Robinson himself kept a journal, it has not been found.

Even today there is a mystery surrounding Robinson's involvement with the expedition. Born January 24, 1782, in Augusta County, Virginia, and only recently arrived in St. Louis, he left his position as acting surgeon's mate at Cantonment Belle Fontaine near St. Louis to join Pike's expedition. In February 1807, Robinson left the expedition and walked to Santa Fe, ostensibly to locate Baptiste LaLande, a Missouri trader who had absconded two years earlier with trading profits belonging to William Morrison, a merchant from Kaskaskia, Illinois. Morrison had asked Pike to present his claim for these profits should the explorer get to Santa Fe. Pike may have decided to use the claim as a pretext to make contact with the Spanish, and Robinson may have volunteered to be the person making this contact. In any case, once he reached Santa Fe, Robinson told the Spanish governor that he was there to collect Morrison's debt, and that he had recently left a party of hunters. The Spanish became suspicious, as Pike may have anticipated, and sent troops. They found Pike's party and escorted them to Santa Fe and then south to Chihuahua. Pike, Robinson, and the others were escorted to U.S. territory at Natchitoches in late June 1807. In his report published in 1810, Pike admitted that he had got lost, for which he was given the sobriquet "the lost pathfinder."

Following the expedition, Robinson served as an Indian agent and merchant at Fort Osage, but from 1812 to 1814 he was a special diplomatic agent for the U.S. State Department. Secretary of State James Monroe unofficially sent the doctor to northern Mexico to ask the Spanish governor to do something about armed bandits causing trouble in U.S. territory. In 1814, Dr. Robinson moved to Mexico and rose to the rank of general in that country's revolutionary army. In 1817, however, while Mexico was still struggling to achieve independence, he returned to the United States.[6]

Lewis and Clark's medical experiences probably would have benefited other government explorers who later went west, but there does not appear to have been any organized effort by the government to share them among the military. Pike's 1805 and 1806 expeditions, however, occurred before Lewis and Clark returned to St. Louis. The lead-

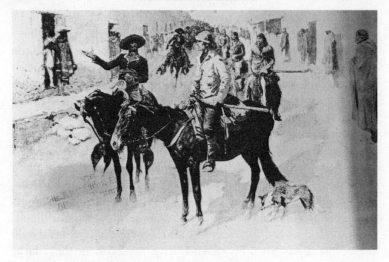

This illustration by artist Frederic Remington shows Zebulon Pike (center) arriving in Santa Fe. The nearest man behind Pike may be Dr. John Hamilton Robinson. The illustration appeared in Collier's Weekly, *June 16, 1906.*

ers of the expeditions who came later may have read the authorized account of Lewis and Clark's journey, but it was not published until eight years after their return in 1806. The diary of Sergeant Patrick Gass, a member of their expedition, was privately published in 1807, but it lacks much detail.

After Pike returned to St. Louis, the next major government expedition into the West did not occur until 1819. Major Stephen H. Long of the Corps of Topographical Engineers was ordered to take a party of scientists to explore the Platte River and the Rocky Mountains. The expedition was apparently well planned, because about a year earlier Long had designed and arranged for the construction of a steamboat called the *Western Engineer* to transport his party up the Missouri and Platte rivers.[7] Long's expedition was well supplied, and, as he observed, all of the gentlemen in the party except Dr. William Baldwin, a botanist, "were in good health." Unfortunately, Baldwin was also the expedition's physician and surgeon. Born in Pennsylvania in 1779, he was educated in rural schools and taught for a while before deciding to study medicine at the University of Pennsylvania. Needing money to pay for his second year of school, he worked as an assistant to Dr. William A. Todd. For one year he served as surgeon on a ship sailing between the East Coast and Canton, China. When he returned to Pennsylvania, he was able to attend the lectures at the University of Pennsylvania and in 1807 received his medical degree. Baldwin, however, suffered from hereditary tuberculosis and moved to Georgia, where he believed the milder climate would improve his health. He then began collecting plants and became a botanist while still practicing medicine. But after Long's expedition left St. Louis and started up the Missouri River in the spring of 1819, Baldwin's health deteriorated. He became so ill that Long had to leave him in the care of a Dr. John Lowry at Franklin, Missouri. There the forty-year-old Baldwin died about a month later.

When Long's steamboat reached a point just south of modern Council Bluffs, Iowa, they learned that Congress had cut the expedition's funding because of the financial panic of 1819. Leaving many of his engineers encamped a few miles south of a second camp with more than a thousand riflemen commanded by Colonel Henry Atkinson, Major Long and a few others in his expedition returned east. Later they would learn that of those they had left behind, 160 soldiers and engineers had died during the winter of scurvy, the cause of which was still unknown. As for Major Long, he soon received orders to go overland to the source of the Platte River and then return to the Mississippi by way of the Arkansas and Red rivers. On this expedition Long took along twenty-three-year-old Edwin James, a native of Vermont who had studied medicine under his two physician brothers. James, tall, erect, and with a bearing of confidence, had also studied botany and geology. Officially appointed botanist and geologist for the expedition, he also served as its physician.

Captain John R. Bell, a West Point graduate, was charged with keeping the expedition's journal, but Bell does not allude in it to any medical matters. Dr. Edwin James, however, kept his own journal and noted that when the expedition was camped near the Platte River in modern Nebraska, three Frenchmen and two Indians arrived in camp. One of the Frenchmen brought a letter and a box containing smallpox vaccine from the War Department. Long and his men were ordered to introduce vaccinations among the Indians. Unfortunately, as the box was being transported west aboard a keelboat, the vessel was wrecked and the box fell into the river. The vaccine was ruined. Major Long and James, however, attempted to explain vaccinations and their value to Pawnee Indian chiefs, but the idea was rejected.

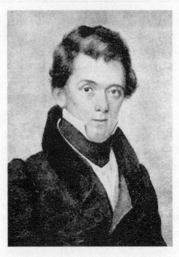

Edwin James (1797–1861) was raised in Vermont, was trained in medicine, and studied botany. After the death of his mentor, Dr. William Baldwin, James joined Stephen H. Long's expedition in 1819. (Courtesy University of Denver Press)

As Long's expedition pushed westward onto the plains, Dr. James wrote in his journal:

> The traveler journeys, for weeks in succession, over a dreary and monotonous plain, sparingly skirted and striped with narrow undulating lines of timber, which grow only along the margins of considerable streams of water. In these boundless oceans of grass, his sensations are not unlike those of the mariner, who beholds around him only the expanse of the sky and the waste of waters.[8]

The almost treeless open spaces with broad horizons were depressing to the men of the expedition. The gloom turned to joy, however, when everyone saw to the west the outlines of the Rocky Mountains. Coming up the South Platte, Long sighted a mountain located northwest of modern Denver that is today called Longs Peak. Many miles south, the party saw another high peak. Convinced that they could climb it, Major Long, Dr. James, and another man made the ascent in mid-July.

James led the climb and the party named it James Peak, but the name did not stick. It was the same mountain discovered more than a decade earlier, though not successfully climbed, by Zebulon Pike. Today it is called Pikes Peak and another mountain located west of Denver is named for James.

The expedition split into two groups as it returned east. Captain Bell took one party down the Arkansas River, while Major Long took the second group south to what he thought was the Red River (it was really the Canadian River). The two groups planned to reunite at Belle Point, the site of modern Fort Smith, Arkansas. As both parties moved east, their accounts tell of numerous problems with mosquitoes, gnats, sand flies, and the "annoyance of innumerable multitudes of minute, almost invisible seed ticks."[9] The "seed ticks" were what we call today chiggers, juvenile mites closely related to ticks usually found in tall grass and areas of brush. Red in color and about the size of a pinhead, they are almost invisible to the unaided eye and they climb on the feet, legs, and then tender areas of the body. They do not burrow under the skin or drink blood, but they do bite and inject saliva, causing the skin to react and create red bumps that itch and cause much scratching.

When the parties met at Belle Point two months later, aside from three men who had deserted Captain Bell's group and disappeared, the health of the men was generally good. Long and his men were delighted to find green corn, melons, sweet potatoes, and other vegetables grown in gardens at Belle Point. But members of the expedition "did not exercise sufficient caution" in indulging in these foods and "we soon found our health beginning to become impaired. We had been a long time confined to a meat diet, without bread or condiments of any kind, and were not surprised to find ourselves affected by so great and sudden a change. It may be worthwhile to remark that we had lost all perceptible saltiness, and the ordinary dishes, which were brought to our mess table appeared unpalatable, on account of being too highly seasoned."[10]

Reports of the next explorer to lead major government explorations west are also thin on medical aspects. Between 1838 and 1846, John Charles Frémont led three different expeditions into the west for the Corps of Topographical Engineers.[11] Frémont's reports of these expeditions include references to flora and wildlife but only passing mention of the health of his men or any medical problems, aside from such things as sore feet and a vague sickness in the mountains. The sickness was probably caused by the altitude, but if a person came down with a fever it more than likely was a viral infection transmitted by the bite of a tick. Mountain fever, as it was sometimes called, usually lasts three days and then occurs again a day or two later and lasts another few days before the person recovers.

Frémont hired experienced guides, including Kit Carson. These men knew how to take care of themselves. Nearly all of them knew something about treating an illness or wounds, though little else about medicine. If Frémont's report of his third expedition to California is complete, his men experienced no major health problems aside from hardship and times of little food. One man, however, François Badeau, died in an accident near the Sevier River, and another man, Alexis Ayot, was accidentally shot through the leg while crossing a stream. Frémont describes the accident as "a mortifying and painful mischance," but provides no details on Ayot's treatment. Although Ayot did recover, he was crippled for life. Another man, Baptiste Derosier, was lost for several days until he eventually found Frémont's camp. But "We were pained to see that his mind was deranged. It appeared that he had been lost in the mountains, and hunger and fatigue, joined to weakness of body, and fear of perishing in the mountains, had crazed him. The times were severe when stout men lost their minds from extremity of suffering—when horses died—and when mules and horses, ready to die of starvation, were killed for food." Derosier remained with the expedition until it reached the Sacramento Valley and Sutter's Fort.[12]

Frémont's fourth expedition, in 1848, was not for the government. Having resigned from the Army, he mounted a private exploring party to locate a central railroad route through the San Juan Range, a rugged region of the southern Rockies. Among his party were the three Kern brothers of Philadelphia—Benjamin, Richard, and Edward. Richard and Edward were artists, but Benjamin J. Kern was a physician. "Old Bill" Williams, an experienced mountain man, was hired to guide the party of thirty-three men and more than a hundred animals. In spite of harsh winter weather, Frémont was determined to cross the mountains. But his expedition got lost and became stranded; their animals died and the men ran out of food and suffered severe hardships. Frémont had no choice but to retreat, and he abandoned his men. Frémont, Bill Williams, and the Kern brothers succeeded in reaching Taos, but about ten men in the expedition died. After the survivors recuperated and the winter's snows began to melt, Dr. Benjamin Kern and Old Bill Williams went back into the mountains to recover a cache that included the doctor's instruments and other possessions, and papers. About March 14, 1849, Ute Indians killed Dr. Kern and Williams. In sum, this fourth expedition of Frémont's was a disaster, due mainly to poor judgment.

While Lewis and Clark paid a great deal of attention to medicine and the importance of maintaining their and their men's good health on the journey, the reports of Pike, Long, and Frémont do not suggest anything like the same concerns.

It is noteworthy that President Thomas Jefferson participated in the planning of Lewis and Clark's expedition, and apparently insisted they do everything possible to preserve their men's health. Such attention to medicine seems to be missing in the planning by later explorers. Pike appears to have been naïve and to have imagined that everyone's

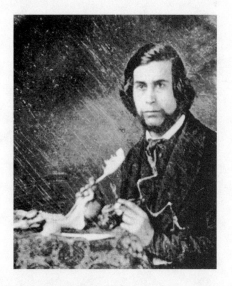

Dr. Benjamin J. Kern, M.D., and his brothers Richard and Edward joined John Charles Frémont's fourth western expedition in 1848 to locate a central railroad route through the San Juan range of the southern Rocky Mountains. Dr. Kern and mountain man Bill Williams were killed by Ute Indians in 1849. (Courtesy Utah State Historical Society)

health would be all right. The reports of Long and Frémont certainly suggest their health concerns were greater than those of Pike, but people other than the expedition leaders kept the journals. These individuals may have failed to mention the men's health and well-being in their records because they believed the subject too unimportant to mention. Certainly Dr. Edwin James, with Long's expedition, did address such matters in his private journal, as might be expected. The explorers who came after Lewis and Clark may have been concerned with the well-being of the men on their expedition but the records do not show it.

CHAPTER FIVE

FUR TRADERS AND TRAPPERS

*I wanted to be the first to view a country on which the eyes of
a white man had never gazed and to follow the course of rivers
that run through a new land.*

—Jedediah Smith

L ONG BEFORE LEWIS AND CLARK returned from the Pacific with
glowing reports about the commercial prospects of the fur trade in
Louisiana Territory, such trade was already well established to the
north in Canada. As early as the 1630s, French-Canadian *voyageurs*, or
"travelers," were paddling along waterways in large canoes and trading
for pelts with the Indians. In 1670, the British chartered the Hudson's
Bay Company, which claimed fur-trading rights in all of the country
that drained into Hudson Bay, on whose shore the company established a trading post. Like the French, the British obtained furs from
Indians. The Seven Years' War interrupted this lucrative practice.
Once Britain won the war against France, the Hudson's Bay Company
gained all fur-trading rights in Canada. Soon, however, the company
faced new competition from merchant fur traders in Montreal, who
in 1784 formed the North West Company. Both companies began
exploring westward across Canada, seeking new sources of fur. In
1793, ten years before Lewis and Clark started west, Alexander
Mackenzie became the first European to reach the Pacific Ocean by
traversing the Canadian Rockies. By then the Hudson's Bay Company
and the North West Company had their men trapping furs all across
Canada. No longer did they rely solely on Indians to supply the furs.

By 1800, the North West Company had 117 trading posts in Canada, and Hudson's Bay had expanded its number of posts into the
interior along the great river networks. When ill or injured, trappers
away from the posts had to doctor themselves as best they could, but
nearly all of the trading posts operated by both companies had well-
stocked pharmacies and surgical chests. Each chest contained manuals

of instruction and lancets and other medical tools, plus an assortment of simple medicines. Each clerk was required to learn how to bleed, and at smaller posts the company's senior officer was responsible for treating the ailments of his men. It is believed that company personnel were generally able to handle common accidents and cure ills through regulation of a patient's diet and by using salts, castor oil, opodeldoc, Friar's Balsam, and phlebotomy.[1]

Keeping fresh medicines in the chests was sometimes difficult. At one trading post in 1796, the chest was described as a "worthless medicine box" because many of the medicines were dry and unusable. The chest contained "one bottle Hartshorne, one bottle Turlington [Balsam of Life], one bottle of lavender, a small bottle tincture of rhubarb, one-pound of jalap, one-half pound of ipecacuanha, two pounds of Gauber salt, two pounds of sulfur, two pounds of basilicon, one-fourth pound of powder of rhubarb, two pounds Spanish juice, four ounces of strengthening plaster, five gallipots, twenty-four small vials, some corks, part of an old sheet, and linen for dressings."[2]

From the late 1760s on, the major posts all had trained doctors on staff, including Thomas Hutchins, John McNab, Edward Jarvis, and John Wright. Later there was Dr. John McLoughlin, who had studied medicine with Sir James Fisher near Montreal. McLoughlin became resident physician with the North West Company at Fort Williams, now Thunder Bay, Ontario. Soon after the North West Company and the Hudson's Bay Company merged in 1821, McLoughlin became chief factor in the region along the Columbia River and built Fort Vancouver on the north bank of the Columbia River near modern Portland, Oregon. In addition to his administrative duties, McLoughlin continued to practice medicine until he retired about 1845.

Another nineteenth-century Hudson's Bay Company physician was Dr. William F. Tolmier, who arrived in Oregon in 1833 and a few years later was appointed chief trader at Fort Nisqually on the southern end of Puget Sound near what is now Tacoma, Washington. He remained there until 1859. Still another company physician was Dr. John Sebastian Helmcken, born in England in 1824. After studying with his family's doctors in London, he went to medical school and in 1847 became surgeon on the Hudson's Bay Company ship *The Prince Rupert*, just before the vessel left for York Factory, a company outpost on the edge of Hudson Bay. Later he served as surgeon for emigrants in the com-

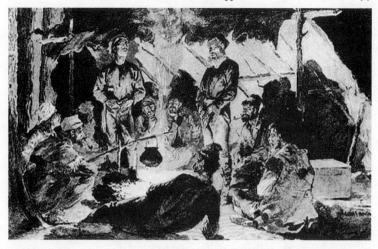

An artist's depiction of voyageurs *in camp. (Courtesy National Archives of Canada)*

pany's colony on Vancouver Island. Dr. Helmcken entered private practice in Victoria, British Columbia, in the 1850s.

Following its establishment in 1784, the North West Company also provided medicine chests for many of its trading stations and assigned physicians to their major posts. Company doctors treated employees and Indians, but some physicians apparently found life on isolated posts difficult. Alexander Ross recounts in his book *The Fur Hunters of the West* (1855) how at Fort George on the Columbia River one ship's physician committed suicide, another became deranged and drowned, and a third had to be shipped home to stand trial for murder.

Early accounts suggest how trappers were treated for their ills. In the fall of 1800 Alexander Henry sought to cure one of his men of colic by using the shotgun approach to medicine, which was rather common at the time. On the first day, Henry gave the man essence of peppermint, sweet oil, jalap, and Glauber's salt. There was no relief, so on the second day Henry gave him an emetic to force him to vomit. When that failed as well, Henry had him try each item in his medicine chest. After nothing worked, Henry put him on a three-day diet of flour, sugar, and tea. The man showed no improvement, but thirteen days later, the man suddenly had a serious attack of diarrhea and fully recovered.[3]

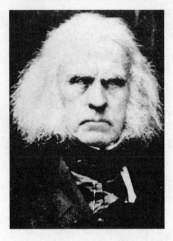

Dr. John McLoughlin (1784–1857), who built Fort Vancouver on the Columbia River near modern Portland, Oregon. (Courtesy Oregon State Archives)

Henry himself had an attack of the colic while crossing Howse Pass, close to the Continental Divide in the Waputik Range of the Rockies in 1811. It made him weak and faint, but Henry recalled that he had some peppermint drops and "a good dose" relieved him. Much earlier, in December 1800, Henry had observed that some of his men were suffering from a rash and itching. He gave them a compound of high wine—distilled spirits containing a high percentage of alcohol—and gunpowder to rub on the outbreak. The compound eased the itching and dried up the rash. At Fort George, Henry recorded that nine of his men were bedridden with venereal disease and were given mercury as a treatment. He added that "two cannot walk. By spring, I fear, at least half our men will be disabled by this disease; at present, a few are free from it and some are far-gone. This foul malady is so prevalent among our people and the women in this quarter that it may seriously affect our commerce."[4]

Frostbite was another problem during the long and cold Canadian winters. In the winter of 1774, Robert Longmoor, a trapper, froze both of his big toes at the newly established Hudson's Bay Company post called Cumberland House on the Saskatchewan River. Samuel Hearne, the English explorer, wrote: "This morning I lay'd Rob't Longmoor's toes open which are froze to the bone, and as the medicine box which ware fitted up at the fort for this place is with Mr. Cocking we have not the least thing to apply to it except the inner rind of the larch tree root which is generally us'd among the natives to stop or prevent a mortification."[5]

Gunshot wounds were also common among Canadian trappers. George Gun was shot in the leg early in 1798 when he accidentally tripped a "set-gun" designed to trap game. William Tomison removed several rounds of shot from his leg but failed to record what else he did to treat it.[6] When another trapper accidentally shot himself while repairing a double-barreled gun in 1814, Alexander Henry recorded that the "contents lodged in his right thigh; though the bone was not injured, he suffered much. The flesh was cut open opposite the wound, and the shot and wadding were removed." Once Henry nearly shot himself in the hip when the horse he was riding stumbled as he was drawing his gun to shoot a buffalo. Another time Henry grazed himself in the buttocks when the cock of his gun caught on a canoe gunwale as he was passing his weapon behind his back. In two other separate incidents, one of Henry's men was killed while playing with a gun in 1804, and another man was killed by his own weapon because it had extremely weak springs and would repeatedly go off when carelessly handled.[7]

The early fur trader and explorer Alexander Mackenzie recalled that in January 1793 he treated an Indian who had lost his thumb when his gun burst. The hand became gangrenous and the thumb dangled by a strip of flesh. Mackenzie washed the wound with spruce-fir bark juice and then put a spruce-fir root bark poultice on it. This was changed three times a day. Within a few days the gangrene cleared. Mackenzie applied a vitriol solution to the loose skin until he was able to remove the thumb. After a month of treatments, the Indian recovered.[8]

Gabriel Franchere, who joined the North West Company after it acquired John Jacob Astor's Fort Astoria and renamed it Fort George, praised the work of the company's physician and the medicine he practiced while at the same time criticizing Indian medicine. Franchere wrote, "As soon as a native of the Columbia is indisposed . . . they send for the medicine man, who treats the patient in the absurd manner usually adopted by these impostors, and with such violence of manipulation that often a sick man, whom timely bleeding or purgative would have saved, is carried off by a sudden death."[9]

It was apparently true that after observing the white man's medicine, some Indians ignored their traditional ways and did not hesitate to trade pelts for medicine carried by trappers or available at trading posts. William Tomison, who first joined the Hudson's Bay Company in 1760 and became head of the company's activities west of Hudson Bay, reported receiving a hundred beaver pelts from Indians for what undoubtedly were large quantities of medicines between 1779 and 1795.[10]

Medicines were important especially if a patient had a fever, or was lethargic or weak. Scurvy was treated with crystallized salt of lemon, essence of malt, port wine, cranberries, and spruce juice. Ointments were produced using homegrown basil, mixed with a wax or glycerin base, and kept in small earthen glazed pots called "gallipots," a slang term for "apothecary." To treat dysentery, the remedy was an elixir made of honey, opium, benzoic acid, licorice, camphor, potassium carbonate, oil of anise, and alcohol. And there were many more medi-

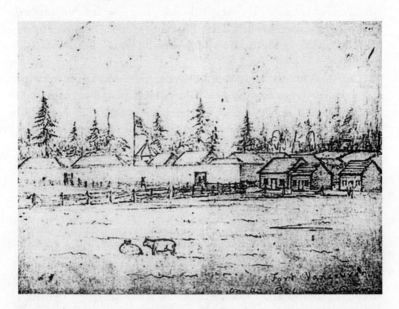

A sketch of early Fort Vancouver on the Columbia River. (Courtesy National Park Service)

cines, either provided by the companies or produced from local herbs and plants.

Medicines, however, could not cure everything. In 1829, a ship sailed up the Columbia River and docked at Fort Vancouver, apparently with someone on board who had contracted intermittent fever and ague. This highly contagious disease soon swept through the fort and wide areas of the region. People suffered from alternating periods of chills, fever, and sweating. John McLoughlin did the best he could to treat trappers and others at the fort, including Indians. He wrote to a Hudson's Bay Company clerk that "we have so much sick that I am quite hampered. We have now forty laid up with Intermittent Fever."[11] Before the outbreak ended, thousands of Indians died. When it began spreading, James Douglas, a trader, observed the Indian villages and wrote: "[T]he living sufficed not to bury the dead, but fled in terror to the seacoast, abandoning the dead and dying to the birds and beasts of prey. Every village presented a scene harroeing [*sic*] to the feelings. The canoes were drawn up upon the beach, the nets extended on the willow boughs, the very dogs appeared as ever watchful, but there was not heard the cheerful sound of the human voice."[12]

Lacking any immunity to the illnesses carried by white men, the Indians were especially vulnerable to such diseases as ague and small-pox, and hundreds of thousands of native people died from them— though the Indians often infected white trappers until vaccinations became commonplace in the early nineteenth century. Otherwise, the major cause of death among the trappers in Canada appears to have been drowning, with accidental gunshots being second. Traditional tales claim that many trappers died from strangulated hernias, but this seems doubtful since most of these men were in very good condition and remarkably healthy. They had learned to take care of themselves.

To the south in the United States, after Lewis and Clark reported Louisiana Territory was rich in furs, Americans responded rapidly to develop the trade. From St. Louis a few men sought to launch the fur trade on the upper Missouri. In New York, John Jacob Astor—who already had made a small fortune from furs in the Great Lakes region and had watched the fur trade grow in Canada—established the American Fur Company in 1808 to compete with the North West Company and Hudson's Bay Company in Canada. Two years later, Astor formed a subsidiary called the Pacific Fur Company to build a chain of small trading posts along the route followed by Lewis and Clark and then construct a large post near the mouth of the Columbia River. His company succeeded in building Astoria, in present-day Oregon, a large trading post, and a handful of smaller posts before the British acquired them in the War of 1812. The Pacific Fur Company then ceased to exist, but in the meantime, in St. Louis fur traders sought to develop their own routes until the American Fur Company made an alliance with them in 1821, which gave Astor a monopoly of the trade along the Missouri River. By then the St. Louis fur men had given up the traditional practice of obtaining pelts from the Indians; it was simply not reliable. They found it easier to have their own men trap beaver for their pelts, and this gave birth to the mountain-man era that lasted until about 1840 in the American West.

Initially, these trappers worked for fur companies that would bring supplies west once a year and return east with the pelts trapped during the previous year. The trappers would meet at a designated point in the West at what became known as the annual rendezvous. Because there were no doctors around, it was at the rendezvous that trappers could obtain a few medicines brought from St. Louis. Some trappers carried nothing more than a dose of salts and a bottle or two of Turlington's balsam, often in the belief that these two items alone would help them overcome most of their ailments. The salts were not of the table variety (sodium chloride) but contained magnesium sulfate—the scientific name of Epsom salts, so called because they came from the mineral-rich waters of Epsom, England. Mixed with water, the salts were used as a purgative. Turlington's balsam was a patent medicine produced in England by Robert Turlington after King George III granted him a royal patent in 1774. Turlington described his bottled product as "The Balsam of Life." British patent office records indicate it contained "twenty-six botanicals, some from the Orient and some from the English countryside, disgested [sic] in alcohol and boiled to a syrupy consistency." Turlington claimed his medicine provided "a Remedy for every Malady," and that it "vivifies and enlivens the Spirits, mixes with the Juices and Fluids of the Body, and gently infuses its kindly Influence into those Parts that are most in Disorder."[13]

Health and well-being were pretty much the responsibility of each trapper, who sometimes had to draw on the knowledge of other trappers. Not known for paying much attention to personal hygiene, they learned to delouse their clothes by spreading them over an anthill. Each man relied on his own experiences, including those learned about home herbal remedies growing up. Many mountain men knew how to use a lancet, spread a plaster, and even give a clyster (enema) when necessary. In all likelihood, though no evidence exists on this point, many mountain men and fur traders either had been inoculated against smallpox or had inherited antibodies to ward off the disease. During the era of the mountain man, there were serious outbreaks of smallpox among Indians in the West, but nowhere has this writer found any reference to smallpox outbreaks among mountain men.[14]

Scattered accounts of mountain men's experiences leave little doubt that most of them learned to survive the hardships, illnesses, attacks by animals and unfriendly Indians, and accidents in the unsettled West. For instance, an 1830 report from the St. Louis trading firm of Smith, Jackson and Sublette observed that among their men in the mountains, sickness and natural deaths were almost unknown. That year, however, the firm listed sixteen deaths at the hands of Indians, three deaths by fighting among their trappers, one drowning, and one death from wounds received from a bear.

Bears could be a problem, as in the case of Hugh Glass, a mountain man who was born about 1800. Little is known about his early life other than that he became a sailor when he was about twenty. Tradition says Glass was sailing on a ship in the Gulf of Mexico when the vessel was captured by a pirate crew of the notorious Jean Lafitte. To save his life he joined the pirates, until one night he was able to jump ship while anchored in a sheltered bay and swam ashore on the Texas coast. He headed inland, wandering north across Texas, only to be captured months later by Pawnee Indians. Glass gave their chief a gift, escaped death, and was accepted as a member of the tribe. Some time later, when members of the tribe including himself visited St. Louis during the summer of 1822, he escaped the Indians. Early in 1823, Glass became one of William Ashley's one hundred men advertised for in the *Missouri Republic* to ascend the Missouri River to the Rocky Mountains and trap beaver.

In early March, Glass left St. Louis with Ashley's expedition and started up the river. The expedition fought Arikara Indians, and Glass was wounded but soon recovered. In August 1823, he became separated from a small party of trappers near the modern town of Grand

River, South Dakota. He came upon and shot a grizzly bear but only wounded the animal. Before Glass could reload his rifle, the bear attacked him, severely slashing him from head to foot. Other trappers arrived and killed the bear, but Glass, bleeding profusely, looked awful. Everyone thought he was going to die, but the men made a litter and carried him. On the assumption that Glass would die at any time, two trappers—John Fitzgerald and Jim Bridger—were told to remain with him until he died, bury the body, and catch up with the others. When Glass went into a coma, Fitzgerald and Bridger suspected death was near. They abandoned Glass, taking his rifle, powder, and gear. Glass, however, did not die. When he came out of the coma and realized he was alone, he got very angry at Fitzgerald and Bridger for abandoning him. His anger may have helped him to survive. Although weak, he discovered he could crawl, and soon realized the wounds on his back had become infected. Knowing something about folk medicine, Glass rolled over onto a rotting log and let the maggots eat the infection out of his back. He then crawled along the Grand River, where he could easily get water. He lived on the meat of dead animals and rattlesnakes. Slowly he regained strength and soon could walk upright. When he reached the Missouri River, some Sioux Indians, who had great respect for anyone who survived a bear attack, befriended him. Glass traveled three hundred miles to Fort Kiowa, near the mouth of the White River, to meet fellow trappers. He later forgave Bridger and Fitzgerald for deserting him. Glass lived another ten years, until 1833, when he was killed by Indians near modern Billings, Montana.[15]

Another story about a grizzly bear involves Jedediah Smith, then traveling with a party of trappers. Smith was attacked in Powder River country in 1824, and the bear mangled Smith's scalp and ear. James Clyman, one of his companions, got a pair of scissors, cut off Smith's hair, and then began to dress the wound. The bear had taken nearly all of Smith's head in its mouth, from the trapper's left eye across the crown of the head to his right ear, laying the skull bare. Clyman dressed the wounds as best he could, using a needle and thread to close them. One of Smith's ears, however, was torn and dangling from his head. Smith told Clyman to stitch it back into place, and Clyman did so, stitching the ear through and through repeatedly and reattaching it. Everyone helped Smith to mount his horse and ride about a mile to water, where they made camp. The trappers pitched their only tent for

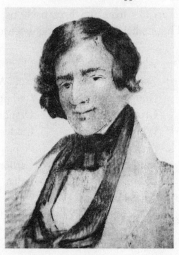

Mountain man Jedediah Strong Smith (1799–1831). During his lifetime Smith probably traveled more extensively in unknown territory than any other single mountain man. (Courtesy Jedediah Strong Smith Collection, University of the Pacific)

Smith and made him as comfortable as possible. To the surprise of some, he recovered.[16]

Most of the trading posts maintained medicines and medical supplies. John Jacob Astor's American Fur Company built Fort Union in 1828, near the junction of the Missouri and Yellowstone rivers in what is now western North Dakota. At its peak the company had nearly a hundred employees to acquire buffalo robes and other furs from various Indian tribes, including the Assiniboine, Crow, Cree, Blackfoot, and Ojibwa. It was the longest-lasting private American fur-trading post. The U.S. Army purchased it in 1867 and tore it down, using the building materials for the expansion of Fort Buford, a military post located a few miles downstream.

We know about Fort Union's medical supplies because an inventory made in March 1833 is on file with the Missouri Historical Society in St. Louis, with the notation that "salts, castor oil, & essence of peppermint are our usual specifics and it requires but little skill in administering them in cases arising from amatory passions; the remedies are equally simple." The medicines listed on the inventory:

Epsom Salts	White Vitriol	Blue Vitriol
Sugar Lead	Copp[er?]	Gum Arabic
Gum Al[oe]	Gum Camphor	Carbonate of Soda
Cream Tartar	Ground Ginger	Orange Peel
[Red Gentian?]	Winter Bark	Calomel
Burgundy Pitch	S ? . . . Sulphur	Henna
Sinna	Rhubarb	Carbonate Magnesia
Mace	Lint	Indian Rubin
Jallap?	Zinc digitalis [foxglove]	Friar's Balsam
Turlingtone	Ess. Spruce	Oppodeldoc
Laudanum	Ink Powder	Tooth Brushes
Lees Pills	Seidlitz Powders	Phials (4, 2, 1 oz.)
Corks	Oil peppermint	Tartar Emetic
Blue Pills	Castor Oil	Balsam Copaine
Linseed Oil	Hartshorn	Tinct. Canthandes Bitters
Sprig lancet	Salt petre	Stone Brimstone
mortar & pestle		

A year before Fort Union was built, a mountain man named Thomas L. Smith was with a party of trappers in North Park on the North Platte River. Smith left the party and set his traps to catch beaver. A wandering band of Arapahos found Smith's traps, and Smith talked with them. When he learned they were unhappy he was trapping beaver, he told them he would leave the area. Smith decided to rejoin his party, but it was a few days before he located them. He then learned that the group's leader, Sylvester S. Pratte, had been killed by Indians and Ceran St. Vrain, a company clerk, was now in charge. For several days the party reorganized and decided to continue trapping while trying to avoid Indians. One morning, as Smith left camp to set his traps, he was shot in his left leg and cried out in pain. The bullet struck him just above the ankle, shattering the bones. He grabbed his gun and fired into some nearby bushes where he'd seen a puff of smoke. Fighting erupted as other Indians fired at the mountain men, who returned fire. The battle lasted for about an hour, during which time Smith took a buckskin thong and ligated his wound to control the bleeding.

When the fighting stopped, the trappers counted nine Indians dead, including the one who had shot Smith from the bushes. In pain, Smith told his fellow trappers to cut off his foot. They refused. Smith then called to Joseph Bejux, the party's cook, to give him his knife. Smith cut the torn muscles at the point where the bones were fractured; the Achilles' tendon was all that was left to hold the shattered foot on the leg. Milton Sublette took the knife and severed it and then suggested using a hot iron to stop the bleeding. Smith refused the iron and again used his buckskin thongs to bind the arteries to control the bleeding. Someone found a dirty shirt and the wound was bound. Everyone now expected Smith to bleed to death, and they assured him they would not leave him until he died.

Smith, however, did not die. Within twenty-four hours the bleeding stopped. By the following day, Smith had regained enough strength to travel. Since it was October and cold weather was approaching, the party decided to spend the winter in a sheltered valley on the Green River some distance away. Two men carried Smith on a litter for a couple of days as the party started out for the river. By then Smith was able to ride his horse. About a month after Smith had been wounded, the party arrived at the Green River. Smith was still recovering, but one bone still protruded from his stump. It was loose and Smith could wiggle it. He used a pair of bullet molds as forceps, and with the help of Milton Sublette, the bone was pulled out.

A few days later, a party of Ute Indians joined the trappers to spend the winter. They knew Smith and respected the courage he had shown in an incident they had witnessed some years before. The Indians said they were sorry to learn that Smith had lost his leg and then began a ritual to heal the wound. They chanted, cried, wailed, and then recited incantations. Indian women and children began chewing roots and soon began spitting upon the wound. This kept up for several days. Smith continued to improve. Soon the last remaining bone fragment protruding from his leg was loose enough to be removed. Smith continued to regain strength. Some of the trappers took their knives and made a wooden leg of either oak or hickory. By March 1828, Smith was walking on this peg and his friends began calling him "Peg-leg Smith." He continued trapping until the early 1840s, when he opened a trading post in Bear Lake Valley on the Oregon Trail. The California gold rush attracted him during the early 1850s, but he apparently found little gold. He ended up in San Francisco begging on a street corner, where an old friend found him and arranged for him to be admitted to a hospital. There Peg-leg Smith lived until his death at the age of sixty-five in 1866.[17]

Indians sometimes came to the rescue of trappers and traders when the white man's medicine failed to find a cure. William Bent, who suffered a mild case of smallpox during the 1830s, later contracted diphtheria at his post, Bent's Fort, in what is now eastern Colorado. Bent could neither swallow nor talk. His Cheyenne wife forced a hollow quill down her husband's swollen throat and fed him by blowing broth from her own mouth. A Cheyenne medicine man was called, and used the handle of a spoon to examine Bent's throat. The Indian went outside and collected several small sandburs about the size of pears, each covered with tiny, sharp barbs. The medicine man then prepared a thread-sized sinew with a knot at one end. Using an awl, he poked a hole through one sandbur and ran the sinew through to the knot. He then rolled the bur in marrow grease and asked Bent to open his mouth. The medicine man forced the bur down Bent's throat. When the fat melted, he pulled it out bringing with it hard, dry matter. The medicine man did this several times until he had removed the diphtheritic membrane. Bent soon found he could swallow soup. Within a few days, he was well enough to eat solid food.

Mountain men sometimes sought Indian cures, but most of the time they were able to cope with illnesses and treat wounds by using their ingenuity and what medicines and other items they carried with them. One medicine carried by some trappers was the painkiller laudanum. John Simpson Smith was one mountain man who put it to unorthodox but effective use about 1833. Having witnessed too many other mountain men lose a year's worth of pelts to gambling and carousing at the annual fur-trade rendezvous, Smith chose to take his pelts, float them down the Missouri River, and sell them at a good price in St. Louis. He built a bullboat of buffalo robes over a willow framework and started downriver. Somewhere downstream his boat struck a snag and turned over. Since his pelts were securely tied to the boat's ribs, he recovered his boat and pelts. He was now, however, chilled and wet. He pulled his boat ashore to dry his clothes and spend the night.

Because he was in Blackfoot country, Smith did not want to attract attention by building a fire. He curled up on the riverbank and went to sleep, but by the next morning he had a severe toothache. His head was racked with pain. He decided to seek help at Fort McKenzie, an American Fur Company trading post located some miles downstream near modern Loma, Montana. When he reached there some hours later, he pulled a few beaver pelts out of his pack and walked to the post and banged on the wooden gate. Someone let him in. He was able to trade his pelts for a jug of liquor and a bottle of laudanum. He immediately took a swig of the laudanum, returned to his boat, and continued downstream. The painkiller worked. In the morning sun Smith became drowsy as his boat drifted down the curving river.

Presently, when his boat rounded a bend in the river, Smith heard a shot and saw five Blackfoot Indians signaling for him to come to shore. Since they could easily kill him if he did not comply, Smith beached his boat where they were standing. He was dragged out of the boat, and the Indians then helped themselves to its contents, including some meat. Next, they slit the bullboat apart with their knives before letting it drift and sink in the river. The Indians took Smith a short distance, stopped, and built a fire to roast the meat. Smith suspected they would kill him after they had eaten. When one of them brought out his jug of liquor, Smith hoped they would get drunk so he could escape. He showed the Indians how to dilute the liquor with water, making it more palatable. About that time the laudanum was wearing off. When he took another dose, the Indians saw the bottle Smith kept in his pocket and tried to take the bottle, but Smith kept it. Perhaps thinking it was liquor, they did not object when he gave each of them a strong dose. Soon the laudanum and liquor took effect. The Indians fell asleep. Smith took the Indians' lead, powder, and buffalo robes, cleaned and reloaded his guns, and then took the best horse the Indians had. Smith filled bags with meat and was preparing to leave when two more Blackfoot rode over a hill and into camp. Smith did not move until the two Indians saw their friends lying on the ground. The newcomers sensed trouble and pulled their weapons. Smith shot one dead. He then shot the other's horse. The Indian fell to the ground, and before he could get up, Smith stabbed him to death. Smith then scalped all seven Blackfoot, wrapping their scalps in a buffalo robe. Atop the best horse, and leading the Indians' horses, he rode south. Using the laudanum to dull his aches and pains, Smith was able to ride day and night toward civilization, stopping only when the horses needed to stop and rest.[18]

When laudanum was not available for killing pain, mountain men used alcohol in any form. Whiskey was a home remedy they themselves had brought west, and they had also learned to make poultices for boils using plug tobacco. Broken bones were sometimes set with splints of sticks and leaves as bandages, or with old pieces of clothing. They made a salve from sugar and soap or beaver oil and cestrum to treat wounds and cuts, and rattlesnake bites were sometimes cauterized by burning small amounts of gunpowder on the open wound. Ingenuity and endurance became their trademarks.

Jim Bridger, a legendary figure in the West, demonstrated these qualities during the early 1830s. Bridger and Thomas Fitzpatrick were leading members of a rival fur-trade company active in Blackfoot country. A party of Indians attacked, and Bridger was wounded by an arrow in the back. After the fight, his companions removed the shank of the arrow and dressed the wound, but they were unable to remove the arrowhead from Bridger's back. Bridger recovered and carried the arrowhead in his back for about three years, until he attended the Green River rendezvous in 1835. Dr. Marcus Whitman, going west to prepare for missionary efforts in the Northwest, attended the rendezvous. Another missionary, Rev. Samuel Parker, was with Whitman and later wrote:

> Whitman was called to perform some very important surgical operations. He extracted an iron arrow, three inches long, from the back of Capt. Bridger. . . . It was a difficult operation, because the arrow was hooked at the point by striking a large bone, and cartilaginous substance had grown around it. The Doctor pursued the operation with great self-possession and perseverance and his patient manifested equal firmness. The Indians looked on while the operation was proceeding with countenances indicating wonder, and when they saw the arrow, expressed their astonishment in a manner peculiar to themselves. The skill of Doctor Whitman undoubtedly made upon them a favorable impression. He also took another arrow from under the shoulder of one of the hunters, which had been there two years and a half. After these operations, calls for surgical and medical aid were constant every hour in the day.[19]

A few other physicians made their way west during the era of the mountain man. One was Dr. Jacob Wyeth, who accompanied his brother Nathaniel Wyeth, a Boston entrepreneur, and a small party to explore fur-trading opportunities in the Northwest in 1832. Dr. Wyeth, however, accustomed to life in Boston and not in the best

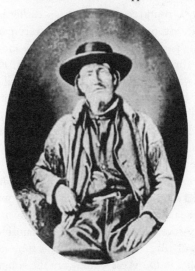

James Bridger (1804–1891) was a native of Richmond, Virginia. He came west as a young man and became one of the most cele-brated mountain men of all, a scout and teller of tall tales. In 1835, Dr. Marcus Whitman operated on Bridger and removed an arrow-head from his back, where he had been wounded three years earlier during an attack by Indians. (Courtesy National Archives)

physical condition, was not prepared for the hardships found in the West. He struggled to keep up with the others in the party. It did not help that Dr. Wyeth became the first member of the group to become ill, with diarrhea, as they followed the Platte River west. Soon others in the party also became ill. But Dr. Wyeth was not able to administer much aid to them. He eventually left the party and with a few others returned east, while his brother Nathaniel continued west with his expedition. At one point on his western journey, Nathaniel Wyeth became ill after smoking too much with Indians who kept passing the pipe.

In 1834, Nathaniel Wyeth organized another trading expedition in St. Louis. He asked Milton Sublette, a seasoned mountain man, to guide him and a party of seventy men to the annual rendezvous. Unfortunately, Sublette was suffering from a fungus infection in one of his legs caused by a wound received ten years earlier in an Indian fight. As they traveled west, Sublette's leg became very painful, and he left Wyeth before the party reached the rendezvous and returned east to seek medical treatment. In St. Louis, Dr. Bernard Farrar treated the leg, but within a year he had to amputate it. Surgical methods in 1835 were still crude. Patients undergoing such operations often died, but Sublette survived the shock and pain of one, possibly two, operations and recovered. He was able to return to the fur trade and attended the 1834 rendezvous with a cork leg that Hugh Campbell, a mountain man friend, had made for him in Philadelphia.

Another doctor who went west was Hugh Campbell's brother Robert, who led a supply train of forty-five men from Missouri to the rendezvous in 1833. Robert Campbell took with him Dr. Benjamin Harrison, twenty-seven years old, son of William Henry Harrison, a hero of the War of 1812. The father paid his son's expenses in hopes that the rugged life in the West would cure the young doctor of alcoholism. The extent of Dr. Harrison's medical contributions on the journey is sketchy, but Charles Larpenteur, a fur trader traveling with the party, mentions him in his book *Forty Years a Fur Trader on the Upper Missouri* . . . (1898). After the rendezvous, Larpenteur, Dr. Harrison, and others started east with pack mules and cattle. One evening, a rabid wolf rushed into their camp and bit one of their cattle, which bellowed madly. The wolf then bit Larpenteur's friend, George Holmes. Moses "Black" Harris and Dr. Harrison searched for a "madstone," a stony concretion something like a ball, taken from the stomach of a deer, that supposedly would cure hydrophobia (rabies). According to legend, the stone had to be ground into powder and then given to the victim. Whether they located the stone is not recorded, but Holmes soon developed hydrophobia. During the next few days his condition worsened, and finally he ripped off his clothes and ran into the wilderness and was never seen again.

Dr. Harrison's experiences in the West apparently did not cure him of the bottle. In 1834, he moved to Texas and later fell into the hands of the Mexican army. After they released him, the doctor returned to Ohio, where he died in 1840, the year in which his father was elected the ninth president of the United States.[20]

Between the early 1820s and 1840, most fur trappers and traders survived their rugged life. One Canadian trapper, Alexis St. Martin, made a significant contribution to medicine after he was accidentally

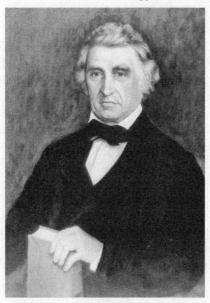

Dr. William Beaumont (1785–1854) was a U.S. Army surgeon at Fort Mackinac, Michigan, in 1822, when Alexis St. Martin, a fur trapper, was shot in the stomach. Beaumont treated St. Martin, but was unable to close the wound entirely. Through the opening thus provided, Beaumont began observing the digestion of food in St. Martin's stomach, and so was able to contribute greatly to our understanding of the digestive process. The doctor was thirty-four years old when this portrait was painted. (Courtesy National Archives)

shot in the stomach in 1822. Dr. William Beaumont, a U.S. Army surgeon at Fort Mackinac, Michigan, treated the wound but was repeatedly unable to close the two-and-a-half-inch hole in St. Martin's stomach. Beaumont put a tent compress and bandage over the hole to keep it closed. Since his patient was unable to return to his work as a trapper, Dr. Beaumont hired him as the family's live-in handyman in 1823. Eventually the doctor recognized the unique opportunity for medical research that St. Martin's condition afforded. Two years later, after being transferred to Fort Niagara, Beaumont began experiments with St. Martin, observing the digestion of food as it was occurring in his stomach. Dr. Beaumont discovered that gastric juice has solvent properties. The experiments continued until the fall of 1825, when the former trapper returned to Canada, married, and had children. After another two years, Beaumont and St. Martin met again at Fort Crawford in Prairie du Chien, Wisconsin, where St. Martin and his family now lived, and Beaumont began a new series of experiments on St. Martin to determine if there was any relationship between digestion and weather. By the spring of 1831, Dr. Beaumont concluded that dry weather increases stomach temperature, humid weather lowers it, and a healthy stomach is a hundred degrees. The doctor also learned gastric juice needed heat to digest, that vegetables are less digestible than other foods, and milk coagulates before the digestive process. Dr. Beaumont also learned that anger hinders a human's digestion. Late in 1832 Dr. Beaumont and St. Martin traveled to Washington, D.C., and conducted other experiments concluding that exercise helps the production and release of gastric juice.

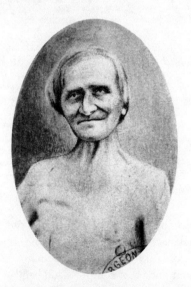

A government photograph of Alexis St. Martin, who died in 1880, outliving his doctor, William Beaumont. St. Martin was in his twenties when he went to work as a voyageur *for the American Fur Company. (Courtesy National Library of Medicine)*

In 1833, Dr. Beaumont's observations and experiments were published and became the greatest single contribution to the knowledge of gastric digestion up to that time, thanks in part to his patient. The Canadian trapper St. Martin died in Canada in 1880 at the age of eighty-six. His family believed he had suffered enough indignities in the name of science and let his body rot in the sun. His remains were then buried in an unmarked grave so no further experiments could be performed. Later a marker was placed near the grave in St. Thomas de Joliette, Canada, relating St. Martin's history and noting that "through his affliction he served all humanity." Dr. Beaumont, considered the "Father of Gastric Physiology," died twenty-seven years before St. Martin after falling on an icy step in St. Louis, Missouri. He is buried there in Bellefontaine Cemetery.

Alexis St. Martin lived longer than the average fur trapper did in the nineteenth century. One authority calculated that of 233 trappers whose dates are known, the average life span was sixty-four years, which was still above the national average of about forty years. Of the mountain men's lives studied, more than half died of old age or associated physical illnesses. Four lived into their nineties, while two lived to be a hundred or more. When the demand for beaver pelts disappeared and the glory years of the beaver trade ended, the mountain men drifted into other occupations including "miner, guide, Indian agent or interpreter, post trader, teacher, sheepherder, carpenter, surveyor, and writer." Nearly all of them maintained active lives, which probably contributed to their longevity.[21]

CHAPTER SIX

ON THE OREGON TRAIL

If a patient dies, the doctor killed him,
but if he gets well, the saints have saved him.

—Italian proverb

THE GREAT WESTWARD MIGRATION slowed about 1820 along a north–south line from where the Missouri River, flowing from the north, turns east at modern-day Kansas City, Missouri. West of that line the major rivers—the Platte, Kansas, and Arkansas—were too shallow for most steamboats. To travel west of this imaginary line, people had to go overland across the unsettled prairies and plains, and onto what Pike and other early explorers labeled "the Great American Desert." Their labeling of this region as a "desert" meant the area had little appeal to settlers who wanted to farm. About the only people who did travel west of the imaginary line were a few explorers, traders traversing the Santa Fe Trail, fur traders and trappers, Indian traders, handfuls of immigrants moving west from Mississippi Territory into Mexican Texas, and a few missionaries taking Christianity to the Indians.

Dr. Marcus Whitman, a physician, and Rev. Samuel Parker were two missionaries who traveled west in 1835 with a fur-trading supply caravan going to the annual rendezvous on the Green River in modern Wyoming. It was there that Dr. Whitman removed the Indian arrow point from the back of mountain man Jim Bridger. From the rendezvous Whitman and Parker continued west to scout mission locations in the Pacific Northwest. Other missionaries followed, including Elijah White, a New York physician educated at the medical college at Syracuse, who was sent west in 1836 by the Methodist Church to be a mission doctor in the Willamette Valley in Oregon. The missionaries made frequent visits east for supplies, and while there gave speeches to raise more funds to support their work, praising Oregon Country and describing its abundance of free land, forests, and water. Government officials in Washington, D.C., aware that the British wanted the region, hoped Americans would settle Oregon Country so the United States could claim it.

After an economic depression struck in 1837 and another followed in 1841, farmers in the Mississippi Valley, frustrated by depressed prices for their crops, imagined that Oregon Country offered everything they wanted. Perhaps a hundred immigrants trickled west beyond the Missouri River in 1841, crossing the prairie, plains, and Rocky Mountains to this new Promised Land. The number doubled in 1842, and in 1843 at least a thousand immigrants headed west from Missouri across what is now northeast Kansas to the Platte River in modern Nebraska, and west through the Rocky Mountains at South Pass in modern Wyoming and then northwest to Oregon. The route became known as the Oregon Trail. In 1845, perhaps 5,000 men, women, and children headed west in the wagons carrying all their worldly possessions. By then, Marcus Whitman had established a mission near modern Walla Walla, Washington, and many immigrants stopped there for supplies and medical services before continuing on to the Willamette Valley. Two years later, however, Indians killed Whitman, his wife, and others at the mission.

The immigrants, like most Americans, had no real understanding of the nature of disease. The idea that microscopic creatures called germs caused disease did not begin to gain scientific credibility until after 1860. Many immigrants did not trust physicians. Even if they had, many did not have enough money to pay doctors. Most immigrants did not reject doctors outright, but usually waited to call upon them for help after home remedies failed. Most immigrants carried with them their home remedies, patent medicines, and self-help medical books such as John Gunn's *Domestic Medicine*. While it is not known how many physicians went west of the Oregon Trail in the 1840s, the most common medical problem on the trail was gastrointestinal illness from chronic bowel complaints to diarrheas and dysenteries, and diseases such as cholera and typhoid fever. Thus, it is not surprising that the larger immigrant companies preparing to travel west tried to get qualified physicians to go along to treat the more serious illnesses and injuries. The larger wagon trains were like small towns on wheels, and common sense told the immigrants that with more people, there probably would be more sickness and more injuries from accidents.

In 1846, 3,000 immigrants traversed the trail. Their diaries and journals tell us there were some physicians, but they also suggest that there were too few qualified practitioners. One notable incident illustrating the point can be found in both the diary of thirty-year-old Nicholas Carriger, a Missouri farmer who set out with his wife and family for California, and the writings of another California-bound immigrant, Edwin Bryant, former editor of the *Louisville* (Kentucky) *Courier*. In his diary, Carriger notes on June 6, 1846: "One boy [seven-year-old Enoch Garrison] fell and two wheels run over one leg and the other foot and ancle [*sic*] near cutting the leg off breaking the bone."[1] The wagon train went into camp and various people did what they could for the boy. Two days later, the company resumed travel, with the injured child carried in the family's wagon. Within a few days his condition worsened, and three men were sent to locate a doctor in one of the other immigrant parties. They traveled back along the trail and apparently stopped at each company and asked if there were a doctor. After traveling about thirty miles, they finally came upon a large company in camp captained by William H. Russell. When asked if they had a doctor, someone pointed to Edwin Bryant. Bryant was well educated and had treated some immigrants in his company as a "good Samaritan," but he was not a doctor. He told this to the three men, but they insisted that he accompany them back to where their own company was camped. Bryant describes what happened next:

After a most fatiguing and exhausting ride, we reached the encampment to which I had been called about five o'clock, P.M. . . . When I reached the tent of the unfortunate family to which the boy belonged, I found him stretched out upon a bench made of planks, ready for the operation, which I would perform. I soon learned from the mother that the accident had occurred nine days previously. That a person professing to be a "doctor," had wrapped some linen loosely about the leg, and made a sort of trough or plank box, in which it had been confined. In this condition the child had remained, without any dressing of his wounded limb, until last night, when he called to his mother, and told her that he *could feel worms crawling in his leg!* This, at first, she supposed to be absurd; but an examination of the wound for the first time was made, and it was discovered that gangrene had taken place, and the limb of the child was swarming with maggots! They then immediately dispatched their messengers for me. I made an examination of the fractured limb, and ascertained that what the mother had stated was correct. The limb had been badly fractured, and had never been bandaged; and from neglect gangrene had supervened, and the child's leg, from his foot to the knee, was in a state of putrefaction. He was so much enfeebled by his sufferings that death was stamped upon his countenance, and I was satisfied that he could not live twenty-four hours, much less survive an operation. I so informed the mother, stating to her that to amputate the limb would only hasten the boy's death, and add to his pains while living; declining at the same time, peremptorily, all participation in a proceeding so useless and barbarous under the circumstances. She implored me, with tears and moans, not thus to give up her child without an effort. I told her again, that all efforts to save him would be useless, and only add to the anguish of which he was now dying.

But this could not satisfy a mother's affection. She could not thus yield her offspring to the cold embrace of death, and a tomb in the wilderness. A Canadian Frenchman, who belonged to this emigrating party, was present, and stated that he had formerly been an assistant to a surgeon in some hospital, and had seen many operations of this nature performed, and that he would amputate the child's limb, if I declined doing it, and the mother desired it. I could not repress an involuntary shudder when I heard this proposition, the consent of the weeping woman, and saw the preparations made for the butchery of the little boy. The instruments to be used were a common butcher-knife, a carpenter's handsaw, and a shoemaker's awl to take up the arteries. The man commenced by gashing the flesh to the bone around the calf of the leg, that was in a state of putrescence. He then made an incision just below the knee and commenced sawing; but before he had completed that amputation of the bone, he concluded that the operation should be performed above the knee. During these demonstrations the boy never uttered a groan or a complaint, but I saw from the change in his countenance, that he was dying. The operator, without noticing this, proceeded to sever the leg above the knee. A cord was drawn round the limb, above the spot where it was intended to sever it, so tight that it cut through the skin into the flesh. The knife and saw were then applied and the limb amputated. A few drops of blood only oozed from the stump; the child was Dead—his miseries were over. The scene of weeping and distress, which succeeded this tragedy cannot be described. The mother was frantic, and the brothers and sisters of the deceased boy were infected by the intense grief of their parent.[2]

Bryant was asked to visit the father of the dead child, who was lying prostrate in his tent suffering from inflammatory rheumatism. The man had been devouring his medicines like food, believing large quantities would produce a fast cure. Bryant advised him to cut back on his daily intake of medication. Next, Bryant was invited to attend a wedding in the camp. It was performed by Rev. Josephus Cornwall of Russell's company in the tent of the bride's father. Bryant recalled, "The wedding-cake was not frosted with sugar, nor illustrated with matrimonial devices, after the manner of confectioners in the settlements, but cake was handed round to the whole party present. There was no music or dancing on the occasion. The company separated soon after the ceremony was performed, leaving the happy pair to the enjoyment of their connubial felicities."

It was dark when Bryant left the wedding. In the distance he saw the torches and lanterns of a funeral procession. From the wedding Rev. Cornwall had gone to the wagon of the dead boy to conduct a funeral service. Now the boy's remains were being taken to the spot where a grave had been dug near the trail. While Bryant was watching the funeral procession, a man approached him and told him a woman in a nearby wagon train had just given birth to a baby and both mother and child were doing well. Bryant walked away and later wrote, "I could not but reflect upon the singular concurrence of the events of the day. A death and funeral, a wedding and a birth, had occurred in this wilderness, within a diameter of two miles, and within two hours' time; and tomorrow, the places where these events had taken place, would be deserted and unmarked, except by the grave of the unfortunate boy deceased!"[3]

The year 1847 saw 4,000 immigrants heading west, including two thousand Mormons bound for their Promised Land in Utah. Early Mormon leaders rejected physicians and viewed their treatments for most conditions as ineffective and sometimes harmful. Prophet Joseph Smith and his successor, Brigham Young, urged reliance instead on faith and priestly blessings and treatment with herbs and mild food. At one point Brigham Young said he regarded doctors and their medicines "as a deadly bane to any community." He said he saw no use for them unless it was to raise grain or to do mechanical work. Initially this pronouncement hampered Mormon acceptance of scientific medicine, but at the same time it probably saved lives.

Dr. Benjamin Cory, a physician who had joined a company bound for Oregon, recalled that one of its members, Wesley Tustin from Illinois, was swept off his horse and killed while crossing the swift upper Platte. Dr. Cory recalled treating immigrants mangled by accidental gunshots, children run over by wagon wheels, and a case of what he described as "prostrate fever" and "bilious remitting fever." He wrote in his journal, "I pull teeth and deal out a pill occasionally free." Near Court House Rock, he delivered a baby girl in a moving wagon as the company followed the Platte River across what is now Nebraska. When Cory's company reached Fort Laramie on June 8, he said they were treated decently by the agent in charge, but the rest of his crew were "scamps, cheats, and liars." Dr. Cory arrived in Oregon in October.[4]

Perhaps 8,000 immigrants headed west in 1848, including 4,000 Mormons. California remained a destination for some because it had been described by travelers as an ague-free land, where everyone enjoyed robust health. One man who was responsible for attracting pioneers to California was Antoine Robideaux, a fur trapper who came east to Missouri in 1840 and related wonderful stories about his home along the Pacific coast. He claimed there was only one man in California who ever had a chill from ague, and this man reportedly was a matter of such wonderment that the people of Monterey traveled eighteen miles into the country to see him shake. When another traveler, Lansford W. Hastings, published an immigrants' guidebook to Oregon and California in 1845, he wrote, "Cases of remittent fevers have scarcely ever been known, in any portion of this country."

There is little wonder, in fact, that so many pioneers sought to leave the fever-ridden Mississippi Valley for California. To get there, most immigrants followed the Oregon Trail into what is now southwest Wyoming and turned south to the new Mormon settlement of Great Salt Lake City. From there they traveled west across the Sierra mountains into California. They apparently were determined to put up with the hardships of the journey in order to reach that healthful paradise. Some immigrants suffered from scurvy on the trip and periods of prolonged thirst, exposure to alkali dust for days on end, plus numerous bites of the mosquito, buffalo gnat, and deerfly, which often caused infection though they were not life threatening. Still, such hardships created medical problems, as did traumatic injuries like being crushed by moving wagon wheels, the accidental discharge of firearms, and stampeding livestock.

Whether bound for Oregon or California, the seasonal travel between spring and fall was more or less orderly. This changed after the discovery of gold in California early in 1848. It took a while for the news to reach the East, but by the spring of 1849, the rush to find gold was on. An estimated 30,000 people headed west over the trail, most bound for California. Unlike the immigrants of earlier years who included many families, the gold-seekers were mostly men on their own, who, if they did have families, had left them behind to rush to the goldfields. Most planned to return East and provide better lives for their families after they struck it rich. While some chose to sail around the Horn to reach California, it was cheaper to go overland, and the populations of Missouri River towns such as Independence and St. Joseph swelled to three or four times their normal size. There, gold-seekers gathered to buy supplies and to prepare to follow the trail west. Some arrived by horseback and in wagons, but others had journeyed by steamboats that kept coming up the Missouri River from St. Louis. It was inevitable that the crowded conditions and poor sanitation in the towns and aboard the river vessels would result in sickness and disease. A cholera epidemic that began aboard some steamboats reached the town of Kansas (now Kansas City, Missouri) on April 25.

Dr. Charles Robinson, a thirty-year-old gold-seeker from Fitchburg, Massachusetts, who would later become governor of Kansas, traveled with the Congress and California Mutual Protective Association party organized in Boston. The group was at the town of Kansas when cholera struck. In one night ten persons died, and cholera quickly spread to nearby Independence and to Westport, located three miles south of the town of Kansas; it soon moved up the Missouri River to St. Joseph and westward into the Kansas River valley.[5]

American physicians were only then beginning to understand what caused cholera. The disease had evolved centuries ago in the Ganges Delta region of India. There it remained isolated until Europeans arrived. Cholera spread to Europe, where it was identified as a specific illness in the late 1700s. By the early 1800s its symptoms and peculiarities were known, and physicians could differentiate it from other fevers such as yellow and typhoid. But it had not been discovered that its cause was an infection with the bacterium *Vibrio cholerae* that spread from drinking water or eating food contaminated by the feces of an infected person. Some physicians suspected that the bacteria could exist and survive for long periods outside the human body in many water sources.

By the middle of the nineteenth century, treatments for cholera were about as numerous as there were physicians, but most physicians agreed that a patient with the disease usually went through four stages of the illness. In the first stage, patients were confined to bed and given a mild aromatic drink such as spearmint, chamomile, or warm camphor julep. Once the patient began to perspire, calomel, camphor, magnesia, and pure castor oil were administered. If the patient had recently consumed food, an emetic such as ipecacuanha or sulfate of zinc was given. If the patient did not show signs of recovery and developed cramps, nausea, massive diarrhea, coldness, physical collapse, and a weak pulse, the physician believed the patient was in the second stage. At this point treatment might include putting the patient's feet and hands in water as warm as he could stand, containing mustard and common salt. A large mustard cataplasm was placed over the stomach and they were given calomel, opium, and camphor every half hour. Should the patient continue to deteriorate, physicians believed the cholera had entered its third stage, often called the "stage of asphyxia." Physicians might bleed the victim, believing it would relieve the internal congestion. The patient would be given small doses of oil of vitriol (sulfuric acid) and an enema consisting of a pint of chicken tea, with a tablespoonful of salt. If the patient did not improve—and one wonders how anyone could have with such treatment—larger doses of calomel and camphor were prescribed, plus quinine and morphine every half hour. The fourth stage usually took place when consecutive fever occurred followed, by coma and death.

Another physician attracted to the gold rush was Charles E. Boyle of Columbus, Ohio, who left St. Joseph, Missouri, in April 1849 with a party of thirty gold-seekers. In his diary, Dr. Boyle mentions treating John Walton, leader of the party, who had been kicked in the head by a mule: "While proceeding to dress the scalp wound, I found suture necessary, and John determined to bear it with patience but promised that if he struck me, I must not take it amiss but go ahead without paying any attention to it. He found however that he could bear the operation very well and I finished dressing the wound as quickly as possible. In another case, after a man came down with cholera the doctor treated him with calomel, opium, and diluted muriatic acid. West of South Pass in the Rocky Mountains, Boyle wrote that his party suffered from "mountain fever," which was probably either altitude sickness or tick fever. When Boyle's party reached a trading post operated by "Peg-leg" Smith on Bear River about 125 miles north of Great Salt Lake City, he met Smith and described him as "jolly." Dr. Boyle noted that he sold Smith a pint of brandy for $4. While at the post, Boyle also prescribed medicine for a Frenchman who was living there with his Indian wife.[6]

The mass of people traveling the Oregon Trail created major sanitation problems that contributed to the spread of cholera and other diseases. Then, too, with more travelers there were more accidents, and doctors were kept busy treating broken legs and arms and other injuries. Some of the physicians who joined the gold rush placed signs on their wagons or used word-of-mouth to advertise their services. As they crossed the prairie and plains, travelers soon came to know which group of wagons carried a doctor. When someone became ill, the sick or injured were often transported in the doctor's wagon until they either recovered or died. New York doctors were in especially high demand because most immigrants figured they were better trained than the others. Some wagon trains paid doctors to travel with them, and each family in the train would pay as much as $5 for having him on call during the journey from Missouri to California or Oregon.

Dr. Jonathan Clark started for California in April 1849, traveling in an ox-drawn wagon with three other men. They crossed the Missouri River at modern Council Bluffs, Iowa, and experienced numerous hardships on their journey. In an apparent accident, Clark was tossed into the icy waters of the Green River. After his rescue, he wrote in his diary, "I was seized with a violent sickness [with] pain of the most excruciating character through my back." He concluded that he had contracted "inflammatory rheumatism," but he did recover before his party reached California.[7]

Another physician, Dr. Dean J. Locke, twenty-six, was hired to go to California from Boston in April 1849 to take care of the medical needs of members of the Boston and Newton Joint Stock Association party of gold-seekers. He treated members of his party and others for cholera, including a deranged man deserted by another company. Locke reached California in September. The California Historical Society in San Francisco preserves his diary. Dr. Locke and his brother, Elmer H. Locke, later owned a ranch and founded the town of Locke-ford, California, where the doctor practiced medicine until his death in 1887 at age sixty-four.

Still another physician going to California in 1849 was Dr. William L. Thomas, who left Kentucky in the spring of 1849, traveling with more than forty other Kentuckians in wagons pulled by mule teams. From letters he sent east we know he arrived in California in August and that he provided medical services to those in his party on the journey. However, he offered few details. At a crossing on the upper Platte River, he wrote that he was appalled at the reaction of other travelers when a young man from Missouri fell into the river and yelled for help. The doctor recalled that the people nearby showed no more interest than if the young Missourian "had been a dog."[8]

Letters written by Dr. Caleb N. Ormsby, who chose in 1849 to go to Oregon instead of California, tell of his treating many patients for cholera along the trail. His letters to his family in the East stopped, however, when he reached the Blue Mountains of eastern Oregon in October. Dr. Ormsby died, possibly from cholera.

Some physicians who joined the gold rush had earned medical degrees, but many either had apprenticed with other doctors or were self-trained. Many of the more educated practiced heroic medicine, but others were herbalists. Still others were homoeopaths, who did not bleed patients as the heroics did. They used a gentler approach, treating patients with minute quantities of drugs. Israel Shipman Pelton Lord was one such doctor. Born in Connecticut in 1805, he began to study medicine in 1826 with Dr. Frederick Fitch at LeRoy, New York, and then in 1828 continued his studies by attending medical lectures. By the early 1830s, he had his own practice, first at Vernal and later at French Creek, New York. Dr. Lord, however, then came down with "ague," which was probably malaria, and was plagued by fever and chills. He moved west to Illinois, believing the change in climate would improve his health. It did not. In 1849 Lord decided to go to California and joined a company of gold-seekers from Elgin, Illinois. Thinking that walking might benefit his health, he chose to walk most of the way to Sacramento. Lord was an observant man and kept a journal detailing his treatment of victims of cholera, gunshots, knife wounds, and stampedes. He wrote in his journal that cholera had caused havoc for doctors along the route. By the time he reached Sacramento, however, he had decided that "ninety-nine out of every hundred who go to California are either madmen, fools, or unprincipled and dishonest." He remained in California until early in 1851, when he took a ship to return east, where he continued his practice of medicine.[9]

Then there is the story of Dr. Augustus B. Caldwell from Missouri, who helped to organize a party of men who fitted out a wagon with four yoke of oxen and carried eight hundred pounds of bacon, eight hundred pounds of flour, two hundred pounds of sugar, a hundred pounds of coffee, and clothing for three years, plus good rifles, pistols, knives, cooking utensils, and everything they thought they would need to get to California. Caldwell's party joined a company with nineteen wagons and sixty men headed by Boone Hays, and started west. Dr. Caldwell did not do much doctoring on the journey, but he did sell some opium to an immigrant near Devil's Gate. The journey was difficult going over the Sierras into California, but when Dr. Caldwell and the others arrived, the physician opened a general store at Beckville to provide supplies, medicines, and medical treatment for the miners. After a new gold strike occurred at Deer Creek Dry Diggings, four miles upstream, Dr. Caldwell opened a second store in the new mining camp that later became Nevada, California. Dr. Caldwell apparently got rich mining the miners. By 1853 he was back in Missouri, where he purchased land in Jackson County near Kansas City and settled down.[10]

Still another physician on the trail in 1849 was Dr. Charles R. Parke, Jr., who traveled with eight other men in three wagons from Como, Illinois. Their Como Pioneer Company traveled overland to St. Joseph, crossed the Missouri River, traveled northwest until they reached the Platte River, and then followed it west. Dr. Parke tried to help four dying Indians at a Pawnee village on the Platte and treated many immigrants for smallpox and cholera. Like Dr. Caldwell and other physicians on the trail, Dr. Parke used opium in his treatments.[11]

Some of the physicians who followed the gold rush to California found gold. Many of these then returned east. Most of those who were not lucky gave up and practiced medicine. Dr. Pierre Garnier, a French physician who left for California from France in 1850, sailed around Cape Horn, and arrived at Monterey in the spring of 1851.

Many of the doctors he met there, he recalled, were quacks and charlatans with no training. In his memoir *Voyage Médical en Californie*, published in Paris in 1854, Garnier said he found eight doctors in Monterey and twelve in Los Angeles. He was distressed at the public advertising and extravagant claims of these "health merchants." He noted as well that surgery was frequently required for knife and gunshot wounds because the Yankees (Americans) had the deplorable habit of settling minor quarrels with their revolvers. At the same time he noted, physicians were often not consulted because the Yankees would turn instead to the apothecary, who served in effect as their doctor. Where Europeans, he wrote, were willing to spend money for doctors, Californians and Indians usually doctored themselves using home remedies and those of Indian medicine men. "[T]hose who would did seek out a doctor when ill would go to anyone with the title, and demand a quick cure for a disease that they themselves had diagnosed. Generally the patients refused a physical examination and simply wished to be provided with medicine."

One doctor who made his home in California was John Frederick Morse, who left his New York medical practice in 1849 believing that the California climate would improve his health. He searched for gold for a time before settling in Sacramento to practice. There he treated many people during a cholera epidemic in 1850 and did so without pay. When the epidemic ended, Dr. Morse had to work at other jobs to support his family. He sold real estate for a time, ran for political office, owned a drugstore, and in 1851 became the editor of the *Sacramento Union* newspaper. He also wrote a history of Sacramento and promoted public health measures to clean up the growing town. In 1863, Morse moved to San Francisco and joined the Medical Department of the University of the Pacific, the first medical school in California. Poor health forced him to retire in 1873, and he died the following year.

More than 50,000 gold-seekers crossed the Missouri River in 1850 from one or another of the jumping-off towns and followed the Oregon Trail toward California. There probably were more self-declared doctors on the trail in 1850 than the previous year, but how many were bona fide physicians with medical degrees is not known. A correspondent for the *St. Joseph* (Missouri) *Gazette* reported in the paper's July 31, 1850, issue that not one wagon train in a hundred had a physician. However, Dr. James Williams, who left Independence in the spring of 1850 and arrived in Sacramento in August, observed that doctors were thick on the road and he had medical competition in his journey west. The truth regarding the number of doctors is probably somewhere between these two accounts.

For men traveling by horseback, hemorrhoids would often bring a rider to the ground. After one traveler, Lemuel Clarke McKeeby, reached California, he had an attack of swollen piles. He asked an old Army officer if he knew a remedy. The soldier told him to use turpentine, but he warned it would make him dance around a bit. That night McKeeby applied turpentine. He recalled that it was some time before he went to sleep, but the next morning he felt much better, and the hemorrhoids gradually went away, so he was able to ride horseback again.[12]

Some doctors kept diaries or journals or wrote letters home, but many make only passing mention of treating immigrants, even though outbreaks of cholera in '49 and again in '50 naturally elevated the importance and need of doctors during those years. One writer, apparently a physician, identifying himself only by the initials R.H.D., wrote from a few miles west of Fort Laramie on June 25, 1850:

> Most physicians along the road believe the disease which has prevailed among emigrants with such fatality, to be epidemic cholera. Of this I am somewhat incredulous, certainly, local causes sufficient exist on the Platte to produce, if not the most violent forms of darrhoea [sic], to incite, at least, the most latent predisposition to cholera into unrestrained action. The entire Platte bottom is covered with saline matter, such as salt-petre, Salaratus, &c. The springs are also strongly impregnated with sulphur, copper, &c. (I have used no analysis but that of taste.) Add to this the first emigrant-sunk wells in the bottom. Into these had accumulated the filth and scum, which 30,000 persons had left along the road. The use of the filthy water, together with exposure and unwholesome diet, are sufficient, in my opinion, to account for all the sickness which has occurred.

When R.H.D. crossed the Laramie Fork with his company, he was asked to treat a sick man traveling with his wife and seven children. "His case I considered then almost desperate, but by close attention might have been saved. Several days after, I chanced to see him again. As I sat by his side with my finger on his sinking pulse, and heard in his throat the death-rattle, that most ominous sign to the physician of approaching dissolution, his wife, with a smothered groan, asked me to tell her precisely his condition, saying she wished to know the worst. I told her she should not flatter herself any longer with hope, but be prepared for the worst. I arose to leave the tent, and as I did so returned the fee I had received on a former occasion, and I let drop a tear in sympathy for her desolate and bereaved condition. God grant I may not, on this trip, be called upon to perform such another duty."[13]

After Dr. George W. Davis arrived in California late in 1850, he sent a letter East that is now preserved in the Beinecke Library at Yale University. Davis wrote that he treated about three hundred people as he made the journey west. He was so busy treating patients in different wagon trains that his work delayed his arrival in California and limited the amount of prospecting he could do before winter arrived. Another physician, Dr. Reuben Knox, recalled treating twenty to forty patients each day for cholera as he followed the trail in 1850. All of the patients were within riding distance of his wagon. In describing a typical day helping people, Knox wrote that he

started at 3 a.m., rode 3 miles from camp, missed my way in the fog and rode a mile in searching for the place, saw a man from Georgia dying, did not live more than half an hour . . . prescribed for 3 more sick in the same camp and some in two other camps on my way back to my own. Breakfasted at 5; got off at 5½ having two men awaiting my departure to conduct me to two camps a mile or two ahead . . . prescribed for two sick in one and three in the other, one nearly gone—before I joined the wagons, had another awaiting for me to come up who had a sick wife and child going along in a train ahead of ours, so rode up and administered medicine as the train was moving along. At about 8 called ¼ of a mile off to see a dying man from Arkansas, would not live an hour. The three remaining members of the company had just buried one of their number; gave medicine to them as one of them was quite unwell and the other two almost frightened to death. Kept away from the wagons by constant application for advice, etc., along the road until 10—found a man there wishing me to go off the road some distance to see a number of sick ones in a train of twenty three or four wagons filled with families from Independence and vicinity—they were burying the sixth— found another dying and 10 to 12 sick. Remained with them until my company had gone so far that I did not reach them until after lunch time and they were about harnessing the mules again. In a mile or so, was called off again. Some distance from the road found a lady from Illinois dying and a young man very sick; ½ a mile from thence and before I reached the road, saw a man dying and his wife quite sick— continued along the road and the river bank among the camps about in the same way constantly trying to relieve the sick and galloping along until 6½ when we camped. Before the mules were harnessed, two messengers came post haste for me, one of whom was cold, purple and pulseless—but who revived about two hours after and . . . sent more medicine and started off in the morning at 3½, finding some out of danger and the other better.[14]

Dr. Samuel Matthias Ayres provided another account of what doctors experienced in a series of letters written to his wife in Pettis County, Missouri. Dr. Ayres left Independence in a small company of eighteen men with five wagons. He reported that cholera was at its worst along the four hundred miles between Fort Kearny and Fort Laramie, where it declined, probably because of cooler temperatures and better conditions. In one letter, he wrote, "[S]ome doctors charge more than at home but not me." Money, Ayres said, was scarce. While one man in his company died from cholera and was buried near the South Platte crossing, the first casualty he saw was a young man who had been shot while in camp: The boy had crept into the sleeping quarters of a young woman, and had been shot by her father. Dr. Ayres, whose letters are preserved in the joint manuscript collection of the University of Missouri and Missouri State Historical Society, reached California safely in mid-September 1850.

Merrill J. Mattes, who spent much of his life studying overland travel, estimated that one out of every ten to twelve immigrants died in 1850. If correct, about five thousand immigrants died that year. Mattes, however, considered his estimate conservative.[15] Whether a greater number of physicians could have resulted in many of these lives being saved is impossible to say with any certainty, because the exact number of qualified physicians who traveled overland with the immigrants in 1850 is not known. Some doctors, moreover, did not have much time to practice medicine. One such was Dr. Thomas Flint, who traveled from Council Bluffs, Iowa, to Great Salt Lake City and then on to Los Angeles with two other men, herding two thousand sheep to California.[16]

Ohio physician Dr. John Hudson Wayman, who headed to California in 1852 with a few companions, wrote in his diary that he did some doctoring along the way. He described two forms of diarrhea: "the pale free watery discharges and the Bilious." After Dr. Wayman and his small party left Fort Laramie, he wrote, he treated patients for dysentery and fever.[17] Another bona fide doctor was Dr. Thomas White from Indiana, who followed the trail west from Council Bluffs, Iowa, in 1852. He delivered babies, and treated immigrants for measles and those wounded in an Indian attack, including one victim who received multiple wounds in his "derriere."[18]

The diaries, journals, and recollections of more than two thousand overland travelers suggest that most physicians they encountered were generous beyond measure with their time and frequently asked for no payment for services. Dr. William R. Allen treated seven hundred patients and received only $150 on his journey west. He recalled that he charged only for the medicine. A few doctors, however, charged $2 to visit a patient with cholera, and $5 to set a fractured arm and dislocated shoulder.[19] By 1850, land that had been initially passed over by whites along the route west was becoming settled. While there were no large cities on the prairie or plains, small settlements sprang up around ferries, bridges, trading posts, forts, and stage stations. The perception of overland travel changed. The government and private entrepreneurs made overland travel easier, but at the same time more expensive.

The guidebooks that started to appear in the early 1840s, and became more numerous after the gold rush began, provided information on main routes, shortcuts, landmarks, and so forth, but contain little reference to health concerns. In 1859, however, Captain Randolph B. Marcy, U.S. Army, wrote *The Prairie Traveler: A Hand-Book for Overland Expeditions*. Unlike earlier guides, Marcy included advice on sanitary considerations, such as: "When camping near rivers and lakes surrounded by large bodies of timber and a luxuriant vegetation, which produces a great amount of decomposition and consequent exhalations of malaria, it is important to ascertain what localities will be least likely to generate disease, and to affect the sanitary condition of men occupying them." He went on to quote extensively from Dr.

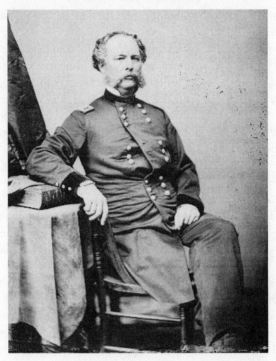

Randolph Barnes Marcy (1812–1887), author of The Prairie
Traveler, *a practical guidebook for travelers about what equipment to carry, methods of organizing a wagon train, techniques
of avoiding Indians, and notes on thirty-four of the most important overland trails. He would eventually attain the rank of
brigadier general and become inspector general of the Army.*
(Courtesy Library of Congress)

Robert Johnson, inspector general of hospitals in the British army in
1845, who had researched the importance of selecting the best camp-
sites. In his guide, Marcy also provided information about treating sick
horses, and devoted several pages to minor medical problems—to
relieve gnat and mosquito bites, for example, he recommended chewing plantain and rubbing the spittle on them. Marcy gave extensive
attention to poisonous snakebites, chiefly in the form of anecdotes
illustrating effective treatments. One story was set in North Texas: "A
small child was left upon the earthen floor of a cabin while its mother
was washing at a spring near by. She heard a cry of distress, and, on

going to the cabin, what was her horror on seeing a rattlesnake coiled around the child's arm, and striking it repeatedly with its fangs. After killing the snake, she hurried to her nearest neighbor, procured a bottle of brandy, and returned as soon as possible; but the poison had already so operated on the arm that it was black as a negro's. She poured down the child's throat a huge draught of the liquor, which soon took effect, making it very drunk, and stopped the action of the poison. Although the child was relieved, it remained sick for a long time, but ultimately recovered."

Then there was the case of a man bitten in the leg by a large rattlesnake near Fort Belknap, Texas. "No other remedy being at hand, a small piece of indigo was pulverized, made into a poultice with water, and applied to the puncture. It seemed to draw out the poison, turning the indigo white, after which it was removed and other poultice applied. These applications were repeated until the indigo ceased to change its color. The man was then carried to the hospital at Fort Belknap, and soon recovered, and the surgeon of the post pronounced it 'a very satisfactory cure.' " Still another case described by Marcy concerned a Chickasaw woman bitten by a rattlesnake near Fort Washita in Indian Territory. The woman, he wrote, "drank a bottle of whiskey and applied the indigo poultice, and when I saw her, three days afterward, she was recovering, but the flesh around the wound sloughed away."

Marcy's advice came from his own experience and those of other overland travelers, but his guide does not contain information on treating diseases. In 1860, when 10,000 to 15,000 people headed west, many of them undoubtedly used Marcy's guidebook as they journeyed to California, Oregon, or the Kansas goldfields in what is now Colorado, or elsewhere in the West. Many were simply trying to escape the threat of the impending Civil War. From the 10,000 to 15,000 of 1860, with the start of the war the number of westward-bound declined to about 5,000 in 1861, but gradually increased again during the conflict. In 1865, perhaps 25,000 people followed the Oregon Trail west from the Missouri River.

That year, John and Mary Louisa Black and their family left Missouri with two wagons bound for Oregon. After John's father died in 1864, and at the urging of relatives living in Oregon, the couple decided to sell out, take their children, and move there. Before they departed, their family doctor gave them a list of medicines—with recommended doses—that he said they should take on their journey. His remarkable list has survived and provides many insights into how medical problems were dealt with on the trail in 1865:

Landanum	4 ounces (dose 25 drops)
Turpentine	16 ounces (dose 1½ teaspoonful)
Castor oil	1 bottle, ½ pt. (dose ½ tablespoonful)
McLeans pills	3 boxes ["Dr. J. H. McLean's Universal Pills or Vegetable Liver Pills," manufactured in St. Louis beginning in 1851]
Calomel	½ drachm
Blue Mass	½ drachm [concoction of mercury and chalk]
Quinine	4 drachms
Sugar of Lead	4 drachms [lead acetate]
Coal oil	1 pint
Eye Water	made of 2 grains of Sulpt of Zinc to one ounce water. Get two ounces made up.
Paregoric	8 ounces and mix one ounce of Tannin with it—for bowel complaint of children—dose your oldest child ½ teaspoon—for the infant give ten drops—for Tillie ½ teaspoonful.
Ipecac	2 drachms—dose 20 grains, 5 grains every 15 minutes [a drug made from the dried roots of a creeping shrub, *Cephaelis* (or *Psychotria*) *ipecacuanha*, native to Brazil but cultivated in other tropical climates]
Epsom salt	¼ pound dose heaping tablespoonful
Mustard Seed	½ pint or 1 box ground mustard
Blister Plaster	3 ounces

One thumb lancet and tooth forceps for the company. One will do the crowd.

Blue Stone	2 drachms [copper sulfate, a blue compound about the color of indigo]
Hartshorn	½ ounce [a leavening agent, and a precursor to baking soda]

With his list of medicines, this unidentified doctor also sent written instructions for the treatment of the Black family:

For Diarhoea [*sic*] give the paregoric and tannin—for an adult, 1 tablespoon is a dose. Or take a dose of tannin with 25 drops of Laudanum and repeat every 3, 4, or 6 hours. Sometimes a dose of the Blue Mass at first is best, then begin on the other.

If you take dysentery or flux (all the same) be sure and not keep the bowels locked up over 12 hours at a time. You must begin on Salts—full dose, after they act two or three times (which you will know by a change in the stools to a more natural character) then quiet the bowels with a full dose of Laudanum and repeat it in six hours. Then at the same time, on the next day that you gave the Salts, you give another dose and give Salts every day at the same time of day, repeat dose in six hours if the first dose not act—then follow it with Laudanum as before. Nearly all of the deaths from flux are from keeping the bowels too much closed.

Mountain Fever—This is the easiest thing treated in the world. You first give a very active purgative, nearly a double dose of McLean's Pills or Blue Mass and Calomel combined, then 40 drops of Laudanum, and sponge the body often with tepid water—repeat the Laudanum from 25 to 40 drops so as to keep the patient under the influence of it 48 hours. Then if there be any fever left, repeat the purgative (a common dose now) followed by the Laudanum.

Colic—give a double dose of Castor oil with ½ teaspoonful of turpentine—repeat every three hours. As soon as it acts your colic is gone.

Cholera Morbus—give oil and Laudanum with mustard over the whole bowels.[20]

John and Mary Black and their three children made the journey to Oregon, but not without tragedy and hardship; their oldest daughter, who had been born in 1859, died from food poisoning soon after they started west. It took the Blacks seven months to reach Oregon. The "Overland Trail," as many were then calling it, continued to be the major route west for settlers until 1869, when the transcontinental railroad was completed and travel overland by wagon began to diminish.

CHAPTER SEVEN

AMONG THE SOLDIERS

I like the dreams of the future better than the history of the past.

—Thomas Jefferson

DURING THE AMERICAN REVOLUTION, more soldiers died from illness and medical treatment than from combat. Many of the soldiers were inexperienced country boys never before exposed to communicable diseases. Dysentery, scurvy, smallpox, typhus, and other diseases took their toll. It did not help that the American soldiers, unlike the British, were poorly clothed and fed, and, in addition, lived in an environment of poor sanitation. Then, too, medical treatments of the day were frequently useless or worse than useless. Doctors did not yet understand what caused most diseases, and their heroic treatments often did more harm than good. On July 27, 1775, Congress authorized the formation of the Continental Army's medical department. By the time the Treaty of Paris was signed eight years later, officially ending the war, most of the doctors who made up the medical department had returned to their homes and their private practices. At the same time all but 80 of the 24,000 soldiers in the Continental Army were discharged.

The pay vouchers for military service given to the discharged soldiers were almost worthless, since the new American government had little money. The vouchers, however, could be used to obtain government land. Many veterans sought to settle west of the Appalachians, especially in former British territory south of the Great Lakes and east of the Mississippi River, which had been ceded to the United States. The Indians living in the region, however, were never consulted about the disposition of their land, and soon came to resent the increasing numbers of American settlers.

As the new nation began organizing a government in 1789, a Department of War was established. It raised a new army, which initially consisted of one infantry regiment of 560 men, including one surgeon and four surgeon's mates, plus an artillery regiment of 260 men, including one surgeon's mate. This army was so small that it did not require a formal medical department. Soon the government established new forts west of the Appalachians in areas where settlers and Indians were likely to come into contact. Army doctors were assigned to the new posts, including Fort Washington, established in 1789 in the Ohio River Valley, near where Cincinnati stands today. The British encouraged Indians in the region to make trouble, and soon more American posts were built, including Fort Hamilton on the site of modern Hamilton, Ohio, and Fort Jefferson near present-day Greenville, Ohio.

The first three years of the campaigns against hostile Indians were ones of failure and included the bloodiest battle in pioneer American history, when General Arthur St. Clair was defeated by Miami Indians in 1791 about thirty miles from Fort Jefferson. Of about 1,400 soldiers, 612 died, including a surgeon, and 264 men were wounded. The Indians scalped many of the soldiers. Two years later, a four-blockhouse post called Fort Recovery was built on the site of the battle, and six months later, in 1794, Fort Defiance was established at the confluence of the Auglaize and Maumee rivers. It was the last post constructed in that early Indian campaign. A few days later, the Battle of Fallen Timbers took place south of modern Toledo, Ohio. The American victory resulted in a treaty with the Indians.

A few months following the battle Dr. Joseph Gardner Andrews, a surgeon's mate, was assigned to Fort Defiance. A 1785 graduate of Harvard College, he was now responsible for the health of about 160 officers and men, plus a handful of civilians, including 5 women and a child. He also cared for sick Indians. In addition, Dr. Andrews kept the weather and medical records at the post and found time to write his own journal.

In January 1795, Andrews recorded that twenty-five men wounded in the Battle of Fallen Timbers were receiving treatment at Fort Defiance. In addition, twelve of the 120 troops at the post were sick with dysentery (which the military called "bloody flux"), "intermit fever" (malaria), sore throats, or colds. In February, the doctor wrote that one wounded soldier had died and another wounded soldier deserted, but he was still treating fifteen battle-wounded men, and nine other soldiers were then suffering from a variety of diseases, including dysentery, rheumatism, and catarrh (runny noses brought on by viral or bacterial infection). In March, Andrews reported that another wounded soldier had died, and that 36, or 11 percent, of the fort's 127 officers and men were sick. Dr. Andrews speculated that the increase in sickness was probably due to the cloudy, snowy winter weather, "together with the bad state of the beef . . . wch [which] is constantly depreciating." In his April report, he noted:

> For every ten well persons . . . there is one invalid, exclusive of the wounded!—The Beef approached the bottom of the Casks appears to be much meliorated & the Diarrae [sic] and Dysentery have ceased; tho' there were several cases of both during the month of March.— The Weather for the last month appears to have been of the species wch [which] gives rise to Intermitting Fever; we accordingly find that two thirds of our sick are afflicted with that Disorder.[1]

By September 1795, Andrews himself had come down with the "fever"—malaria—and he had "not a particle of Hospital Stores" to treat himself or his patients. He turned to the bark of the dogwood tree to produce a drink to treat himself and his patients. The post's officers and Andrews finally obtained eight gallons of liquor for the hospital by promising to pay for it with their own money should the government refuse to do so. Andrews later acquired a keg of wine and thirty pounds of brown sugar. From October through November, two-thirds of the ninety-four people at the post were suffering from the fever. When colder weather arrived in December, illness subsided, but the lack of medicines, hospital stores, and, in some cases, surgical instruments created problems at Fort Defiance and at other posts. Because the Army supply system was so poorly organized, it was often up to doctors to locate needed supplies on their own.

While the Army medical service was struggling to do its job, Indians were determined to stop the westward advance of American settlers. The Shawnee chief Tecumseh sought to create a great Indian confederacy to resist the white men. He traveled through the Mississippi Valley as far south as Tennessee seeking support from other tribes. At the same time, Tecumseh's brother, a medicine man called the Prophet, exerted much influence, telling tribes they should return to their old ways and give up the customs and evil habits they had acquired from the white men. Gradually warriors from different tribes gathered at the Prophet's town on the Tippecanoe River, about seven miles north of modern Lafayette, Indiana. Disturbed by the news, Indiana territorial governor William Henry Harrison sent for U.S. Army troops and called out his militia. He was shortly marching with a thousand men toward the Prophet's town.

As Harrison's troops neared the village, they made contact with the Indians and arranged for a meeting. The Prophet, however, attacked the Americans while they were sleeping in their camp. The Americans rallied and fought back, routing the Indians and burning the Prophet's village. During the battle 37 of Harrison's soldiers died and more than 150 were wounded, including a surgeon's mate serving with the militia. At least three physicians, a surgeon, and two mates were with Harrison's troops. The wounded were taken to a hospital at Vincennes and supervised by Dr. Josiah Foster and another physician, but the wounds received by 25 men proved fatal by the time they arrived, and three more died later. Foster reportedly performed two amputations at the shoulder, a type of surgery then not often undertaken. Because many wounds were slow to heal, Foster suspected that the Indians had used poisoned ammunition. When balls found in soldiers' wounds were examined, they were seen to have been "chewed before they were inserted into rifles for the purpose of enlarging the wound and lacerating the contiguous flesh."[2]

When Tecumseh returned to his brother's village, he was angry with the Prophet, whose actions had shattered Tecumseh's plans. After the War of 1812 began, Tecumseh and a small group of followers headed north to Canada and joined with the British against the Americans. Tecumseh died in battle during the war.

THE PERIOD BETWEEN the American Revolution and the War of 1812 was the low point in the history of the U.S. Army's medical service. It lacked organization, a system to distribute medical supplies to surgeons, and focus. It was not prepared when Congress, recognizing the likelihood of a second war with Britain, ordered the creation of a volunteer army of 50,000 soldiers five months before the War of 1812 began. Congress was reluctant to spend money, but eventually, nine months after war broke out, it created the offices of Physician and Surgeon General and Apothecary General. In May 1813, President James

Madison issued new rules and regulations for the Army. Until then Army surgeons and surgeon's mates had been permitted to conduct private medical practices in addition to meeting their military responsibilities. The new rules and regulations, however, forbade military physicians to engage in private practice. The government also established the following pay scale:

POSITION	MONTHLY SALARY
Hospital Surgeons	$75.00
Hospital Surgeon's Mate	$40.00
Steward	$20.00
Wardmaster	$16.00
Surgeon	$45.00
Mate	$30.00

In addition, all of the above received rations. Surgeons and mates also received forage allowances for their horses.

Late in 1814, the Army introduced higher standards of cleanliness and sanitation. In its hospitals, close stools (chamber pots) were to be cleaned at least three times a day and each had to contain either water or charcoal. Beds and bedclothes were to be aired each day and exposed to sunlight when possible. The straw in each bed sack was to be changed at least once a month. When a patient died or was released, the straw from his bed sack was burned. Each patient was to be washed once a day, and his hair combed. In addition, at least one female attendant was to be assigned to each hospital or infirmary to clean or wash bunks, floors, bedding, and cooking utensils, for which she was paid no more than $6 a month plus one ration a day. When necessary, commanding officers could hire civilian doctors, who were paid the same salary as surgeon's mates.[3]

Fevers, digestive ailments, and respiratory ills were the most prevalent diseases among soldiers during the War of 1812. Some doctors began to question the value of mercury and opium in certain treatments, but many continued to use them. When healthy soldiers tried to avoid duty by going on sick call, one surgeon found that the suggestion of blistering would often cause a soldier to return to duty rather than submitting to that painful treatment. Many doctors concluded that discipline was a key to keeping the sick population down and that improved hygiene could prevent disease. They also learned that vaccinations could control smallpox and made them mandatory in the U.S. Army. It became obvious that proper clothing was important for the health of soldiers, including footgear to keep their feet warm and dry, "with woolen socks and laced shoes, reaching at least to the ankle." In hot weather, however, some doctors concluded those soldiers should wear "pantalets & shoes, without stockings."[4]

Following the war, some Army physicians wrote articles about their professional experiences, but since the Army's central organization was now disbanded, there was no formal process to gather, organize, and study their conclusions. Within months, American political leaders realized there was a need for a permanent and efficient professional army in peacetime that could be ready to expand in case of war. In 1818, permanent Army departments were established, including one for medicine. This change laid the foundation for what would become a much stronger Army medical service, which became heavily involved in scattered conflicts from the Seminole Wars in Florida and Georgia to the Black Hawk War of 1832 in Iowa and Wisconsin, which resulted in the deaths of seventy settlers and soldiers and hundreds of Indians. Unfortunately, many veterans of the Black Hawk War unwittingly spread cholera across the nation as they returned home. Active-duty soldiers also carried the disease with them when transferred to new posts. For instance, there were 16 deaths out of 150 cases of cholera at Fort Gibson in Indian Territory. Throughout the Army, nearly 200 soldiers died out of nearly 700 reported cases.

The southern border of Indian Territory was the Red River, then the international boundary between the United States and Mexican Texas. When Moses Austin sought to colonize Texas in 1821, he was accompanied by an Irish-born doctor named James Hewetson, who treated the colonists. After the Texas Revolution began in the fall of 1835, an untold number of doctors in the United States answered the call for help and volunteered their services working alongside Texas doctors. Seven of the fifty-nine men who signed the Texas Declaration of Independence were physicians. Before the revolution ended with the battle of San Jacinto on April 21, 1836, several doctors had lost their lives. Six died at the Alamo, and others in the Goliad Massacre. Mexican army officers spared the lives of some Anglo physicians at Goliad after they treated wounded Mexican soldiers at La Bahía, where the mission served as a hospital. One Texas doctor of note, Alexander W.

Ewing, treated President Sam Houston, whose right leg had been fractured by gunfire in the battle at San Jacinto; he served as surgeon general of the Republic of Texas's army until June 1837. Before the revolution, American doctors apparently had to obtain licenses from the Mexican authorities to practice medicine.

Back in the States during this period, efforts to certify civilian physicians were faltering, but in 1834, the Army medical service established a board of examiners to give written and oral exams to doctors seeking commissions as medical officers. The exams lasted two or three days. Many doctors failed, and many of those who passed often had to wait until positions opened up. A few of those who passed but for whom no positions became available were hired as contract civilian physicians to care for Army personnel. The certification of doctors elevated the Army's standards above those of civilian physicians.

When thousands of eastern Indians were moved west during the 1830s in advance of more and more white settlers coming from the East, the War Department built new forts to defend the western frontiers. Isolation was a problem because of the vastness of the West. At each fort the post surgeon was charged with providing medical care for all officers, enlisted men, laborers in the service of the federal government, and their families. Each post was required to have a hospital directed by the post surgeon, who conducted all sick calls, supervised the pharmacy, and gave medical exams to all recruits and prisoners. Most post hospitals were small. A surgeon was lucky if he had an enlisted man to act as steward, nurse-cook, and general assistant. The post surgeon also monitored all living areas, the water supply, and cooking for proper sanitary measures, was responsible for financial accounts, the requisitioning of medicines and other supplies, and for a voluminous amount of paperwork, including quarterly reports to the surgeon general. Because physicians realized that climate in certain ways influenced health and disease, they also took twice-daily readings of temperature and wind conditions, measured rainfall, and recorded other such information.

The life of a post physician was not easy, because he shared in the boredom, dull routine, hardships, and sickness of everyone else. Some doctors turned to alcohol and others pleaded for transfers, but most made the best of their difficult surroundings. Some trained themselves to be competent naturalists, particularly ornithologists, and even provided specimens to the Smithsonian Institution in Washington.[5]

The 1835 diary of Leonard C. McPhail provides insights into the life of an assistant surgeon in the West. Although little is known about McPhail's early life, he became an Army physician late in 1834 and was assigned to the Regiment of Dragoons, a newly created unit of soldiers on horseback at Fort Gibson, Indian Territory. Gibson, established about a decade earlier, was nothing more than a wretched collection of log and frame huts when Dr. McPhail arrived in 1835 and found the hospital unfinished and unfurnished. He had to lay his sick on the puncheon floors, cursing the unhealthy dampness. Such conditions gave Fort Gibson a reputation as the "charnel house of the frontier." Dr. McPhail reported to the surgeon general that only one room in the hospital under construction had a floor, and that this was installed only because it was used as a ballroom. McPhail noted that dysentery and malaria were the most common and most fatal diseases among the soldiers. Opium and ipecac were the medicines used, since quinine and cinchona bark were not available. He also observed that a great variety of herbaceous species of plants grew everywhere. Indians, he wrote, used a decoction of one whole plant, unidentified, to treat intermittent fever, and used slippery elm bark (*Ulmus fulva Michx*), sometimes called "Indian meal," to make poultices to treat burns.[6]

The medical problems McPhail faced on the frontier were not unique. Surgeons found alcoholism a problem in nearly all posts and frequently went searching for the infamous cask of liquor hidden in bushes near isolated posts, and they fought the clandestine whiskey-sellers and the operators of nearby "hog ranches," brothels that military doctors constantly condemned. The women at the hog ranches also carried venereal disease, a common illness among soldiers. Sporadic outbreaks of scurvy were another problem, since the diet of the frontier very often lacked fresh fruit and vegetables. Soldiers spending long winters at some isolated posts without fruit and vegetables often had their teeth drop out from scurvy. In addition, fevers such as typhoid and malaria, numerous gastrointestinal ailments, including chronic diarrhea, were common, especially at posts where sanitary conditions were poor. The close proximity of the water supply to pit toilets and "honey wagons" was a major contributor to disease. Lax regulations concerning personal hygiene—including infrequent bathing by soldiers, especially in the winter, when facilities were limited—

contributed to the problems. It is no surprise that disease produced more casualties than wounds and trauma resulting from sporadic fighting with hostile Indians, accidents with horses and wagons, or even soldiers' frequent use of knives and firearms to settle disputes among themselves.

When the United States went to war with Mexico in the spring of 1846, the medical department of the Army consisted of the surgeon general, twenty surgeons, and fifty assistant surgeons. Two more surgeons and a dozen assistants were added during the course of the war, which involved more than 100,000 American soldiers. About 1,500 died in combat, but more than 10,000 died from disease. There were not enough doctors: At most there were a hundred American doctors in Mexico at any given time, and many of them were inexperienced volunteer and contract surgeons. Because the medical service was short-handed, at times the patients ran the hospitals. Dysentery and other digestive ills took their toll, but doctors were able to stop outbreaks of smallpox with vaccinations before they became epidemic, and malaria was treated with some measure of success by large doses of quinine. One doctor, William Roberts, an assistant surgeon, became an unsung hero during the Mexican War. He treated a wounded company commander under fire at Molino del Rey, and then voluntarily took charge of the unit until he himself was killed. His body was returned to the United States, and he was the first person buried in the now famous Bonaventure Cemetery in Savannah, Georgia.

One American Army unit in the Mexican War was the Mormon Battalion, made up of five hundred volunteers. While it never engaged in battle, it did make the longest sustained march in U.S. history, from the Missouri River to California. Dr. George B. Sanderson of Platte, Missouri, who was not a Mormon, was assigned as the unit's assistant surgeon. He earned the sobriquet "Dr. Death" from his reluctant patients, who thought him a tyrannical quack and distrusted his medicines. Those medicines consisted primarily of calomel powder and arsenic, plus bitters made of bayberry bark and chamomile flowers. Brigham Young, president of the Mormon church, had warned the soldiers, saying, "If you are sick, live by faith, and leave the surgeon's medicine alone if you want to live, using only such herbs and mild food as are at your disposal. If you give heed to this counsel, you will prosper; but if not, we cannot be responsible for the consequences. A hint to the wise is sufficient."[7]

By the time the Mexican War began, the War Department was establishing forts along the Oregon Trail to protect travelers. Each post had an army surgeon. Immigrants found the forts oases of relief and comfort if they were ill, injured, or needed medicines. The demands upon the physicians at the posts increased dramatically after the California gold rush began in 1849 and continued into the early 1850s. Fort Kearny, located about forty miles southwest of modern Grand Island, Nebraska, boasted a four-room frame hospital that was finished in the fall of 1849. Farther west on the Oregon Trail at Fort Laramie, in modern-day southeast Wyoming, the hospital was housed in an old adobe fort, but as the number of sick increased, tents were set up nearby to accommodate the overflow in patients, both military and civilian. Dr. S. P. Moore, assistant surgeon at Fort Laramie during 1849 and 1850, later reported, "I presume I saw and prescribed for every sick emigrant passing the fort, and many were necessarily left under my charge." In 1850 four immigrants left with Dr. Moore for treatment of cholera died.[8]

Because the War Department in 1849 sold pistols, rifles, and ammunition at cost to immigrants going to California and Oregon, many became victims of gunshot accidents and ended up in post hospitals. In June 1849, there were several victims of accidental shootings in the hospital at Fort Kearny being cared for by a Dr. Hammond, the post surgeon. Hammond also amputated the arm of a man bitten by a rattlesnake. In 1852, the hospitals at forts Kearny and Laramie filled with sick immigrants, many suffering from cholera. At Kearny, there were so many ailing immigrants that many had to be housed in soldiers' living quarters. One account relates how a sick immigrant was turned away from the post and left nearby in a tent with fifteen days' supply of food. The post surgeon apparently visited him regularly. At The Dalles, near the western end of the Oregon Trail, the Army established Fort Dalles in 1850 to protect travelers following the Whitman massacre. Fort Dalles was the only military post between Fort Laramie and the Pacific coast. Its doctor treated his share of sick and injured immigrants, although the post hospital was described as miserable.[9]

One future military physician who followed the Oregon Trail west about 1849 and then took a cutoff to California was Alexander T. Augusta, a black man born free in 1825 at Norfolk, Virginia. He was secretly taught to read as a boy and was educated by an Episcopal bishop at a time when it was against the law to teach black people. By the early 1840s, he was studying medicine with private tutors while working as a barber. Augusta went to California during the gold rush in hopes of making enough money to attend medical school. He apparently did and returned East, only to be denied admittance to the University of Pennsylvania medical school in Philadelphia. He then went to Canada, where he was admitted to Trinity Medical College at the University of Toronto. There he earned his medical degree and became director of the university's hospital. Late in 1862, after the Civil War began, he returned to the United States. He sent a letter to President Abraham Lincoln requesting appointment as a surgeon or physician for one of the black regiments formed by the Union Army. Commissioned a major, Dr. Augusta holds the distinction of being the first black surgeon in the Union Army. Following the Civil War he was brevetted a lieutenant colonel for meritorious and faithful service. Dr. Augusta moved to Washington, D.C., where he practiced medicine and served on the faculty of Howard University's department of medicine. He died in 1890 at the age of sixty-five and is buried in Arlington National Cemetery.

During the 1850s, scurvy remained a serious problem at many western posts. At Fort Laramie, Dr. Edward W. Johns, assistant surgeon, used watercress to supplement the hospital diet as long as he had a supply. He also administered cactus juice to soldiers to treat scurvy, but most troops would take it only if it was mixed with whiskey. In the Dakotas during the 1850s, a soldier named Augustus Myer, who later wrote *Ten Years in the Ranks, U.S. Army* (1866), recalled that he and other soldiers suffered from scurvy until they imitated the Indians and dug up roots to eat. Army doctors meantime learned that wild onions, berries, and raw potatoes could cure or prevent scurvy.

During the fifties, soldiers in the Southwest saw much military action against Apaches and Navahos. One military physician of note was Lieutenant Bernard John Dowling Irwin, a native of Ireland. He treated soldiers wounded by Cochise's band at Fort Buchanan under miserable conditions. At one point Irwin traveled to a stage station where a man had lain for almost a week after an ax blow nearly severed his left arm. The wound was maggot-infested when Dr. Irwin arrived. He immediately amputated the arm while his patient lay on an operating table consisting of sacks of grain. The patient recovered. Just before the start of the Civil War, Dr. Irwin volunteered to lead a rescue party after word reached Fort Buchanan that Cochise and his band of

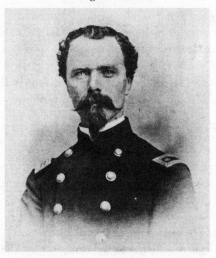

*Bernard John Dowling Irwin, M.D. (1830–
1917). For his actions as a surgeon in battles with
Apaches in the Southwest during the 1850s, Irwin
became the first recipient of the Congressional
Medal of Honor. (Courtesy National Archives)*

Chiricahua Apaches had besieged a detachment of five or six men of
the Seventh Infantry commanded by Second Lieutenant George N.
Bascom. Dr. Irwin and fourteen men set out in a heavy snowstorm on
a forced two-day march. Not having horses, they rode mules. Their
sudden appearance drove the Indians away, and Dr. Irwin treated the
wounded soldiers. Later he joined in an attack on the Apache camp
and supposedly suggested the execution of six Indian prisoners in
retaliation for the six soldiers killed. President Abraham Lincoln proposed the creation of the Medal of Honor on July 12, 1862, and Irwin's
heroic act was the first for which the coveted badge of valor would be
awarded, but it was not presented to Irwin until 1894.

When the Civil War began in 1861, the U.S. Army medical department was unprepared. Surgeon General Dr. Thomas Lawson, who
had served in that position for twenty-five years, had slashed the medical service's budget during the 1850s and had done little planning for
the war so widely anticipated. The seventy-two-year-old Lawson,
however, died soon after the war began, and Dr. Clement A. Finley was

appointed surgeon general. The medical service had shrunk because eight of its thirty surgeons and twenty-nine of its eighty-three assistant surgeons left because they supported the South. One of them, Dr. Samuel Moore, became Confederate surgeon general and organized the southern army's medical service along the lines of the Union's service. During the war's early months, there were not enough doctors and medical personnel to treat and evacuate the wounded and to set up hospitals as Confederate troops defeated Union troops. Meantime, patriotism attracted many prominent civilian physicians to the Union medical service, and their enrollment in turn attracted many young doctors just out of medical school. The younger doctors also realized that the practical training they would receive in the medical service would be far more comprehensive and valuable than anything they might experience in private practice.

During a battle at Winchester, Virginia, in May 1862, Major General Thomas J. "Stonewall" Jackson's forces captured the Union's hospitals there, but Jackson took the position that the surgeons staffing them did not make war and should not suffer its penalties. This was the first time the neutral status of doctors was recognized. Jackson unconditionally returned the doctors to their own lines. Subsequently Union general George McClellan and Confederate general-in-chief Robert E. Lee formally agreed on this neutral status for doctors, although the agreement was briefly suspended later in the war. The principle met with popular support in both the North and the South, and the practice spread to Europe and later was made official under the Geneva Conventions.

By 1862, the Union medical service had improved its chain of evacuation from battlefield to hospital after line officers began to understand the problems facing the doctors and the fact that speedy evacuation and efficient care of the wounded were essential. Success in these respects, however, depended upon the tide of battle. Another problem developed when a northern or southern state assembled the necessary number of volunteers to form a regiment. In the North, Congress then authorized the governor of that state to appoint a regimental surgeon and an assistant surgeon, often someone fresh out of medical school. These doctors were required to pass a medical competency review by a medical examining board, but in too many cases the senior regimental officer made the selection, which often had little to do with their medical competency. Their abilities, or lack thereof, became evident once the regiment went into battle. When the troops took their positions on a battlefield, the established procedures called for the assistant surgeon, his hospital steward, and several helpers to find a sheltered spot a few hundred yards behind the front line to serve as the regimental emergency and ambulance depot.

A red flag marked the depot and guided the wounded to the spot. Once the battle began, wounded soldiers who could walk would go to the depot while the more severely injured would be carried there on stretchers by the helpers. The assistant surgeon would control any hemorrhages, put splints on fractures, give pain medicines, and provide other forms of first aid. The seriously wounded would be transported by ambulance to a makeshift regimental hospital farther behind the front lines, where a surgeon would remove bullets, amputate, and stitch lacerations, among other surgical tasks. The success of following

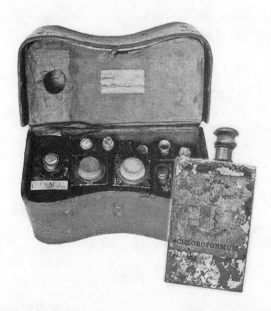

Collidge's Field Surgeon's Kit (1863). Designed by U.S. Medical Inspector R. H. Collidge, the kit was created for field surgeons to use during the Civil War. The leather case includes tins for chloroform, opium, quinine, sugar, and tea. When new, the kit would also hold bandages, needles, and whiskey. In the kit shown, the whiskey has been replaced by Hamlin's Cholera Mixture containing laudanum. (Courtesy Wood Library Museum)

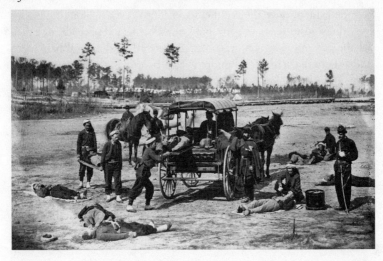

A unit of the Union Army's ambulance corps, shown in a training exercise during the Civil War. (Courtesy Library of Congress)

these guidelines, however, depended upon the regimental surgeon's skills and organizational ability. Too many regimental doctors were surgeons in name only. Back home in their private practices many had had few opportunities to practice surgery. Often the assistant surgeons, fresh out of medical school, used their position as a patriotic way to become experts in surgery.[10]

One assistant surgeon, S. H. Melcher, of the Fifth Missouri Volunteers, was present at the first major battle in the western theater of war among the rolling hills and densely covered gullies near Wilson's Creek, south of Springfield, Missouri, on August 10, 1861. He provides a firsthand description of battlefield medicine:

> The wounded were sent to the rear in wagons as the fight progressed. The attendance they received was trifling, consisting of water dressings or adhesive plasters. . . . The flies were exceedingly troublesome after the battle, maggots forming in the wounds in less than an hour after dressing them, and also upon any clothing or bedding soiled by blood or pus. The wounded left on the field in the enemy's hands were swarming with maggots when brought in. After several ineffectual attempts to extirpate these pests, I succeeded perfectly by sprin-

kling calomel freely over the wounded surface. When the sloughs separated, clean granulating surfaces were presented, and by using balsam [of copaiba] as a dressing, smearing the bandages with this oleoresin [a mixture of an oil and a resin extracted from various plants], I could keep the wounds free from maggots.[11]

Military doctors from both North and South left countless accounts of how they treated wounded soldiers. The repair of wounds was always a slow, painful, and exhausting process. Doctors did not even imagine healing wounds without inflammation. There were no antiseptics. The cleanliness of wounds was considered of little or no importance except when there was a great deal of foreign matter. Even the dressings carried into action were few and scanty. A wounded man covered his wounds as best he could, often with a soiled handkerchief or piece of cloth torn from a sweaty, dirty shirt. When the wounded man reached a surgeon, the wound was often packed with astringent, coagulant, and generally harmful chemicals. Medicines were carried in either pill or liquid form. Soluble tablets were unknown. Doctors car-

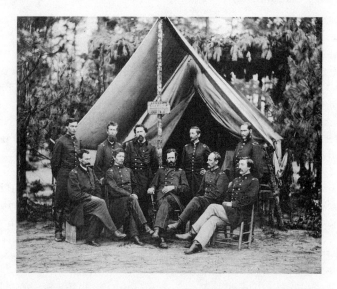

Union surgeons of the Third Division pose before a hospital tent in the vicinity of Petersburg, Virginia, during the Civil War. (Courtesy Library of Congress)

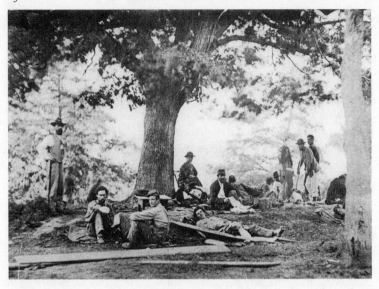

Wounded Union soldiers being treated in the field after the Battle of Chancellorsville near Fredericksburg, Virginia, in May 1863, where Union forces were defeated by Confederate troops. (Courtesy Library of Congress)

ried drugs like opium in their natural form, instead of in a concentrated form like morphine. Some doctors carried chloroform, but surgical anesthesia was so new to medicine it was scarce. Hundreds if not thousands of major operations, including untold numbers of amputations of arms and legs, were performed with no anesthetic. In many cases, patients received only whiskey for pain relief while being operated on.

Union doctors had a better supply of medicine than did their Confederate counterparts. After the Union naval blockade began working in 1862, the South found it difficult to obtain manufactured medicines. The Confederacy turned to natural remedies and published a pamphlet listing herbs and plants that could be used to treat patients. The list includes snakeroot, sassafras, partridgeberry, lavender, dogwood, tulip trees, and the leaves and bark of white oak trees.

As during the American Revolution, in the Civil War more soldiers on both sides died from disease than from combat. Of at least 618,000 soldiers from the North and South who died, about 414,000 succumbed to disease. As also in the Revolution, large numbers of soldiers on both sides came from rural areas where they had never been exposed to common diseases such as chicken pox, mumps, and measles. In the Union Army alone, more than 5,000 soldiers died of measles during the war. The main killer, however, was unsanitary living conditions that promoted the spread of typhoid, dysentery, smallpox, malaria, and diarrhea. Interestingly, regular Army soldiers who had been trained to be careful about their food and water were far less likely to suffer from intestinal disease than volunteers. Often following battles, large numbers of soldiers suffered from muteness, deafness, and loss of mobility in their arms and legs. Most doctors diagnosed them as suffering from mania or dementia and sent them home to recover. In truth, these men were suffering from what later generations would call combat fatigue or shell shock, a condition not then identified.

Neither regular nor volunteer medical officers were immune to disease and death. Among northern doctors, 32 died in battle or at the hands of guerrillas, 9 died in accidents, 83 were wounded in action (10 of whom died), 7 died of yellow fever, 4 died in Confederate prisons, 3 of cholera, and 271 of other diseases.

When the Civil War ended, the doctors with the northern and southern armies were probably the best surgeons in the United States because of their experience. The field of medicine, however, was still evolving. The war did see improvements in the organizational management of the Union medical department. At the war's end it had become the model for other armies around the world, and its organizing methods are still the American standard in time of emergencies and war.

During the Civil War, physicians in the medical service realized that disease could be reduced by improved sanitation. Scurvy was reduced by providing soldiers a diet rich in fresh fruit and vegetables, and quinine was used effectively to treat malarial fevers. Surgeons, however, were frequently frustrated because civilian communities located near military posts paid little attention to their water supplies, disposal of human waste, and garbage until an epidemic occurred. Both military and civilian doctors were helpless during the years just after the Civil War in their primitive attempt to prevent disease. One physician observed, "The treatment of disease is the weak spot in our profession." Another doctor noted that "the history of medical pro-

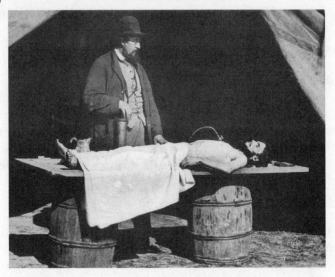

An embalming surgeon prepares an unidentified soldier's body for burial during the Civil War. (Courtesy Library of Congress)

gress [is still] a history of men groping in the darkness." Charles W. Eliot, the president of Harvard, complained about "the ignorance and incompetence of most American doctors who have graduated at American Schools. They poison, maim, and do men to death in various ways, and are unable to save life or preserve health."[12] Most physicians, military and civilian, did not abandon the heroic practice of medicine whereby they purged and bled patients regardless of their conditions or specific disease. The extensive use of opiates prescribed by military doctors during the Civil War continued among many veterans afflicted with chronic dysentery and extended to others who believed they would relieve whatever ailed them. By the late 1860s the popularity of medicinal alcohol taken internally continued, as did the use of aspirin and similar drugs to reduce fever. Such drugs cost less and had fewer side effects.

THE SURGEON GENERAL in Washington, D.C., experienced numerous administrative problems following the Civil War, but they did not significantly affect the work of military doctors at widely scattered posts in the West. The doctors still endured long hours of physical labor under miserable conditions treating soldiers ravaged by disease. Corruption and wrangling between government and private contractors did not guarantee the prompt and reliable delivery of proper foodstuffs needed to preserve the soldiers' health. Most military doctors accepted the need for good sanitation because the surgeon general stressed that need, although many still did not understand the relationship between poor sanitation and disease. After 1885, sanitation was important enough that the post surgeons had to send regular reports to the surgeon general detailing conditions at their posts. The surgeons also encouraged new vaccinations, whereas immunization was often discouraged in the civilian population. The military blamed an outbreak of smallpox among black soldiers in 1866 on what they believed was bad vaccine. Soldiers received new vaccinations.

In 1866, after the close of the Civil War, Congress reorganized the nation's peacetime regular Army. Many of the 186,000 black soldiers who had fought for the Union looked with favor on military service, since it offered shelter, education, steady pay, medical attention, and a pension. Congress authorized two segregated regiments of black cavalry and six infantry regiments commanded by white officers. Congressmen and senators realized that southerners and people in the East did not want to see armed black soldiers in or near their communities, and the lawmakers made certain they were sent west to fight Indians.

Another interesting story concerns a black soldier who enlisted in February 1867 at St. Louis and gave the name William Cathey, occupation cook, age twenty-two. An army surgeon examined Cathey and declared the recruit, who was five feet nine inches tall with black eyes, hair, and complexion, fit for duty. Cathey was assigned to the Thirty-eighth U.S. Infantry Regiment at Jefferson Barracks just outside of St. Louis, and was soon mustered into the regiment's Company A with seventy-five other black recruits. About two months later, Cathey's company marched first to Fort Riley and then to Fort Harker, both in Kansas. By July, they were marched to Fort Union, New Mexico Territory. In September the company marched to Fort Cummings, New Mexico Territory, where it remained for eight months. Although Private Cathey had been treated for illness in at least three Army hospitals and had withstood the marches, he was admitted to the post hospital at Fort Cummings in January 1868 complaining of rheumatism. He was soon returned to duty and marched with the company to Fort Bayard in modern-day Grant County, New Mexico. Again Private Cathey was admitted to the post hospital and remained one month. On October 14, 1868, William Cathey was honorably discharged from the Army at Fort Bayard. The surgeon's certificate said it was for disability. The surgeon was apparently unaware that the soldier was a woman, her true name being Cathey Williams. She was born into slavery to a wealthy farmer in 1842 near Independence, Missouri. If her secret had been discovered at any time during the twenty months she spent in the military, she would have been instantly discharged. She apparently had never fully undressed during her hospital stays or doctors' examination, which raises a general question about the thoroughness of Army medical exams during this period.

From the American Revolution through much of the nineteenth century, dental care was something that soldiers usually had to seek out their own from civilian dentists or itinerant tooth-pullers. True, many Army physicians and hospital stewards did have rudimentary training in dentistry so they could treat soldiers' teeth when time permitted. Although the first dental school was established at Baltimore College in 1840, strengthening the argument that the military should recognize dentistry as a medical field, the Army ignored dentistry. Yet during the Civil War, recruits were turned away if they did not have six opposing upper and lower front teeth with which to bite off the end of the powder cartridges used with muzzle-loaded weapons. It was not until 1872 that William Saunders, a hospital steward at the U.S. Military Academy at West Point, where he provided dental service for cadets and staff, became the first soldier to be recognized as a U.S. military dentist. Not until early in the twentieth century did Congress formally establish the U.S. Army Dental Corps.

UNLIKE THE CIVIL WAR, which had been fought in a conventional manner using the rules of the white man, the Indian wars of the nineteenth century were unorthodox. Only occasionally were soldiers involved in actual fighting with the mobile Indians. For the post doctor, the principal work was often caring for the sick rather than patching wounds. At some posts, there was little demand of any kind on physicians and many spent the major part of their time hunting and fishing. While proud of their medical training, many also loved the outdoors and the camaraderie of the frontier posts. One Army surgeon, David Powell, who had worked in an Omaha, Nebraska, drugstore before going to medical school, would later become friends with William F. "Buffalo Bill" Cody. The gregarious and flamboyant Powell was stationed at Fort McPherson in western Nebraska. He enjoyed saloons and drinking, and after his military service ended he practiced medicine in Wisconsin.

Another Army doctor, R. H. McKay, was mustered into service as an acting assistant surgeon early in 1869 at St. Louis and ordered to Fort Leavenworth, Kansas, for duty. Dr. McKay later wrote:

> I was on waiting orders at Fort Leavenworth for something over a month, during which time I got my first impression of the rank and file of the Regular Army. The officers impressed me as very self important, exceedingly courteous and cordial, and charming in their broad-gauge views of current events and their unreserved candor in discussing all subjects. I must except one subject, however, and that was politics. An army officer is supposed to have no politics, or if he has he keeps them in reserve. . . . While at Leavenworth, the officers gave a hop. I never knew why it was called a hop instead of a dance, but it was always so designated in the army. Officers came from other places, particularly Fort Riley, among whom was General Custer of cavalry fame during the Civil War, and a noted Indian fighter on the frontier. I watched him with a good deal of interest, for at that time he was a distinguished man in the service, and I must say that I was rather disappointed in his appearance. He seemed to me to be undersized and slender, and at first blush to be effeminate in appearance. Maybe his long hair, almost reaching to his shoulders, gave this impression, but the face was something of a study and hard to describe. . . . He was a very graceful dancer.[13]

Dr. McKay went on to serve nearly seven years as a physician at posts in New Mexico, Indian Territory, and elsewhere. Except at Fort Sill in what is now Oklahoma, McKay served at no post with more than two companies of soldiers. When assigned to a temporary military camp in Colorado, he spent a great deal of time hunting and fishing because he had only two patients in his tent hospital, one a civilian blinded in a premature mine detonation, and the other his own dog, a pointer, accidentally shot on a hunting trip. Dr. McKay was never assigned to a major expedition against the Indians.

Not all Army doctors had assignments like McKay's. Others had to care for soldiers in unsettled and often rugged country where conditions created new problems for surgeons who were far distant from a post hospital and without adequate medical supplies to treat the wounded. The rough terrain they often encountered prohibited the use of wheeled vehicles to evacuate the sick and wounded. Sometimes horses were used, but for a seriously wounded soldier the surgeons used a horse or mule litter requiring two animals and four soldiers. One man led each animal; two more walked beside the litter to keep it from swaying. Another mode of evacuation was an Indian-style travois, a litter-like device, fastened to a horse or mule and dragged upon the ground. Two men guided it; one led and another steadied the patient and carried the free end over streams or rough terrain. During the Modoc War in southern Oregon and northern California during 1872–73, the lava beds were so difficult to traverse that a surgeon devised a litter similar to a reclining chair that was borne on the back of a single mule.

When soldiers were wounded in Indian fights, most military doctors could perform surgery under primitive conditions if they had Civil War experience. For most, however, arrow wounds were new, and removing an arrow without leaving its head in the patient's body required much skill. Once an arrow struck a human, body fluids tended to soften the animal tendons that the Indians used to fasten the arrowhead to the shaft. This made the arrowhead difficult to remove, and many surgeons did leave it embedded in the wound. While serving in the West just before the Civil War, an assistant surgeon, Lieutenant Joseph H. Bill, familiarized himself with the designs used by many different tribes. He learned that most Indians placed the head either parallel to the slit in the shaft that accommodated the bowstring or at right angles to it. Dr. Bill published an article in 1862 noting that it was therefore easy to determine how the head lay in a wounded soldier. He then explained, once that was done, how to insert a looped wire along the shaft to snare the arrowhead and then remove it and the shaft at the same time. If an arrowhead embedded itself in a man's skull, Bill instructed that it could be used to raise any piece of bone that the arrowhead had depressed in removing it from the skull. Other surgeons expanded on Bill's work after the war, and their observations were published by the surgeon general in 1873.[14]

Many military physicians, like their counterparts in the civilian world, sought every opportunity to advance their knowledge of the human body. There are accounts claiming that some Army surgeons used the corpses of Indians to further their anatomical studies. Colonel Virgil Ney, a military historian, relates in *Fort on the Prairie* (1978) how in 1821 at Fort Atkinson, in what is now eastern Nebraska, Private John Shepherd was hanged for the murder of a Sergeant Siemens. Shepherd's body was given to the surgeon at the post for dissection. Since the Civil War, Army surgeons had been directed to collect samples showing different types of wounds and diseases for the Smithsonian Institution and the Army Medical Museum that opened in Washington, D.C., in 1887.

There is not enough space here to relate the countless stories about surgeons in the Indian wars, but a few examples will demonstrate the kind of lives they led. During a raid on an Arapaho village in July 1874, a contract surgeon named Thomas McGee was applying a dressing to a wounded soldier when he saw an Indian about to shoot a nearby soldier. McGee grabbed his patient's gun, shot the Indian, and calmly returned to his bandages. Another contract surgeon was Dr. Leonard Wood, a recent Harvard Medical School graduate. His infantry unit, assigned to the Southwest, began chasing Geronimo and his Apaches. Assistant Surgeon Wood volunteered for field duty, and in the spring of 1886 carried dispatches through a region filled with hostile Indians. He made a journey of seventy miles in one night and walked thirty miles the following day. Also for several weeks, he rode in close pursuit of Geronimo's band, constantly expecting an encounter. When the commander of the detachment of infantry was lost, Dr. Wood requested and received command. For his action, Dr. Wood was awarded the Congressional Medal of Honor in 1898. Wood went on to command the Rough Riders during the Spanish-American War and later served as governor of Cuba. Major General Wood served as Chief of Staff of the U.S. Army from 1910 to 1914.

Dr. Wood was only one of several surgeons and medical personnel awarded the Congressional Medal of Honor. The story of Dr. Bernard J. D. Irwin has already been related, but there are others. On Jan-

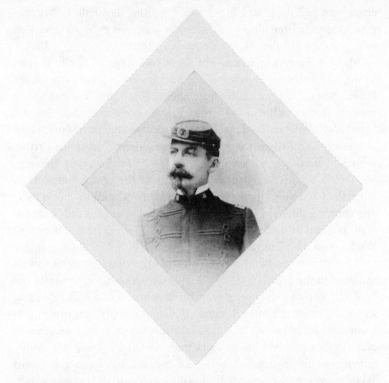

John O. Skinner was a contract surgeon with the U.S. Army in Oregon in 1873. He rescued a wounded soldier during an assault on a Modoc Indian stronghold, and later received the Congressional Medal of Honor for his action. (Courtesy National Archives)

uary 17, 1873, John O. Skinner, a contract surgeon, rescued a wounded soldier who lay under close and heavy fire during an Army assault on a Modoc Indian stronghold in Oregon. Two soldiers had attempted to rescue the man, but both were wounded. Three years later, William C. Bryan, a hospital steward, accompanied a detachment of cavalry in a charge on a village of hostile Indians on the Powder River in Wyoming. Bryan, a native of Ohio, fought through the engagement and had his horse killed under him. He continued to fight on foot. Under severe fire and without any assistance, he took two wounded soldiers to places of safety. The following year, 1877, Dr. Henry R. Tilton, a major and surgeon, risked his life rescuing and protecting several wounded men in a battle with Indians at Bear Paw Mountain in Montana. The last

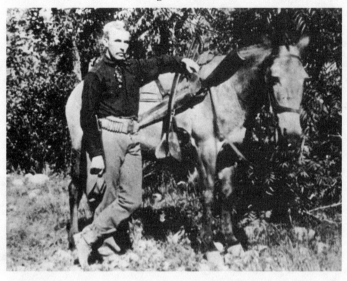

Leonard Wood, M.D. (1860–1927), a native of New Hampshire, was educated at Harvard Medical School. He was appointed an assistant army surgeon in the Southwest, and pursued Geronimo and other Apaches in the 1880s. When his commander was lost, Wood was given command. (For his actions, Wood would be awarded the Congressional Medal of Honor in 1898.) Later he served as a physician to presidents Grover Cleveland and William McKinley and commanded "The Rough Riders" in Cuba during the Spanish-American War. (Courtesy National Library of Medicine)

Congressional Medal of Honor awarded during the Indian wars went to Oscar Burkard, a private in the hospital corps. He showed distinguished bravery during an uprising of Chippewa Indians on Lake Leech in northern Minnesota in October 1898.

A military doctor who received honors of a different sort was Walter Reed, a surgeon. In 1876, he was stationed at Fort Lowell, located where Tucson, Arizona, stands today. A Private Kelly suffered constantly from diarrhea and spent much time in the post hospital. Dr. Reed tried every medicine in his dispensary without success. One day, he noticed that the castile soap he placed in the hospital washroom kept disappearing. Since Private Kelly frequented the washroom more than any other patient, the doctor confronted him and the soldier admitted he had been eating the soap to keep his diarrhea flourishing to avoid work. He was soon returned to duty.[15]

It was also at Fort Lowell that Dr. Reed theorized that the sharp

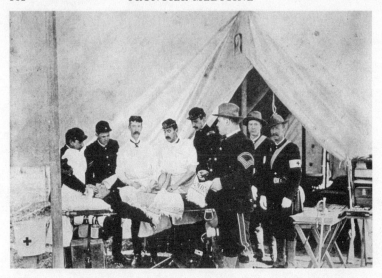

U.S. Army surgeons treating a soldier in a hospital tent during the Spanish-American War. (Courtesy National Library of Medicine)

differences in temperature between day and night caused malaria. He accordingly advised the post commander to delay reveille until after sunrise to lower the malaria exposure of the men. The soldiers were delighted, but continued to contract malaria. Eventually, however, Reed would score a signal success in medical research: In 1900, he led the team which proved the theory first set forth in 1881 by Carlos Finlay, a Cuban doctor, that yellow fever is transmitted by mosquitoes rather than by direct contact with other humans.

CHAPTER EIGHT

ON HOMESTEAD AND RANCH

*Healing is a matter of time, but it is sometimes
also a matter of opportunity.*

—Hippocrates

AFTER LEWIS AND CLARK returned east in 1806 and related stories
about the rugged country they had crossed on their journey to the
Pacific, President Thomas Jefferson concluded that it would take
Americans "a hundred generations" to settle the vast region west of the
Mississippi River. Jefferson apparently did not grasp the pull that the
West would exert on the American spirit. Although much of the plains
and prairies between the Missouri River and the Rocky Mountains was
declared Indian Territory in the 1830s and was bypassed by immigrants
going to Oregon and California, the sheer vastness of the nation's
lands strengthened the belief that the public domain rightfully
belonged to the people. Distributing public land became difficult
because small farmers had to compete with larger and more wealthy
concerns. Missouri senator Thomas Hart Benton championed the
Pre-emption Act of 1841 giving farmers the right to squat on plots of
public land not yet surveyed, with the option then of later buying the
land from the government. Tennessee congressman Andrew Johnson,
however, believed working people had a right to land free of charge,
and made this his cause. Southerners opposed the idea because they
feared working-class whites would not support slavery in new states.
Once the Civil War began and the southern states left the Union,
Congress passed and President Abraham Lincoln signed the Homestead Act in the spring of 1862. It became law in 1863.

The Homestead Act declared that any person could file for 160
acres of federal land if he or she was an American citizen, or had filed
papers of intention to become a citizen. The person filing had to be

twenty-one years old or the head of a family, or have served fourteen days in the U.S. Army or Navy and never have fought against the United States. This excluded some Mexicans, Canadians, and Britons, and many residents of the South; but Congress altered the law in 1866 to make Confederate veterans eligible for homesteads. After paying a nominal filing fee, the person could secure a fee simple title to the land by residing on or farming the claim for five successive years, and provided, if originally a foreigner, he or she had since become a citizen of the United States. If a homesteader did not wish to wait five years, a commutation clause in the filing papers allowed for the purchase of the land at $1.25 an acre after six months' residence and rudimentary improvements. The Homestead Act opened 270 million acres, or about 10 percent of the continental United States, to settlement by private citizens.

People in eastern portions of Kansas and Nebraska Territory filed for homesteads as soon as the act became law in 1863, but the real surge did not begin until after the Civil War, extending into the 1870s. In the timbered areas west of the Missouri River, many homesteaders built log cabins and many prospered, but farther west, beyond the 100th meridian on the arid plains, there were few trees. Homesteaders turned to constructing dugouts or sod houses made by cutting blocks of sod from the ground. At first, they used spades to cut one brick at a time. Later, in the mid-1880s, a new plow, called a "grasshopper" or "breaking" plow, was invented that cut sod into strips twelve inches wide and four inches thick. The strips were cut into three-foot lengths with a spade or corn knife. The sod bricks were then stacked lengthwise, and the home constructed. The walls were usually two feet thick.

Sod houses were cool in the summer and warm in the winter; however, the dirt floors left much to be desired. Disease germs were everywhere. You could not scrub a dirt floor, and sweeping it only raised dust, which contaminated the air and everything inside the homestead. Wooden door and window frames let in some sunshine, but the sod invited vermin such as fleas, lice, and other insects, and occasional snakes attracted by the presence of mice.

When homesteaders could not claim land near rivers, streams, or springs, they had to dig water wells. Such water was usually drinkable to begin with, but since a well was usually dug close to the house and outbuildings, in time human and animal waste would contaminate the water. Some homesteaders built cisterns or used barrels to collect rainwater. During hot weather, however, a barrel of rainwater usually became infested by mosquitoes, flies, and other bugs, and acquired a fine layer of wind-blown dust. Such things had to be skimmed from the surface before the water was used. In the winter, melted snow supplemented the family water supply. On many homesteads, the scarcity of water might compel six or more family members to take turns bathing, usually not more than once a week, in a single tub of water. The bathwater was often saved and used for washing workclothes or cleaning. To save water, food dishes and cups were usually not washed or rinsed. When the homesteader's wife told her children to clean their plates, she meant it literally.

For many homesteaders, the simple and seemingly lenient requirements for obtaining their land claim free and clear were too much. Many people with little or no farming experience took claims. But even experienced farmers found it difficult to grow crops on the arid plains west of the 100th meridian, and a farm of 160 acres was in any case too small to produce profitable crops even in wet years. Of more than two million individuals who filed claims, less than half "proved up" on their claims and obtained deeds to their homesteads. Their sod houses withstood hailstorms, blizzards, prairie fires, and relentless wind, but often their crops suffered, especially between 1874 and 1877, when swarms of locusts consumed just about everything in sight as they darkened the skies. With accumulated debt and a lack of cash, poor crops, and little to show for their efforts, many farmers simply pulled up stakes and left.

Even before the Homestead Act became law, significant numbers of people settled in the new territories of Kansas and Nebraska. A few of the settlers were physicians. Most of them were not well educated in medicine and had no medical degree. Most became doctors by studying books and apprenticing to older physicians. One pioneer who arrived in Kansas Territory in 1854, James R. Stewart, a young bachelor from New Castle, Pennsylvania, settled in what is now Burlingame in Osage County in eastern Kansas. On May 31, 1858, Stewart made a bargain with Dr. E. P. Sheldon to become an apprentice to him to learn medicine. Stewart kept a diary, and the following selected entries suggest what his apprenticeship was like:

Thursday, June 24 Warm through the day, heavy rain after
night.

Read [on medicine] . . . went to the woods
with Dr. Sheldon and got good mess
mulberries.

Sunday, Sept. 5   High wind. Read CYClopedia of practical
medicine [*The Cyclopedia of Practical
Medicine*, published 1845].

Saturday, Sept. 11   Fine with good breeze. Read Meigs all day
[*Obstetrics: The Science and the Art* by
Charles D. Meigs, 1849].

Monday, Sept. 13   Fine & pleasant. Read Meigs all day. Played
Euacher in the evening.

Sunday, Sept. 19   Very fine. Read—went to the woods in the
evening and got lot of Paw paws.

Monday, Sept. 20   Fine all day. Read Bedford all day
[Gunning S. Bedford's *A Practical Treatise
on Midwifery*, 1847].

Tuesday, Sept. 21   Fine all day. Read all day.

Monday, Sept. 27   Fine day—Read Druitt on Surgery [Robert
Druitt's *The Principles and Practice of Modern
Surgery*, 1842].

Saturday, Oct. 9   Pleasant but windy. Mixed up medicine &
made pills—

Monday, Oct. 11   Cloudy in forenoon. Clear and pleasant in
afternoon.
Made pills and prepared for a trip down
Neosho [River].

Sunday, Oct. 31   Rained hard last night. Rainy all day—very
high water.
Higher than ever known here. Read
medicine up in Dr. Sheldon's new office.

Monday, Nov. 1   Cloudy and rainy—muddy. Read Neil &
Smith [authors of a series of handbooks on
chemistry, physiology, and the practice of
medicine].

Saturday, Nov. 27   More moderate. Read Draper's Physiology
[John W. Draper's *Human Physiology*, 1856].

Wednesday, Dec. 1   Little rain—windy. Finished reading
Physiology and commence Materia
Medica.

James Stewart continued to read medicine and work as an apprentice to Dr. Sheldon until August 25, 1859. That day he wrote in his diary, "Took a notion this morning to turn my attention to the Study of Law." He provides no explanation but has apparently decided that medicine is not for him. In all probability, many other young men who apprenticed with a physician also changed their minds, for any of a variety of reasons.[1]

The hardships of homesteading contributed to poor health. Scurvy was a common problem, often caused by a diet of salt pork, dried food, cornbread, and other foods lacking in vitamins and minerals. What they ate also gave some homesteaders what they called "bilious fever," better known today as gastritis; but in the nineteenth century it was sometimes called "remittent fever," especially during the summer and autumn, and the term was loosely applied to certain intestinal and malarial fevers. The illnesses found to the east in the Mississippi Valley, such as typhoid fever, diphtheria, cholera, smallpox, and malaria were not unknown, and occasional epidemics took the lives of many homesteaders. Some believed malaria was caused by poison gases omitted from the ground as they plowed the rich soil. Others blamed the heavy dew that covered the ground during certain times of the year. Some mothers would not let their children play outside until the morning dew had dried for fear they would become ill.

When homesteading began early in 1863, it attracted some physicians who liked the idea of free land. They claimed homesteads in Kansas and Nebraska, but many eventually gave up and moved away, or moved to new settlements and opened practices. They learned quickly that practicing medicine in homestead country had many drawbacks. One was the fact that most settlers had little money. As in the East, physicians accepted produce, animals, and merchandise as payment. To survive financially, some doctors had to engage in other moneymaking ventures. Another difficulty was the long distances that a physician had to travel at all hours of the day or night to reach patients. There were the hardships of long hours in the saddle or a buggy without rest or food. If called to visit a patient on a dark night, the doctor might get lost.

John W. Thompson, a doctor in western Nebraska, got so lost one night going to visit a patient that he drove his buggy around aimlessly for several hours searching with his lantern for familiar landmarks. He finally stopped to get his bearings. Suddenly an angry man surrounded by several frightened children challenged him. "Get out of here," the man shouted. "What do you think you're doing! Get off my house." Only then did Dr. Thompson realize he had stopped his team on the roof of a dugout, which happened to be the home of his patient.[2]

Homesteaders often struggled to survive. In 1864, following Indian raids that extended as far east as Jefferson County in Nebraska Territory, the First Nebraska Cavalry was mobilized at Meridian to drive the marauders across the Colorado border. A Dr. Thomas from Alexandria, Nebraska Territory, was regimental surgeon. While the regiment was following the stage road between Meridian and Hebron, the fourteen-year-old son of a homesteader appeared along the trail and pleaded for food, saying he and his folks had not eaten in two days. Dr. Thomas replied that the soldiers were chasing Indians and that it would be a violation of orders to divide the group's rations with anyone. The doctor added, however, "These soldiers are a careless lot and if you follow our trail, perhaps some of them will lose something that may be of help to you." A few yards down the trail, the doctor cut loose from behind his saddle all of the rations he was carrying. A minute or two later he looked back and saw the boy pick the package up and hurriedly start for home.[3]

Following the Civil War, many military doctors returned to civilian life and a great many moved west to practice medicine. Like their civilian counterparts, only a few had medical degrees, but nearly all had gained considerable experience during the war. By the 1870s, many of the more conscientious physicians who had been practicing for ten or twenty years began to enroll in one of the increasing number of medical schools to meet changing requirements in many states to practice medicine. A common school diploma showing the holder had passed at least the eighth grade was the only requirement for entrance to many of these new schools, where most students received medical degrees after a two-year course. Like veteran physicians, the new doctors were expected to preside over difficult births, perform surgery on kitchen tables without proper anesthetics, treat wounds, and remove Indian arrows, a surgical procedure not taught in most medical schools. In the territories, many new doctors started practicing with little or no training, since there were no restrictive laws for years after they opened up.

Nebraska enacted its first law regulating the practice of physicians in 1880, fourteen years after it became a state. The law provided that after June 1, 1881, all practicing physicians should place their names and credentials in *The Physician's Register* kept in the office of each county clerk. All physicians first beginning practice had to be graduates of a reputable medical school; those who had practiced for at least two years before the law took effect were able to continue, even though their training was deficient.[4]

In Kansas Territory, the territorial legislature incorporated the Kansas Medical Society early in 1859, five years after the territory was formed, and gave the society the right to grant licenses to all respectable physicians. But the society was distracted from this task by the outbreak of the Civil War. By the time the war ended, Kansas was a state and physicians were divided into a number of different organizations, each comprising the adherents of one particular medical theory. These different organizations could not agree on uniform

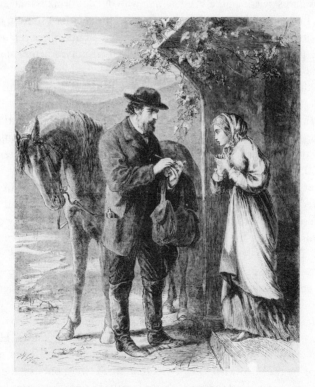

"The Country Doctor," a drawing by A. R. Waud, appeared on the cover of Harper's Weekly, *March 6, 1869.*

procedures until the establishment of a State Board of Health in 1885. Although the measure establishing the Board of Health contained no reference to medical practice, someone discovered a forgotten law, the Medical Practice Act of 1870, which remained on the statute books. It required doctors in practice less than ten years to have a certificate from a medical school or medical society. In 1890 the Kansas Supreme Court upheld the law and the new Board of Health began a vigorous campaign to drive out quack doctors.[5]

The first law concerning physicians in Dakota Territory was passed by the first territorial legislature, and it dealt with the liability of a practitioner. If a physician poisoned a patient or otherwise put a patient's life in danger while intoxicated, the doctor could be found guilty of a misdemeanor. If the patient was killed by the poison, the physician could be found guilty of manslaughter in the second degree. During this period in the West, a man who did not drink was an exception. Because of their often long hours, fatigue, and hardships in treating patients in scattered areas, many physicians drank. Some reportedly had a glass of whiskey to relax and steady their nerves before starting an operation.

Other doctors drank for other reasons. In the case of Dr. Brewster Higley, a native of Ohio, he was driven to the bottle by the loss of his first three wives to illness or injury. When he married a fourth time in Indiana, things did not go well and Dr. Higley again took to drink, left his wife, and headed west. While his fourth marriage was later dissolved so he could take a fifth wife, Dr. Higley ended up in Smith County, Kansas, where he practiced medicine in Gaylord, a small town located on the Solomon River. Soon after, the doctor filed a claim to a homestead on the banks of West Beaver Creek. On July 4, 1872, his friends gathered for a cabin-raising and that day his new home was constructed. In his spare time, Higley played the violin and wrote poetry. Some weeks after his house was completed, he put some words on paper to capture his feelings about his new home. He titled the composition "My Western Home." He placed it in a book and forgot about it until a patient visited him some time later, found the composition, liked it, and encouraged the doctor to put it to music. Higley asked a young musician friend from Rhode Island, Dan Kelley, a carpenter by trade, to write the music. The words were published in two local newspapers and the song played locally. In time, it became highly popular across the nation under the title "Home on the Range." Nei-

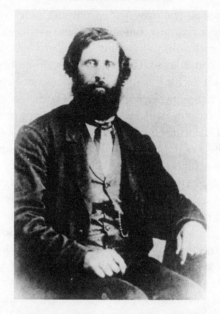

Dr. Brewster Higley, a native of Ohio, who fled the East and his fourth wife and homesteaded in Smith County, Kansas, in 1872. He is best remembered for writing the words to the song "Home on the Range." (Courtesy Kansas State Historical Society)

ther Dr. Higley nor Kelley lived to see its success, however. Kelley moved to Iowa in 1889 and died there at age sixty-two in 1905. Meantime, Dr. Higley found the winters in Kansas too severe and in 1886, his health failing, moved to Arkansas and later to Shawnee in modern Oklahoma, where he died in 1909 at the age of eighty-six. Today Dr. Higley is remembered more for "Home on the Range" than for his doctoring.[6]

Often when called to see a patient, a doctor had no idea what was wrong. He had to go prepared for anything, carrying a few instruments and medications, not knowing if he was to treat an infection or to deliver a baby. When a bolt of lightning struck a homesteader in Turner County, Dakota Territory, during the 1880s, the nearest doctor was twenty miles away. When he finally arrived and examined the patient, he found the lightning had badly burned one leg and side.

The doctor applied poultices made from sour milk mixed with clay. The homesteader regained consciousness and lived.

Another story involving lightning was related by Dr. E. E. Morrison of Great Bend, Kansas. The setting, he said, was the town of Millard in northwest Barton County, Kansas, where one Sunday afternoon "three or four men were playing cards in the kitchen of a settler's home when a thunderstorm occurred. A bolt of lightning struck the stovepipe, followed it down to the stove, and struck the foot of one of the young men who was sitting near it. The foot was torn open. The pious women of the neighborhood said that the event was a providential punishment for playing cards on Sunday. The members of the family dressed the foot for a long time." There was, Morrison continued, a former captain of a sailing vessel living in the area at the time who had told neighbors how years earlier a tropical disease had struck almost everyone on his ship and killed its doctor; using the doctor's medical literature and medicines at hand, the captain had said, he had done what he could to care for his stricken crew. Dr. Morrison and the family now sent for this seafaring man. When he arrived and examined the foot, he found the wound filled with maggots. Dr. Morrison said the captain told everyone "to leave the maggots alone, that they are carrying out the dead flesh and dead bone. They never attack anything that is living. They are the best scavengers that you can have. Let them alone." The family was astounded at the advice, said Morrison, but he knew the captain was correct. The young man struck by lightning recovered.[7]

While the dreaded triad of heroic medicine—bleeding, purging, and emetics—was still used extensively in the West during the 1850s, it was less used during the 1860s, and began to disappear in the 1870s. By then many physicians favored medicines and in particular calomel, although other popular medicines were quinine, jalap, opium, bismuth, nux vomica, castor oil, and whiskey. Doctor William Browner in Jefferson County, Nebraska, was different from most. He prescribed "August Flower Bitters" for each patient, regardless of the illness. It was manufactured in Woodbury, New Jersey, by G. G. Green beginning in the 1870s. Green, who liked to call himself "Dr." Green, claimed his concoction contained a weed with a yellow flower that usually grows along creeks and in sandy and rocky places, and that blooms only in August. He described "August Flower Bitters" as good for dyspepsia and biliousness, as a remedy "for irritation of the nucous [*sic*] membrane of the stomach and bowels, kidneys, and bladder." How successful Dr. Browner was in curing his patients with Green's concoction is not known.

When new doctors arrived in homesteading country, they quickly learned that some settlers expected free medical service. In 1876 a new doctor came from the East and opened an office on the main street of Fairbury, Nebraska. Some days later a homesteader from nearby Bower rode into Fairbury and asked where he could find a doctor. He was directed to the office of the new doctor. Entering the doctor's office, he said, "Doc, an emigrant is at my home with a broken leg. I will take care of him and his team until he is able to travel again, but I want a doctor to set his broken leg." The doctor replied, "Well, if you guarantee my fees, I will go with you." The homesteader replied, "No, I will care for him and his team without any pay, but I want a doctor who will assist him without a fee." The doctor said, "I am not practicing my profession for my health." To that the homesteader said, "I supposed you were a human being, but I see my mistake." Without another word, the homesteader walked out of the office. He soon found another physician, a Dr. Kinnemon, in Fairbury. Fifteen minutes later the new doctor met the homesteader and Dr. Kinnemon on the street. The new doctor stopped Dr. Kinnemon and said, "You're a damn fool to go out there gratis." Kinnemon replied, "Possibly, but I'd rather be a damn fool than a damn brute." The homesteader then warned the new doctor, "Now, Doc, don't ever have any business at or near Bower. If you do, I'll kill you if I'm there. Such skunks as you ought to be run out of Jefferson County with a coat of tar and feathers. You're a disgrace to the frontier." At that the homesteader and Dr. Kinnemon left for Bower, where the doctor took care of the injured man and stayed with him until he was able to resume his journey. Dr. Kinnemon never asked for a fee.[8]

When a patient was seriously ill, doctors usually remained at the patient's bedside until the crisis passed. If the patient was dying, the doctor then became a clergyman caring for the person's spiritual needs until death and then calming the family members. For most doctors it was particularly difficult when a baby died at birth, and even worse when the mother died, as in the case of Martha "Mattie" Oblinger, the thirty-six-year-old wife of a homesteader. Mattie married Uriah Oblinger, a Civil War veteran, in 1869 in Case County, Indiana. For several years the couple farmed some rental property and then decided to go west and get a free homestead. Leaving Mattie and their daughter Ella in Indiana, Uriah, his brother, and Mattie's two brothers headed west. Uriah homesteaded in Fillmore County in south-central Nebraska, where he built a sod house and began farming. In the spring of 1873 Mattie and Ella traveled from Indiana and joined Uriah on the homestead, where two other daughters were born—Estella and Maggie. Early in 1880, a doctor was called when she was expecting another child. Mattie died. Her brother, Giles Thomas, related the story to his parents in a letter written late in February 1880, and now preserved by the Nebraska State Historical Society. It reads in part:

> The Lord called for sister Matt this evening at 4:15 o'clock. She indeed was taken away unexpected to us but her master said come and she now is resting with the angels. She was confined Tuesday evening about 4 o'clock and about 8 o'clock she took a fit very sudden and never spoke after the first one—the spasms come on about every hour and last until about 18 hours before her death. The doctors were compelled to perform a surgical operation by relieving her of the child. The child [a son] is also dead and will be buried with her some time Sunday. There has been nothing left undone that could be done in her case. The doctors worked with great skill but to no good. . . . Uriah said he could not stand it to write now. Don't know what he will do yet. It has left his three little girls in a sad condition—with out a Mother.

Countless babies were born without doctors being present. When a woman was about to deliver, the usual routine was to send for a doctor and then to call women living nearby to help. The children, if any, were usually sent to stay with a neighbor. Because the closest doctors might be twenty or more miles away, the baby often arrived before the doctor. But at least one woman in each neighborhood had some skill in the art of midwifery and often ended up delivering the baby and acting as nurse before the doctor could get there. Such occurrences were common in the early days when doctors were scarce and people had to rely on themselves and home doctoring.

On western homesteads, the woman of the house had many responsibilities. She did the cooking, washing, and housekeeping, cared for the children, and carried water and fuel. On the treeless plains, fuel was often limited to buffalo or cattle chips gathered by women and children. To doctor her family she used or devised all types of home remedies from materials at hand. For instance, she used coal oil to cure dandruff, while warm urine was sometimes poured into the ear to treat earaches, and sometimes used to treat sunburn. Snakebites were sometimes treated with warm manure. For injuries and wounds more generally, one home cure was to tear a live chicken apart and place a piece of the meat on a wound. Still another treatment was to pour turpentine over the wound, give the victim enough whiskey to get drunk, and see what happened. Also a common cure was a mixture of goose grease and turpentine, rubbed on children's skin to squelch a cold. Sassafras tea was used to cure a fever, and buttercup tea to treat asthma. Folk beliefs dominated in some families. For instance, some homesteaders thought carrying a potato in a man's pocket would reduce rheumatism. Throwing a bean over the left shoulder into a well was thought to cure warts. Because cuts were extremely dangerous in a time without antibiotics, people worked hard to keep infections away. Sometimes they put salt pork on a cut to draw out the poison. Another treatment was the use of bread-and-milk poultices. Even manure was used. Pitch, turpentine, spiderwebs, and "puffballs" (dandelion seed balls) were employed to stop bleeding and to prevent infections.

One early homesteader in Iowa recalled:

Every family had a "doctor book" which advised a treatment for every ill and injury to man and beast. Many wild plants were used as medicines, most of them steeped and drunk as tea. They included "Culver's root" [*Veronica virginica L.*] taken "for the liver." The dandelion, both as extract and as wine, was used for the same purpose. Tonics were made from the butterfly weed, sweet flag root, sassafras bark, and boneset. Of course, sulphur and molasses were taken nearly every spring. For colds, pennyroyal, prairie balm, and horse mint were popular remedies. Mullen was used externally for pleurisy. Mullen seeds were among those mother had brought with her from Hoard County [Missouri]. Smartweed was used externally for boils. Cubeb berries were smoked for catarrh. Castile soap was used to cleanse wounds on stock as well as for hand and shaving soap. Dry baking soda was also applied to barbed wire cuts on the stock.[9]

Because doctors' fees were viewed as excessively high, little wonder that homesteaders did as much home doctoring as possible. One

Nebraska doctor charged 50 cents a mile to visit a patient on a homestead and added $1 to his fee for any medicine he gave them. In
Kansas, charges were similar, but prescription-writing started at
50 cents. Delivering a baby cost $10, as did tonsillectomies. Because
most homesteaders were poor and did not have cash, if they called in a
doctor for a serious illness, they often gave him a colt or calf in payment. Homesteaders who did have some money often ended up supplying the major share of the neighborhood doctors' livelihood.

Because so many doctors found it difficult to make a living in their
chosen profession, they often engaged in other work, such as real
estate or politics. The first governor of Dakota Territory, William
Jayne, was a physician. Born in 1826 at Springfield, Illinois, Jayne
graduated from the University of Illinois and the Missouri Medical
School. He practiced medicine in Springfield and became the family
physician of Abraham Lincoln. When Lincoln became president in
1861, he appointed Jayne governor of Dakota Territory. Jayne was
chosen to be the territory's delegate to Congress in 1863, but later
resigned and returned to live out his life in Springfield, where he
served as mayor, practiced medicine, and became wealthy. Jayne died
in 1916.[10]

Winters were often bad on the plains, as Dr. S. V. Moore learned.
Moore was living in Illinois when he learned a doctor was needed in
York County, Nebraska. He brought his family west and took a homestead north of modern Bradshaw and built a sod house on a hill. One
day he was called to the bedside of a young woman who was very sick
with pneumonia.

A storm was raging and lighted lanterns were hung outside the door
of the house to guide the doctor. As he entered the little room where
the woman lay he found her bed surrounded by weeping friends who
believed her to be dying. The doctor left the door wide open and
someone in the room suggested that it be closed. "No, leave it open,"
commanded the doctor as he made his way toward the sick woman.
When she had recovered the power of speech the patient told the
doctor that she heard his command and blessed him for it for she was
perishing for lack of oxygen and the air in the little room was rendered the more impure by the number of people who were crowded
in. All of these friends save the husband and a woman to serve as a
nurse were banished by the physician and since it was too cold to

send them to their homes he told them to make themselves as comfortable as possible in a sod annex to the house. To those who insisted that the patient was dying he said, "She is not dead yet," and she did not die.[11]

The Homestead Act of 1862 was revised by subsequent congresses, and homesteading spread into most areas of the West. Because what is now Oklahoma had been designated Indian Territory, homesteading came late there, after Congress changed the law regarding some of the land. In the spring of 1889, 50,000 people swarmed into a portion of what was now designated Oklahoma Territory in a land race to stake a claim. The following year, "No Man's Land," what is today the Oklahoma Panhandle, became part of Oklahoma Territory, and in 1892 it was opened to homesteading. One doctor who practiced medicine in the Panhandle was Dr. Lindsey L. Long, who was born in Kansas in 1875. Long worked in a drugstore owned by a doctor and later earned his medical degree in 1898 from University Medical College in Kansas City, Missouri. After practicing in Alva, Oklahoma Territory, he moved to the Panhandle settlement of Beaver.

Dr. Long was on call twenty-four hours a day, seven days a week. He saw about 80 percent of his patients on house calls and the rest in his office, which was located in his home. In his recollections he described many treatments but also the difficulty of getting wounds to heal in the stale air and unsanitary dugout houses where many of his patients lived. One morning he was called to visit a family of seven living in a dugout about 16 by 24 feet that was poorly ventilated. Four of the five children and the father had pneumonia. Telling them he would be back, the doctor returned to Beaver, explained the problem to some businessmen, and asked to borrow a tent, a stove, mattresses, blankets, and a nurse. The businessmen delivered the supplies to the dugout that day and later brought a nurse. As Long recalled:

In due time . . . they all recovered and moved back into the unventilated dugout. . . . There had been a lot of criticism among the man's neighbors on the day I moved them out. They all thought that exposure to air was what produced pneumonia in the first place, and that the move would kill all of them. I explained that they must have fresh air, they needed oxygen and I did not have an oxygen generator at the time. . . . After futile explanations, I finally became exasperated and said, "This is my responsibility, not yours." After their recovery, the neighbors changed their attitude. . . . It was a real satisfaction to save such cases, a fine feeling of accomplishment.[12]

Dr. Long, like many other doctors, paid attention to minor things in his practice. One day he was invited to dinner in the home of one of his patients, a wealthy farmer. He had noticed when he arrived that the farmer's four-month-old grandchild had gained only a half pound since birth. Long told his host, "I can tell you what the trouble is. . . . It is too much papa, too much grandfather, too much grandma, too much mama, too much uncle, and too much auntie. Do you know how many times that baby has been taken out of its crib since I have been in the house—sixteen times." Long told the parents the baby was not getting enough rest and sleep, that a baby should sleep about twenty hours a day until it was six months old. The doctor told the family that only the mother should touch the baby, and then only to feed and bathe it. A week later, the grandfather told the doctor that the baby had gained a pound; in four weeks it gained four pounds.[13]

When the Homestead Act was modified in 1909, thousands of settlers were attracted to free land in Montana. The earlier story of doctoring on the plains was repeated in Montana and elsewhere in the West. At first, physicians were scarce and most homesteaders engaged in home doctoring. Homesteaders in Montana were successful growing wheat until a severe drought began in 1917 and continued into the early 1920s. The drought ruined many homesteaders, and was not kind to doctors. Homesteading, however, continued in the West until 1935, during the Great Depression, when remaining public lands were withdrawn and closed to homesteading.

When the homestead act of 1862 was passed, the act did not apply to Texas (then part of the Confederacy). In fact, unlike other states, when Texas joined the Union in 1845, it retained control over its vacant and unappropriated lands, something that continues today. Texas made land available to settlers between 1845 and 1898. Much earlier, when American settlers were first attracted to Mexican Texas in the 1820s, land was plentiful. Each head of a family—male or female—could claim more than 4,600 acres at a cost of 4 cents an acre, payable in six years. At the time, Mexico and the United States had no reciprocal agreements enabling creditors to collect debts or to return U.S. citizens. Thus, Mexico was a safe haven for American farmers who had defaulted on their loans when agricultural prices declined at the end of the War of 1812 and bankers had demanded payment.

Between the 1820s and about 1850, the practice of medicine in Texas was not a profession. The few American doctors who had gone to Texas became farmers or merchants. When the need arose, they did treat bullet wounds, set bones, amputate limbs to prevent gangrene, and prescribe drugs to relieve pain, reduce fever, or induce vomiting, sweating, or bowel movements. Among the most widely used drugs were calomel and various forms of opium. As elsewhere, the common diseases were malaria, cholera, and yellow fever.

One of the earliest American doctors in Texas was James Aeneas E. Phelps, who may have been born either in Connecticut or in Mississippi. He arrived in 1822 and soon cultivated land in modern Brazoria County. In time he owned a plantation, where he resided with his wife, two sons, two daughters, one servant, and fifteen slaves. Little is known about Dr. Phelps's medical qualifications, but in 1833 he treated Texans for cholera at San Felipe. Three years later, he joined the Texas army fighting for independence, serving as a surgeon.

Another early Texas doctor was Johnson Calhoun Hunter, a native of South Carolina, born in 1787. Hunter earned a diploma in medicine in 1805, soon married, and set up a medical practice in Circleville, Ohio, where he made ends meet. He also taught school and opened a mercantile business. Hunter moved to New Madrid, Missouri, in 1817, but four years later settled in Texas, where by the late 1820s he had established a plantation on Oyster Creek in modern Fort Bend County, southwest of Houston, but continued to practice medicine.

Another doctor, Anson Jones, was the last president of the Republic of Texas. Dr. Jones, a native of Massachusetts, obtained a medical degree from Jefferson Medical College in Philadelphia in 1827. After his medical practice failed, he became a merchant in New Orleans in the early 1830s. Again he failed, and drifted into Texas, where he opened what became a prosperous medical practice at Brazoria. He served in the Texas army as its apothecary general for a brief period before returning to Brazoria and his medical practice, but medicine soon took a backseat as he became involved in politics and public service. As a leading advocate of Texas being annexed by the Union, he gained the title "Architect of Annexation" when this step was taken.

Because doctors were scarce during the first half of the nine-teenth century in Texas, many Texans, like others elsewhere on the frontier, relied on home remedies and patent medicines. The home remedies, similar to those used elsewhere in the West, included coal oil, soda, sugar, whiskey, turpentine, soot from wood stoves, and vine-gar, which was employed to soothe sunburn or treat high blood pres-sure. Some made use of camphor, Epsom salts, paregoric, sulfur, and alum, plus plants with medicinal qualities such as sassafras, pennyroyal, anise, oregano, senna, and the barks, roots, and leaves from native plants. Catnip tea was used to treat colic, and corn-shuck tea and ice to treat measles.

Unfortunately, the trained physicians could not provide any con-vincing evidence that their remedies were any better than those sold over the counter or touted by quacks traveling through the country. To capture trade, some doctors opened drugstores to sell not only patent medicines brought into Texas from the East but their own concoctions compounded from local plants and trees. Many commercial and homemade medicines contained large amounts of alcohol and occa-sionally morphine. By the 1860s, most Texas doctors practicing heroic medicine had abandoned bloodletting in favor of bottled medicine. One favorite was Daly's Aromatic Valley Whiskey for Medicinal Pur-poses and another was Sachem Bitters and Wigwam Tonic. Both con-tained much alcohol.

Like settlers elsewhere, many Texans were superstitious and be-lieved humans could transfer an illness to an animal, an object, or an-other person. The folk beliefs found elsewhere also existed in Texas. For example, some thought that a person could get rid of a crick in the neck by watching a hog and rubbing the neck where the animal rubbed its neck. Some people believed if they rubbed a wart with a slice of potato or stolen dishrag and then buried the object in the ground, the wart would disappear as the object in the ground rotted. There were even Texans who believed if they kept a "Mexican hairless" Chihuahua dog in their house, the dog would get their asthma and they would be cured. Other popular beliefs included rubbing a gold wedding band in the eye to remove a sty, placing an ax under a bed to "cut" labor pains, wearing a copper bracelet to cure rheumatism, or wearing a lead fish-ing sinker around the neck to cure nosebleeds.

In Texas and in what is now New Mexico, Hispanics often used *curanderos*, male or female folk healers who were well established, so much so that they even specialized. A *yerbero* specialized in the use of herbs. A *partera* was a midwife, concerned chiefly with delivering babies. Still another was the *sobador*, or masseur. The *curandero* had the skill to treat many illnesses, but he or she was the only healer who could treat *malpuesto*, illnesses caused by witchcraft or supernatural causes. Unlike a conventional physician, the *curandero* might, depending upon the illness, prescribe an herb as a cure or conduct a religious ritual.

Apparently no *curandero* was available to a Mexican man found in the late 1870s by Dr. Henry F. Hoyt in a shack near Tascosa, a crossing of the Canadian River in the Texas Panhandle. As Dr. Hoyt later recalled, the Mexican was in much pain, having dislocated his shoulder while chasing buffalo. Since the doctor had no anesthetic with him, he pulled off one of his boots, used his heel as a fulcrum, and by hard pulling reduced the dislocation. Hoyt then improvised a bandage and bound his patient's arm to his body, leaving instructions for him to keep quiet and visit him the next day in Tascosa. The next morning, however, the Mexican tore the bandage from his arm to see whether it was ready for use. Again the shoulder was dislocated. The doctor had to repeat the painful resetting of the shoulder.

Earlier in Tascosa, Dr. Hoyt had been called to the bedside of the daughter of Don Casimiro Romero, who came from Mora County, New Mexico, in 1876. Romero had become wealthy as a sheep rancher. His daughter, Piedad, was very ill with smallpox—there was not a spot on her body without a pustule. To relieve the itching, Dr. Hoyt experimented by mixing gunpowder with water and spreading it over the girl's entire body. The doctor had concluded that since gunpowder consisted of charcoal, saltpeter, and sulfur, it should help. It did and Piedad soon recovered.[14]

Dr. Hoyt undoubtedly charged a fee, since it was the normal practice of a physician to do so at the end of a medical call. Ranchers usually paid, but doctors found it more difficult collecting fees from poorer settlers. The *Denison* (Texas) *News* of July 3, 1873, reported the following case:

> A Texas doctor recently rode fifty miles to attend a patient. After he cured the patient he presented a bill for fifty dollars, and completed his preparations for the journey back to the post, thinking no more about the matter. As he was about to mount, the patient's husband

put in an appearance, trusty rifle in hand. "Doctor," said he, "I reckon we'd better settle this matter right now;" and taking him aside, "You wan't going off without a settlement, was you? I don't want to owe no man nothing. Here's a ten, which is about a square thing, I reckon. Now if you ain't satisfied just git yet [*sic*] weppin and come behind the hill thar, so's the old woman won't be riled up, and we'll settle it. I don't want no man to go away from my home dissatisfied; especially you, Doc."

The fact that the doctor reported the incident to the newspaper suggests that he accepted the $10 and quickly rode away.

One doctor who had no set fees was Thomas W. Henley, a Texan, who had once been a schoolteacher. He had gone to medical school in St. Louis but had to quit before he received his degree because he ran out of money. He returned to Texas and practiced with another doctor. In 1881 Henley took a homestead five miles west of Fort Stanton on the Rio Bonito. His daughter, Edith L. Crawford, later remembered, "In those days there were very few doctors and most of the farmers that lived around close to us always sent for father. They paid him whatever they felt like giving him as he never set a price."[15]

When Dr. P. C. Coleman opened his practice in January 1883 at Colorado, Texas, he soon learned the area he was to cover was forty miles to the south, or about halfway to San Angelo, but not as far to the east because another doctor had moved to Sweetwater, Texas. To the west, however, his practice extended for a hundred miles. Late in life Dr. Coleman recalled the time when a young boy rode up to his office and told him a baby was sick at home. The young boy, on his horse, led Dr. Coleman in a wagon forty miles south of town over hills and through valleys. Dr. Coleman later wrote:

After we had made a long and tiresome journey with many turns the boy said, "this is the place." In the darkness it seemed to me that there was nothing whatever in the vicinity except a bank or bluff set back a short distance from the [Colorado] river bank proper. But I hitched my team, took my medicine and followed him down this bluff. Near the bottom of the steep incline we found a door opening into a dugout. After I had seen to the wants of the baby (suffering from some temporary trouble) the family gave me the choice bed. This was on the ground under the bed on which the sick baby lay.

This dugout was about fifteen feet square, with low ceiling, but twelve persons occupied it that night.[16]

Most early settlers in Texas came from the South and had their roots in southern culture, where farming predominated. However, the land policies of Mexico and the Republic of Texas were favorable to raising livestock, especially cattle. Beginning in the 1830s many Texans recognized the importance of the lush rangeland where cattle could thrive with minimum care. Many Anglo Texans soon became cattle raisers, supplying beef to Texas settlements and towns, and even to New Orleans and places north of Texas, where the cattle could be fattened and later sold in Philadelphia and New York. The Texans borrowed the Spanish word *rancho*, meaning a farm devoted to the breeding and raising of livestock, and called their home a ranch and their occupation ranching. In time, the ranchers hired hands who became known as cowboys.

Professional doctors were scarce in ranching country. When home remedies did not work, physicians like Dr. Coleman at Colorado, Texas, were called to ranches to treat injuries, set broken limbs, adjust fractures, and remove bullets. Most doctors used ether and chloroform, since local anesthetics were not known.[17] One Texas rancher, Charles Goodnight, relied on home remedies. In fact, he came up with a remedy for hemorrhoids, a homemade suppository containing pure salt in a base of buffalo tallow. Goodnight, who raised buffalo, believed in the medicinal qualities of buffalo fat and even devised a buffalo soap that he claimed stopped soreness in a corn on his foot. It might even, he thought, relieve rheumatism.

When Texans drove thousands of longhorn cattle north to railhead markets in Kansas and elsewhere following the Civil War, they did so over what became well-known trails like the Western Trail running from Texas north across Indian Territory to Dodge City, Kansas. Jonathan Doan and his nephew Corwin established a store at a crossing of the trail on the Red River near modern Vernon, Texas, in the late 1870s. It was the last chance for cowboys to buy supplies before entering Indian Territory. In 1880, Jonathan Doan became very ill with the fever, i.e., malaria, as earlier indicated. The nearest doctor lived in Henrietta, Texas, about seventy miles to the southeast. Doan's people sent a covered wagon to Henrietta to get the doctor. Three days later the doctor arrived and found Doan so sick that he remained three

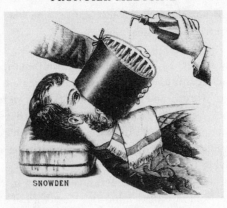

A drawing of an Allis Ether Inhaler being used on a patient. Invented by Oscar H. Allis (1836–1931) in Philadelphia in 1874, it became a popular means of administering ether during operations. The device contained an artificial sponge that absorbed the ether administered from the dropper. (Courtesy National Library of Medicine)

weeks. After Doan recovered, the doctor charged Doan $25 for the visit and Doan's people returned the doctor to Henrietta in the same covered wagon.[18]

In the early years of the great cattle drives, most cowboys had to be their own doctors. Jack Bailey, who trailed a herd of cattle north from Texas in 1868, kept a journal in which he noted that the pain in his side was due to pleurisy. He also complained about rheumatism and treated himself for fever and pneumonia. He wrote that he suffered diarrhea on two occasions, once after eating the meat of a badly boiled yearling, and again after consuming too many wild berries he had picked. On September 22, 1868, he wrote: "I am sick to day. You bet I would like to be at home. My side and shoulder kept me awake all night. I took some pills last night, which operated finely. Hope I will be better when they work off."[19]

By 1870, as trail-driving became more organized, the cook usually carried medicine in the chuck wagon and treated cowboys for cuts and bruises, common illnesses such as an upset stomach, constipation, and diarrhea, or for an occasional broken bone. Such simpler medical problems were usually treated successfully on the trail drives, but the daily hardships of cowboying—sleeping under the stars, working long hours in sun or rain, heat or cold, and not eating well—were responsible for numerous more serious—and longer-term—health problems. One cowboy who suffered was James Emmit McCauley, the son of an East Texas farmer, who left home at age fifteen to become a cowboy. He got a job as a horse wrangler on a trail drive to Kansas and for the next fifteen years broke broncs at $5 a head, trailed countless longhorns north, and even punched cattle on a train. When he was almost thirty, his body was so battered and his health so poor that he had to quit cowboying. He was "stove up," as cowboys described the condition.

McCauley remembered: "I have done as most cowpunchers do after they have got too stove up to ride. For a man to be stove up at thirty may sound strange to some people, but many a cowboy has been so bunged up that he has to quit riding that early in life. Now at thirty I went back to my early raising." McCauley, with less than $500 that he had saved, got married and bought 320 acres of land in Texas and returned to farming. "All I got out of cowpunching is the experience. I paid a good price for that. I wouldn't take anything for what I have saw but I wouldn't care to travel the same road again, and my advice to any young man or boy is to stay at home and not be a rambler, as it won't buy you anything. And above everything stay away from a cow ranch, as not many cowpunchers ever save any money and 'tis a dangerous life to live."[20]

Certainly most experienced cowboys knew their work was tough, especially on the northern plains, where vicious winter weather occurred. But the plains of Wyoming are hardly where one would expect to find a cooperative health care program, the first in America, in the late nineteenth century. It happened in the spring of 1885, when cattlemen and cowboys realized they needed such a program, and the only way to obtain it was through a cooperative approach. A few dozen cattlemen and cowboys organized at that time the Fetterman Hospital Association. One rancher, Ephraim Tillotson, loaned a former two-story Army barracks he had purchased when Fort Fetterman was closed in 1882. It was to be a hospital. The Association's officers hired Dr. Amos Barber, a graduate of the University of Pennsylvania Medical College, at a salary of $100 a month, and agreed to pay his moving expenses to Wyoming. They also hired a man named Mortinson as hospital steward and later a cook. Cowboys who signed up paid $1 a month and ranch owners paid considerably more for full medical service. Initially 219 cowboys and cattlemen signed up as subscribers.

During the Association's first year, Dr. Barber treated 149 patients. All but 14 were subscribers and they paid $2.50 per treatment, plus more when surgery was required. The doctor dealt with a wide range of complaints, including broken bones, the effects of cold weather, asthma, gunshot wounds, respiratory diseases, rheumatism, and alcoholism.

That first winter, the Association found it difficult to heat the hospital and voted to close the building during the cold months. During the Association's second year, the salaries of Dr. Barber and the steward were increased and a full-time nurse was hired. By March 1887, however, ranchers were feeling the financial pinch of the vicious winter of 1885, a drought in 1886, and the blizzards that began sweeping over the northern plains from November 1886 into April 1887, which killed untold thousands of cattle. The cattlemen's financial hardships and the arrival of the Fremont, Elkhorn and Missouri Railroad at Douglas, eleven miles from Fetterman, caused the town to die, and many of its buildings were sold or moved. The Fetterman Hospital Association faded into history. Dr. Barber moved to Douglas and established a private medical practice. Later he became the first secretary of the state of Wyoming. America's first health cooperative is all but forgotten today.[21]

CHAPTER NINE

IN WESTERN TOWNS

Don't live in a town where there are no doctors.

—Jewish proverb

TOWNS SPRANG UP on the prairies and plains near where homestead-ers, ranchers, and others settled because these people needed places to purchase goods and supplies and to sell what they produced. More towns appeared after the iron horse arrived, and some established towns themselves moved to the railroad to capitalize on the better trans-portation. As towns grew in size, most acquired one or two stores sell-ing general merchandise, including groceries, a blacksmith shop, a small hotel, livery stable, lumber dealer, one or more restaurants and saloons, a post office, a weekly newspaper, churches, a school, an attor-ney, and a doctor. Having a doctor was as essential to the community's status as its weekly newspaper, churches, and schools. All these things helped towns erase their raw frontier character and made them appear more civilized, like established communities in the East.

The story of what is now Waco, Texas, is typical of many western towns. At some early point an Indian tribe built a village along the Bra-zos River and lived there until 1830, when another Indian people, the Cherokees, forced them to move. In 1844 George Barnard, a white Indian trader, established a trading post in the area. In 1846, soon after Texas joined the Union, a blacksmith set up shop nearby. A town site was laid out in 1849 and lots were sold for $5 each, while farming lots went for $2 to $3 each. A post office, a hotel, and two churches were constructed by 1850, when the area was organized as McLennan County, named for an early settler, Neil McLennan. Waco Village, as the town was called, became the county seat.

Dr. Alexander Montgomery arrived in November 1851, figuring it was a good place to set up his medical practice because the town showed promise of growth. He may have been the first physician to settle in Waco, though this is not certain. Dr. Montgomery came from Ohio, where he had graduated from a medical school. He brought his wife and seven children to Waco Village in a two-horse wagon. This was unusual, since most people in Texas traveled in ox-drawn wagons. A few weeks after arriving, Mrs. Montgomery traded two bed quilts and a Kentucky-made rag carpet for ten acres of wooded land. The town got its first newspaper in 1854, and in 1856 Waco Village was incorporated as the town of Waco. By then, Dr. Montgomery had built a comfortable home and had a growing medical practice. Waco prospered as settlers in the area turned to raising cotton along the Brazos River. By 1859, the town had a population of 749, and Montgomery had gained the reputation of never turning down a call, day or night, fair or stormy weather, to visit patients by horseback. Those who knew him said he was an old-time botanical doctor who made most of his medicines out of herbs that grew in the area. Dr. Montgomery thought it almost a crime to treat patients with calomel.[1]

Other physicians settled in Waco, including Dr. James C. J. King, a native of Tennessee. His parents moved to Texas in 1846, when King was four years old. He received a good common school education and joined the Confederate service in April 1861 and served as a soldier in Arizona, New Mexico, Texas, and Louisiana until the Civil War ended. Following the war he went to Henderson County, Texas, and taught school for nearly a year. It was during this time he began reading medicine with Dr. W. E. Buie of Milford, Texas. King then took a medical course at Tulane University in New Orleans, graduating in 1871, the year the twenty-nine-year-old doctor began practicing in Waco. By then there were at least ten physicians in Waco and the town had its own medical society, organized in 1866. Dr. King became a leading physician in central Texas, was considered an able, conscientious, and successful doctor, and spent much of his life there.[2]

Waco's pattern of growth, with the arrival of the early doctors, was similar in other towns on the prairies and plains. But doctors were individuals and their stories varied. Soon after the village of Omaha, Nebraska Territory, was founded in 1854, Dr. George L. Miller crossed the Missouri River from Iowa, announced he had come to stay, and became the first doctor in the tiny settlement. Dr. Miller, who was born in 1830 at Boonville, New York, had a good medical education by the standards of the time. He began to study medicine at the age of seventeen with a physician at Syracuse, New York, and then entered the College of Physicians and Surgeons in New York, where he earned his medical degree in 1852. He practiced medicine in Syracuse for two years before coming west in 1854, settling in the struggling village of Omaha.

Indians living in the area were among the first to learn of the doctor's arrival, and his first visitor seeking medical aid was a tall Indian, who made signs indicating he wanted the white medicine man to go with him. At first, Dr. Miller hesitated but then decided to go. They walked a couple of miles over the prairie to the Indian's village, where the doctor found the man's baby very ill. Although his efforts to save the baby failed, the Indians maintained faith in the doctor, and during the weeks and months following he made frequent trips to Indian camps in the area. When a government boat passed Omaha on the Missouri River and cholera broke out on board, Dr. Miller accompanied the soldiers upriver, helping as many as he could.

Because there were few people in Omaha and patients even scarcer, Dr. Miller sought other ways of adding to his income. About a year after he arrived, he entered politics and was elected to the Territorial Council. He served three years in that body and was the presiding officer during the last year. While his income had improved, his financial rewards from medicine and politics were meager. After about four years in Omaha, Dr. Miller left and moved about 140 miles down the Missouri River to St. Joseph, Missouri. He opened his medical practice, and to generate more income got a job writing editorials for the *St. Joseph Gazette*. His success as a journalist caused him to think about turning to full-time newspaper work, but he gave up the idea when the Civil War began. Dr. Miller became sutler at Fort Kearny, Nebraska Territory, where he remained until 1864. He then returned to Omaha and started the *Omaha Herald* newspaper, serving as editor until the spring of 1887, when, at the age of fifty-six, he retired.

There were many other doctors in the West who eventually gave up medicine for other careers, but it appears that a majority of the physicians who came stayed the course and found success, happiness, and satisfaction practicing medicine in new western towns. Most built good practices and gained the trust and respect of people in their communities. The success of any physician seems to have depended upon the person's intellect, skill, dedication, and understanding of medicine and not the medical degrees held. Early in the 1870s, there were 474 medical schools in the United States, more than today. Most schools were owned by the teachers, whose profits and salaries were usually paid by student fees, and most had no admissions standards other than the student's ability to pay tuition. Formal American medical education often consisted of nothing more than two four-month terms of lectures, and students were not allowed to routinely perform autopsies or see patients. Few American medical schools were then associated with a university, and few had ties to a hospital where students could learn by experience. European medical schools were far superior to those in America and required and gave rigorous scientific training. They were, moreover, generally supported by the government of their country.

During the middle of the nineteenth century not many towns between the Mississippi River and the Pacific attracted foreign-trained physicians. One exception was the sleepy village of San Francisco, with a population of about 700. It changed rapidly after gold was discovered in the area and the rush began. By 1850, San Francisco became a cosmopolitan city of 35,000 people. Several foreign-educated doctors were among the thousands of gold-seekers heading west in 1849. By early 1850, there was one doctor for every hundred people in San Francisco, though many were quacks. Some doctors went west overland to California (the experiences of some of these are told in Chapter Six), but other physicians who were more affluent traveled by ship.

Dr. Jacob David Babcock Stillman was among those who arrived by ship in San Francisco. Born in 1819 in Schenectady, New York, Stillman earned his medical degree from the College of Physicians and Surgeons in New York, and he practiced there until he decided to go to California in January 1849. He arrived in San Francisco in August and set out for the gold fields near Sacramento with five friends. After several weeks the party's dreams of riches faded and they voted to return to Sacramento, where Dr. Stillman set up a medical practice with another newly arrived physician, Dr. John Frederick Morse, who has already been spoken of in Chapter Six. They opened a drugstore and established a small hospital. Unlike Dr. Stillman, who sailed around Cape Horn, Dr. Morse sailed to Panama, crossed the isthmus to the Pacific, and then came north in another ship. Without pay, he did the work of the ship's doctor as they traveled up the California coast, and even organized the passengers to clean up the filthy ship. Arriving at

San Francisco in August 1849, he immediately headed for the gold diggings, where he soon met and became friends with Dr. Stillman.

Another physician of note was Dr. Thomas Muldrup Logan, who left New Orleans and traveled by ship around Cape Horn to San Francisco soon after the gold rush began. He was an experienced and highly qualified doctor, not one of the numerous quacks attracted to California by the gold rush. He was then about forty-one years old, having been born in 1808 in Charleston, South Carolina. Logan was a third-generation physician. His grandfather, Dr. Thomas Logan, had earned a degree in medicine at Edinburgh in 1773 and had practiced in Charleston, as had Thomas Muldrup Logan's father, Dr. George Logan, who received his medical degree in 1802 from the University of Pennsylvania. Thomas Muldrup Logan earned his medical degree in 1828 at Charleston, married, and spent several years practicing medicine in Clarendon, North Carolina. In 1832, he went to Europe to soak up the professional culture of physicians in England and France. He then returned to practice again in Charleston, where he also produced color engravings in two editions of a book on surgery. In 1843, he moved to New Orleans to practice medicine there. In 1847 he participated in organizing the American Medical Association. Dr. Logan remained in New Orleans until gold was discovered in California in 1849.

Dr. Logan set up a medical practice when he arrived in San Francisco in January 1850, but a few months later decided to search for gold around Coloma. There, in October 1850, he learned that Asiatic cholera had broken out in Sacramento. He gave up mining and rushed to Sacramento to help. Having studied cholera during earlier travels in Europe, he was eminently suited to treat patients and to provide leadership in ending the epidemic. In November 1850, Dr. Logan wrote:

> As I apprehended, our worst fears have been realized—for never, in the history of this cosmopolitan disease, since its first appearance in the Gangentic delta in 1817, and its subsequent progress around the globe, which it has at last encompassed, has any visitation been so destructive and appalling. . . . The like mortality is unprecedented, and only to be surpassed by the Black Death and awful plagues of the fourteenth century. Even in Paris, in 1832, when I first encountered the disease, and where the mortality was regarded as excessive—

amounting to 18,000 out of a population of 800,000, the proportion-
ate number of deaths was not so great, by more than one-half; there
only one in 44 died; but in Sacramento City, one out of 17 inhabitants fell victim to the scourge and this is a most moderate calcula-
tion, based solely upon the mortuary record of the two coffin-makers
and undertakers. Of the ninety physicians embraced in the population not one fled; all remained and performed their duties with an
unflinching firmness and fidelity worthy of all honorable mention.[3]

Dr. Logan liked Sacramento, settled there, and soon became
prominent as a physician and leader in public health. He was friends
with doctors Stillman and Morse and for a time was a partner with
Morse. All three physicians were active in the founding of the Sacramento Medical Society in April 1855. Later, in 1871, Dr. Logan
brought the first national meeting of the American Medical Association west to San Francisco, and the following year he was elected president of the AMA. During his presidency, Dr. Logan introduced a
resolution supporting the right of women to study and practice medicine, but it was not approved. Dr. Logan died in Sacramento on February 13, 1876.

The Sacramento–San Francisco area was rich in highly educated
physicians like doctors Logan, Stillman, and Morse. Of the thirty-two
doctors who established the first, short-lived San Francisco Medical
Society in June 1850, almost a third had received foreign training.
Three held certificates from the Royal College of Surgeons, two from
French schools, and one each from Scottish, Belgian, and German colleges. Four had graduated from the New York College of Physicians
and Surgeons, three from Bowie Medical College in Maine, two each
from the universities of Pennsylvania, Maryland, and Harvard, and
Berkshire Medical College in Pittsfield, Massachusetts, one from the
Philadelphia Medical College, one from Transylvania in Kentucky,
and one who listed his authority to the "Army Medical Board, 1813."
For any area in the West during the mid-nineteenth century to have so
many doctors with such impressive credentials was unusual.

The first San Francisco Medical Society collapsed about four
months after it started because it represented the "regular" physicians
in the city, a term that ignored countless quacks, cultists, and a group of
self-appointed doctors who had little or no formal training in medicine.
Those not considered regular doctors had flocked to San Francisco to

make their fortunes by mining the miners and anyone else ignorant enough to seek their services. Sixty-three physicians attempted to organize another medical society in San Francisco in 1853 but it died after the start of the Civil War. It was not until early 1868, following the war, that fifty-seven physicians reorganized the San Francisco Medical Society, an organization that continues today. By then gold fever had been replaced by permanence and stability, and San Francisco claimed a population of nearly 150,000 people. The city had a medical school, an opera house, theaters, and many permanent buildings including homes, and the telegraph had arrived linking the East to the West. The local medical press freely questioned the veracity and honesty of questionable practitioners and used such terms as *charlatan*, *quack*, and *seller of quack medicine* to do so in their editorials.

San Francisco was struck in the summer of 1868 with infectious diseases. Scarlatina and measles came first, followed by more than thirty cases of smallpox each month, with a 35 percent death rate. Members of the San Francisco Medical Society finally persuaded the city fathers to construct a shack south of the county hospital. Smallpox patients were forcibly confined there.[4]

News of the California gold rush had attracted countless Chinese to San Francisco as they sought to escape poverty and ruin in their home country. By the late 1860s thousands of Chinese had arrived, and many found work with the Central Pacific Railroad being constructed east from Sacramento to join up with the Union Pacific being built west from Omaha to create in 1869 the transcontinental railway. It was dangerous work, and at least 1,200 Chinese workers died building the Central Pacific. Since the Chinese did not trust Western doctors or Western medicine, the laborers turned to their own doctors, who specialized in herbal medicines derived from plant, mineral, and animal substances.

Chinese medicine was actually far more sophisticated than Western medicine of the day, and far more effective in dealing with chronic disease. For example, the Chinese created a compound of whiskey and opium to relieve influenza and diarrhea, and they learned to use common baking soda to treat a skin infection caused by poison ivy. They also used molds to cure infection long before the invention of penicillin. It was not surprising that the Chinese then spreading into most areas of the West should use their own doctors for medical treatment.

One such doctor was Fong Dun Shung, who came from southeast

China, bringing with him his second and third sons. Soon after arriving in San Francisco in 1867 they went to work for the Central Pacific
as laborers. When not working, Fong Dun Shung treated many Chinese and promoted the traditional, balanced Chinese diet of rice, fish,
and vegetables and the drinking of hot tea. White laborers often
laughed at the Chinese for drinking tea, until many whites became ill
from dysentery after drinking unboiled groundwater. About 1870,
Fong Dun Shung quit working for the railroad and opened an herbal
shop called Kwong Tsui Chang (Success Peacefully) in Sacramento,
and practiced Chinese herbal medicine. One account suggests he also
treated Chinese men who were sick or seeking sexual prowess, and
Chinese women, mostly prostitutes, who fought venereal disease,
tuberculosis, and pregnancy. Fong Dun Shung returned to China in
1871, leaving his sons to run the business.[5]

The year Fong Dun Shung arrived in California, the Central
Pacific Railroad in Sacramento established a prepaid medical plan for
its employees. The plan was so successful that in 1870 Central Pacific
built a hospital in Sacramento devoted exclusively to serving its
employees. The plan was soon adopted by other railroads across the
nation, who also hired physicians and surgeons and built hospitals. By
1899, Central Pacific had fifty-five physicians under contract to treat
sick or injured employees of the line. Those who worked full-time for
the railroad were paid salaries. Others who saw only a few patients
were given passes to travel on the line in exchange for their medical
services.

During the late 1800s more Chinese arrived on the West Coast and
soon journeyed to countless other places where gold was discovered,
including Montana and its boomtowns like Alder Gulch, Virginia City,
Billings, Anaconda, and Butte, which claimed Montana's largest Chinese community. It was there that Dr. Huie Pock, another Chinese
physician, became wealthy practicing herbal medicine, acupuncture,
and surgery. He became highly respected after successfully treating the
ulcers of the daughter of William Andrews Clark, one of the famous
"Copper Kings" of Butte and one of the wealthiest men in America.
Dr. Pock developed an effective herbal poultice that used banana
stalks. In 1918, he was able to save many lives in Butte during an outbreak of influenza. Dr. Pock continued to practice medicine there until
his death in 1927.

Virginia City, Nevada, was another western mining boomtown created by an 1859 gold and silver strike that attracted several Chinese physicians, including Wai Tong, who became prominent. Virginia City even had a Chinese phrenologist who claimed to determine character traits from natural lumps on the head. Virginia City also attracted Dr. Charles Lewis Anderson, who arrived in 1861. He left his wife and two daughters with friends in Wisconsin and crossed the plains and mountains by wagon train and stagecoach. Dr. Anderson practiced medicine briefly in Virginia City and then moved to Carson City and set up an

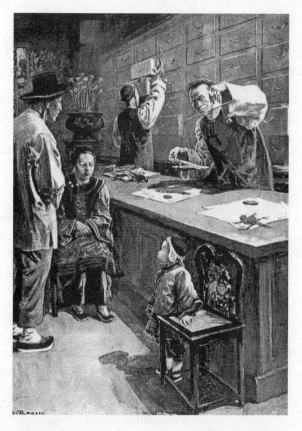

"Weighing Out Medicines in a Chinese Drug-Store, San Francisco." This illustration by W. A. Rogers appeared in Harper's Weekly, *December 3, 1899. By the end of the nineteenth century, such drugstores were common in western cities with large Chinese populations.*

office in a drugstore. He charged patients $5 per visit plus $5 a mile if he had to travel outside of Carson City. These charges were high, but then everything cost more in the mining town.

Like many other doctors in the West, Dr. Anderson came from the East. He was born in Virginia, but at the age of ten moved with his parents to Indiana, where he worked his way through medical school. He then practiced medicine in Minneapolis, Minnesota. When he opened his practice in Nevada, he did not have a great many patients, perhaps because of the healthy, dry climate. He also was a botanist and enjoyed studying Nevada flora. Two eastern Sierra plants are named for him: the Anderson's buttercup (*Ranunculus andersonii*) and the desert peach (*Prunus andersonii*). In November 1862, a few months before his family joined him in Carson City, Dr. Anderson wrote his wife in Wisconsin telling her of his plans and aspirations:

> The height of my ambition is to have a pleasant quiet cottage of 5 or 6 rooms, one for a library where we could read and converse evenings or enjoy other amusements, a small garden of vines and fruits with a few choice flowers. A business that would yield a comfortable living and a few select friends to come and see us. Out of debt so that what I earned I could call my own, my motto could be to 'owe no man anything.' In the study of Nature, and Nature's God, we could be enabled to live nearer to Him, and with greater happiness to ourselves.

Dr. Anderson became involved in Carson City civic affairs, and after Nevada was given statehood in 1864 he was appointed state surgeon general. In 1867, however, he decided to move his wife and daughters to a milder climate, with a more stable society, than he had found in Nevada. They settled in Santa Cruz, California, where he died in 1910.[6]

Another easterner who arrived in Virginia City in 1861 was Samuel Langhorne Clemens. After he failed to find gold, he got a job reporting for the Virginia City newspaper, the *Territorial Enterprise*. (This was before he wrote under the pen name "Mark Twain.") The newspaper received a letter from a man named William in Springfield, Missouri, asking about Virginia City's climate, whether or not it was healthy, and "What diseases do they die of mostly?" The paper's editor asked Clemens to answer the letter. His reply, which would later appear in his book *The Celebrated Jumping Frog of Calaveras County and Other Sketches* (1867), reads in part:

It is mighty regular about not raining. . . . It will start in here in November and rain about four, and sometimes as much as seven days on a stretch, after that you may loan out your umbrella for twelve months, with the serene confidence which a Christian feels in four aces. Sometimes the winter begins in November and winds up in June, and sometimes there is a bare suspicion of winter in March and April, and summer all the balance of the year. But as a general thing, William, the climate is good, what there is of it.

"Is it healthy?" Yes, I think it is as healthy here as it is in any part of the West. But never permit a question of that kind to vegetate in your brain, William; because as long as Providence has an eye on you, you will not be likely to die until your time comes.

"What diseases do they die of mostly?" Well, they used to die of conical balls and cold steel, mostly, but here lately erysipelas and the intoxicating bowl have got the bulge on those things, as was very justly remarked by Mr. Rising last Sunday. I will observe, for your information, William, that Mr. Rising is our Episcopal minister, and has done as much as any man among us to redeem this community from its pristine state of semi-barbarism. We are afflicted with all the diseases incident to the same latitude in the States, I believe, with one or two added and half a dozen subtracted on account of our superior altitude. However, the doctors are about as successful here, both in killing and curing, as they are anywhere.

No gold or silver rush was responsible for the rapid growth of Leavenworth, Kansas Territory, in 1854. It was politics. That year Congress passed the Kansas-Nebraska Act, which called for the respective residents of each of the two new territories to determine if it would be slave or free. Southern supporters assumed Nebraska would be free, and they wanted to make sure Kansas would be a slave state. People on both sides of the question rushed to Kansas Territory in May 1854. Three ministers, four lawyers, two printers, four merchants, one surveyor, two Army officers, one Army clerk, eight farmers, and five doctors crossed the Missouri River from Missouri and organized the Leavenworth town company close to Fort Leavenworth, established in 1827. Some men in the group had southern sympathies, but most, including the doctors, seem to have been more interested in promoting the town, in selling lots, and in commerce generally, than in politics, or, for the doctors specifically, in practicing medicine. All the men realized the slavery issue would quickly attract new residents and generate business. Two of the doctors opened drugstores: Dr. Samuel Norton, who built the first frame building on the town site in the fall of 1854, and Dr. R. E. Allen, newly arrived from Liberty, Missouri. Both doctors apparently sought thereby to capitalize on the settlers' preference for using home remedies and patent medicines instead of relying on doctors, who many settlers believed charged excessive fees.[7]

Perhaps the most prominent doctor to settle in Leavenworth was Dr. Cornelius Logan, who in 1858 organized the Leavenworth Medical and Surgical Society, the first medical society in Kansas. A native of Illinois, Dr. Logan was one of the new breed of doctors who looked at medicine as a science and were actively concerned with medical research and scholarship. In fact, in 1861, Dr. Logan wrote and had printed in Leavenworth a nineteen-page booklet titled *An Essay on the Remote and Proximate Causes of Miasmatic Fever.* Logan founded the first civilian hospital in Kansas and cofounded the first medical journal in Kansas, *The Leavenworth Medical Herald,* which urged doctors to "wake up and seize hold of your pen . . . your practice doesn't require your whole time, if it does you have more patients than we do. . . ." Early in 1867, Dr. Logan also introduced the clinical thermometer to Leavenworth doctors as a diagnostic instrument.* In January 1866, he was elected president of the Kansas Medical Society, which had been incorporated by the legislature in 1859. In the early 1870s, Dr. Logan sought to locate the proposed state medical school at Leavenworth, but was unsuccessful. He left Kansas about 1873, when he was appointed the U.S. minister to Chile, a position he held from 1873 to 1876 and again from 1882 to 1885. Between 1876 and 1882 he served as minister to several Central American countries. Dr. Logan died in 1899.[8]

Kansas attracted other prominent eastern physicians, including Dr.

---

*The thermometer was invented by Galileo Galilei in 1592, but it was a friend of his named Santorio Santorio who first used it for medical purposes. More than two and a half centuries later, in 1866, Thomas Clifford Allbutt, an English physician, invented the clinical thermometer. It was much smaller than the earlier ones, which were more than a foot long and required twenty minutes to display a reading. Allbutt's clinical thermometer could take a temperature in only five minutes.

Charles Robinson, who became the state's first governor; Dr. Joseph Root, the first lieutenant-governor; and Dr. John W. Robinson, secretary of state. All three were medical doctors by profession. The professionalism of these and many other early Kansas physicians elevated the importance of medicine in Kansas. These and other doctors were influenced by Louis Pasteur's research, which confirmed in 1862 that microorganisms infected animals and humans and could cause disease. While Pasteur did not develop the germ theory, he proved it was true, and proposed the use of systematic measures to prevent microorganisms from entering the human body. English physician Dr. Joseph Lister took Pasteur's idea and developed antiseptic methods in surgery, including the use of germicides such as carbolic acid. Dr. J. W. Brock of Leavenworth, who kept abreast of the latest medical advances, borrowed Lister's idea and introduced carbolic acid paste as an antiseptic soon after it was proposed. Lister's approach, along with improved methods of binding up wounds, had a great impact on the practice of medicine in Kansas and elsewhere.

The history of Kansas is not only unique because of the many

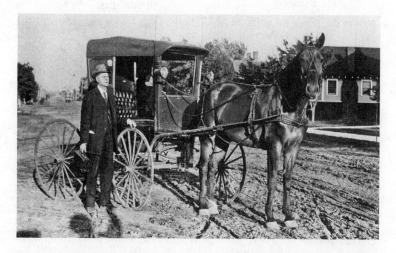

Dr. J. D. Pate of Francis, Oklahoma Territory, was typical of physicians attracted to railroad towns. Francis, then located on the Frisco Railroad just south of the Canadian River, was a division point with a roundhouse. Dr. Pate treated railroad employees and others in and around the farming community in south-central Oklahoma Territory. He made his rounds in this horse and buggy. (Courtesy Western History Collections, University of Oklahoma Libraries)

highly educated doctors who settled there during its territorial and early-statehood years, but because for two decades (1867–1887) it could claim railhead cattle towns. The Texas longhorns were to the Kansas cattle towns what gold and silver were to the mining towns farther west. At first, these towns did not attract well-educated physicians but as the communities grew after the cattle trade departed, better-qualified doctors arrived. The cattle-town era began when the Union Pacific Railroad, Eastern Division (it became the Kansas Pacific in 1868) pushed west from Kansas City across Kansas and reached the tiny settlement of Abilene in 1867. Abilene became the first Kansas railhead cattle town in 1867, and anxious Texans soon arrived seeking to sell their herds of longhorn cattle. Although the cattle trade was seasonal, between the spring and fall, merchants flocked to these towns and opened stores, and saloonkeepers saloons, to provide the Texans places where they could spend their money after weeks on the often dusty Chisholm Trail. The wild and woolly cattle towns also attracted characters with get-rich-quick schemes, gamblers, prostitutes, con artists, and others seeking something for nothing. It was only natural that the towns also attracted doctors looking for business.

Charles C. Furley may have been Abilene's first physician. He arrived in 1869. Born in New Jersey in 1838, Furley grew up in the shadow of New York City. In 1850, when he was twelve, his parents moved to California, where young Furley finished his education, studied medicine, and earned his medical degree in 1860. When the Civil War began, he was commissioned assistant surgeon of the Second California Cavalry and served until 1863. He left to become a surgeon with the Pacific Mail Steamship Company for one year. He then returned to the military, serving in the Army of the Potomac, Departments of Virginia and of the Gulf, until the war ended. He spent a year in Wyoming Territory and then moved to Abilene in 1869 but two years later moved again, to Wichita, Kansas. He was appointed to the first board of examiners after the Kansas Medical Society was given the authority by the legislature to regulate physicians. In 1880, he was elected president of the Kansas Medical Society and continued his practice in Wichita into the twentieth century.[9]

About a year after Furley came to Abilene, another physician named Lucius Boudinot arrived and set up practice. Like Furley, Boudinot was a native of New Jersey. Whether Dr. Furley encouraged him to come west to Abilene is not known, but Boudinot had enlisted

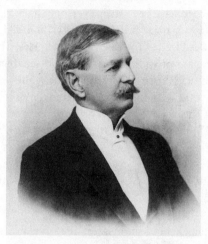

Dr. Charles C. Furley, perhaps the first doctor in Abilene, Kansas. He arrived there in 1869, the year after Abilene became a railhead cattle town. Furley had earned his medical degree in California in 1860 and served as a doctor in the Union Army before coming to Kansas. (Courtesy Kansas State Historical Society)

at the age of forty-five for a hundred days of service in the Forty-fourth Regiment, Iowa Volunteer Infantry, as a hospital steward. His position suggests that he lacked a strong medical education; otherwise he probably would have been a surgeon. In Abilene, Boudinot was elected to the town council on a platform favoring a moderate saloon license fee of $100 a year. When the council approved a $200 annual fee, Boudinot announced he was resigning. Little else is known about Boudinot other than he died in Abilene in July 1873 at the age of fifty-four from a kidney disease. His widow remained in Abilene for many years.[10]

During Abilene's wildest cowtown years (1867–1871), doctors Furley and Boudinot apparently found it difficult to make a living. The Texans probably gave them some business when they were in town, but the town lost population in the late fall and during the winter, because the cattle trade was seasonal. Abilene's year-round residents preferred to rely on patent medicines and home remedies when illness hit, and some townspeople provided free medical attention. Mrs. Edward

McCollam seems to have been such a person. She ran a boardinghouse
in Abilene, and it was there that James B. "Wild Bill" Hickok made his
home after he was hired as the town's lawman. Mrs. McCollam apparently was so good at providing medical assistance that she earned the
nickname "Doctor." When Thelphilus Little's nine-year-old son Will
accidentally cut off two of his fingers, "Doctor" McCollam dressed the
boy's hand. As she was doing so, "Wild Bill" came in and saw the
injured boy. "Ah, that is too bad, too bad, and such a fine manly little
fellow too." Hickok then patted Will on his head, according to the
boy's father, who later wrote an account of the incident.[11]

Stuart Henry, who moved to Abilene as a boy with his parents in
1868, later recalled:

> Everybody thought he or she must eat three stout meals a day or they
> were really sick, and mysterious stomach troubles became not
> uncommon. Some guessed they could be mainly ascribed to the hard
> drinking water. You saw how many residents dosed themselves with
> patent medicines since physicians, like experts and lawyers, seemed
> much scowled upon as ignoramuses more skilled in harming than in
> helping, and ordinarily described as quacks. A chronic complaint was
> sometimes regarded as a manifestation from Jehovah and, hence, to
> be borne with resignation as incurable and sacred.[12]

Doctors in Abilene began to build good medical practices only after
the cattle trade moved farther west and Abilene grew into a stable
farming trade center. Because longhorns spread Texas fever among
local settlers' cattle, the Kansas legislature prohibited Texas cattle from
being driven through settled areas; and as more homesteaders moved
west across Kansas, the quarantined area, or "deadline," as it was
called, was also moved farther west to accommodate them. New cattle
towns, including Newton, Ellsworth, and Wichita, developed along
either the Kansas Pacific pushing west toward Colorado or the Atchison, Topeka and Santa Fe Railroad pushing southwest across Kansas.
By the late 1870s, only one settlement on a railroad west of the quaran-
tine line could receive Texas cattle driven overland—Dodge City, the
last Kansas railhead cattle town.

Located close to Fort Dodge, the town of Dodge City began about
1872 as a supply point for buffalo hunters and dealers in pelts. When
the Atchison, Topeka and Santa Fe Railroad reached it in 1877, the set-

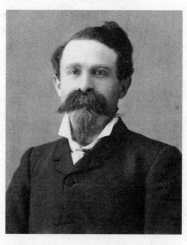

*Dr. T. L. McCarty, a graduate of the Jef-
ferson Medical College in Philadelphia in
1876, came west and opened his practice in
Dodge City, Kansas, in 1872. (Courtesy
Kansas State Historical Society)*

tlement became a cattle town. For nine years it catered to the cattle
trade. While residents of Dodge City could call on the military surgeon at nearby Fort Dodge, the town did have an experienced and
educated physician. He was Dr. T. L. McCarty, who settled in Dodge
City in November 1872 and opened a medical office. Born in Illinois,
he graduated from Jefferson Medical College in Philadelphia in 1870
and then practiced in St. Louis before moving to Dodge City. In 1877
he opened a drugstore there, and also served as a contract surgeon for
the Atchison, Topeka and Santa Fe Railroad for several years. Dr.
McCarty was described as

> the only man in Dodge City in the early days of the town to hold on
> to the habits of civilization, day in and day out. Always there was the
> daily shave, white collar, white tie. In fact, he never adopted the fron-
> tier way of living. He could not adopt their approved style of dress
> but he liked their western spirit. He had high ideals. He liked the
> infectious spirit of adventure in the West, the western genuineness,
> and freedom from sham, the way they took their changing fortunes.
> He had . . . an inborn dignity that conditions of frontier life could

not break down. He had unfailing courage and a tender regard for humanity, and accomplished professional achievements under difficult circumstances, no questions asked. It was Dr. T. L. McCarty who plugged the bullet holes, and every rough and ready man would fight for him at the drop of a hat. Cowboys said his heart was where God put it; "his blood was allus red; his mouth, he alluz shut it when troubles were ahead." In their mind's eye an early day patient could see him—neatly trimmed blond mustache, finely featured face, and clear Irish-blue eyes, and always anyone would notice his massive gold watch chain, a legend in Dodge City.[13]

Another early physician in Dodge City was C. A. Milton, who opened a small hospital, the first in town, and had a trained nurse, Miss Hollipeter, known as "Hollie" by townspeople who loved her. The town had another well-known physician, but Dr. S. Galland never practiced medicine there. He gave up the profession before moving to Dodge City. Born in Germany in 1822, he earned his medical degree in Berlin, practiced there for two years, and then came to America in 1849. He practiced medicine in New York City for two years before going to California, where he was a physician until 1857. He then practiced in St. Louis and New Orleans before moving to Kansas City, Missouri, in 1868, and then Topeka, Kansas, in 1870. In 1878, when he was fifty-six years old, he retired from medicine and moved to Dodge City, where he ran the Great Western Hotel. Dr. Galland established a hotel rule that required guests to be in by ten o'clock each night or else they did not get in until the following morning. He made sure the hotel was locked up tight at ten. Tradition has it that Dr. Galland's guests obeyed this rule because the hotel had good beds and service.

Robert M. Wright, an early Dodge City merchant, told the story of another doctor who claimed to be a specialist in venereal and other "intimate" diseases. This unidentified doctor from Illinois saw Dodge City as a disease-ridden town and wrote to its postmaster and others, wanting to know if it might be a good place for him to practice. Wright later wrote: "Some of the gang got hold of his letters and wrote him that the town was overrun with disease, that even our ministers were not free, and that more than half the people were suffering. Anyhow, they made out a frightful condition our people were in and that it had got beyond our physicians, and to come at once if he wanted to make a

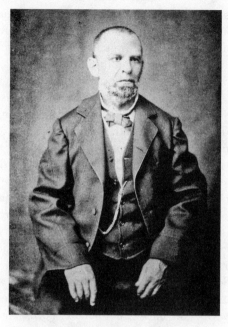

*Dr. S. Galland, a native of Germany and a gradu-
ate of the Berlin School of Medicine, came to the
United States in 1840. He practiced in St. Louis,
New Orleans, Kansas City, and Topeka, Kansas,
before retiring from medicine in 1878. He then
moved to Dodge City, Kansas, a rough-and-tumble
cattle town, and ran the Great Western Hotel.
(Courtesy Kansas State Historical Society)*

fortune. They signed one letter, 'Sim Dip,' 'Ed Slump,' and another,
'Blue Pete.'

"Now, if the man had had any gumption, he would have known
these were fictitious names, but he took the bait and away he came. On
his arrival, he hunted up Sim Dip and Blue Pete. Of course, he was
introduced to these gentlemen. They came to me for the key and the
loan of the Lady Gay Theater, a large old building. At first I refused,
but they promised to do no harm, or only to scare the fellow and have
some fun. They printed and put out their notices and in the afternoon
started two boys with bells to ring up the town, which they did effectu-
ally, judging by the crowd assembled that night.

"The house was crammed and jammed from the door to the stage. Bat Masterson was on one side of the doctor and Wyatt Earp on the other, with Jack Bridges and other gunmen sitting around on the stage in chairs. The doctor had only got on a little way in his lecture when some one in the audience called him a liar. He stopped and said to Bat, 'What is that? I don't understand.' Bat got up, pulled his gun in front, and said, 'I will kill the first man that interrupts this gentleman again.' The lecturer had not gone much farther when some one again called him a vile name. Bat and Wyatt both got up and said: 'This gentleman is a friend of ours, you want to understand that, and the next time he is interrupted we will begin shooting and we will shoot to kill.' He had not gone much further in his talk when some one in the audience said, 'You lie, you s— of a b—!' Bat, Wyatt, and Bridges all arose and began shooting at the same time. First they shot out the lights and my! what a stampede began. The people not only fell over each other, but they tumbled over each other, and rolled over, and trampled each other under foot. Some reached the doors, others took the windows, sash and all, and it was only a short time till darkness and quiet reigned in the Lady Gay. Only the smell of powder and a dense smoke was to be seen, coming out the windows and doors.

"There was a broken-down, tin-horn gambler by the name of Dalton, a total wreck from morphine and whiskey, whose avocation was a sure-thing game, and his specialty was robbing the stiffs (as the dead bodies were called), and he was an expert at this. Dalton happened to be asleep when this occurred, in a room back of the stage, but the noise and shooting awakened him. He located the place at once from the pistol smoke coming through the windows, and was sure there must be stiffs in the building after so much shooting.

"I must interpolate here, there was scarcely anyone of that big audience who were wise to the lecture, but nearly all thought everything was straight and, when the shooting began, thought, as a matter of course, it was a genuine shooting scrape, and they could not get away from the scene of action fast enough or far enough, but kept on running in the opposite direction and never looking back. Now this lecturer thought as the audience did and, as soon as the firing began, he ducked down under a table in front of the platform and there he lay, as still as a mouse, for fear someone would find him and kill him yet.

"Mr. Dalton crawled along the floor on his belly, hunting the stiffs. When he came to the table, of course he felt the stiff underneath and [attempted] to divest him of his wealth. But the lecturer gave one mighty spring, threw Dalton over to one side, and jumped up and ran for dear life holloing, 'Murder! Thieves!' and everything else, as loud as he could bawl. Dalton, equally scared to have a stiff come to life and pitch him off, just as he was about to rob him, took to his heels the other way. That was the last seen of the lecturer that night; he sneaked off and hid out. The next morning Sim Dip and Blue Pete waited on him and told him a fine story—how sorry they were, but if he would stay over that night, they would assure him a fine audience and ample protection to his meeting, and he, never dreaming but what it was all on the square, stayed.

"The gang wanted to know of me if ten pounds of [gun]powder would hurt him. I told them a pound would kill him if it were rightly confined. This put me on my guard and, just before dark, [I] found out they were going to place a big lot of powder under the box on which he was going to lecture, and I knew it would blow him up and maybe kill him. So I went to him privately and said: 'My friend, you don't know what you are up against. Get on the local freight, which leaves here inside an hour, and never stop until you get back to your own Illinois, because you are not fit to be so far away from home without a guardian.' When the gang was certain he was gone, they touched a match to the fuse they had connected with the powder under the box, and blew it to kingdom come. It went way up in the air and came down a mass of kindling wood. When the boys saw the result, they were glad they did not carry the joke any further."[14]

THE HEALTH COMPLAINTS, sickness, and disease that regularly plagued people in larger western communities during the latter half of the nineteenth century were essentially the same found among home-steaders, ranchers, and others in less populated areas from the Mississippi River west. Cholera, smallpox, typhoid fever, and diphtheria occasionally came in epidemics in larger communities where people lived close together. There were fewer epidemics among people living in less populated areas as a general rule. Scattered records suggest that pneumonia was particularly deadly among old people regardless of where they lived, while malaria (ague or fever) killed more young people than any other disease. Diphtheria probably was a close second in taking young lives. Most physicians treating patients in towns on the prairie and plains were the same ones who treated homesteaders living nearby. By the 1860s, most were trying to cure illness with medicines like calomel, and those of the "patent" variety.

Dentists began arriving in many western towns in the latter half of the nineteenth century. One of the more prominent was Oscar H. Simpson, born in 1861 in Decatur County, Indiana. He received his education at the Ohio College of Dental Surgery in Cincinnati. After completing the six-month course, he practiced dentistry about a year in his hometown of Warrensburg, Indiana. In 1885, he went on vacation to visit a friend in Dodge City, Kansas. He took a liking to the place and stayed. He opened an office with an old cycloid dental chair and a $3 table on which he spread his instruments, many homemade. He married and became nationally known when he invented the gold inlay process for filling teeth, which he patented in 1912. In time, he was invited to give clinical demonstrations before dental associations in most major cities.[15]

Dodge City also claimed another dentist, but only for one summer: John Henry Holliday, a native of Georgia, born in 1851. He earned the degree of Doctor of Dental Surgery from the Pennsylvania College of Dental Surgery at Philadelphia in 1872. He set up his practice in Atlanta, Georgia, and was considered a good dentist. Before his first year of practice ended, however, he discovered that he had contracted tuberculosis. Several doctors told him he had only months to live, but that a dry climate might prolong his life. Holliday headed west to Dallas, Texas, where he went into practice with another dentist. But coughing spells wracked his thin frame and often interrupted his work. He changed professions and became a gambler. One day he got into a fight with a saloon keeper and killed the man. This was the first of several men to be killed by Holliday, who fled Dallas for Jacksboro, a frontier town in north-central Texas.

As a gambler, Holliday carried a gun on his hip, another in a shoulder holster, and a long knife, and in the months that followed became involved in other gunfights as he drifted from Texas to Wyoming and then New Mexico before returning to Texas. From there he went to Kansas. About 1878 he spent a summer in Dodge City gambling and making friends with Wyatt Earp. In the summer of 1879 he tried practicing dentistry again in Las Vegas, New Mexico. His practice was short-lived after he bought a saloon. He then shot and killed another man. Holliday fled to Tombstone, Arizona, where in 1882 he was involved in the gunfight at the O.K. Corral. He later spent time in Colorado but never practiced dentistry again. "Doc" Holliday died at Glenwood Springs, Colorado, in 1887, a victim of tuberculosis.[16]

Eastern medical ideas about good sanitation and cleanliness for improved health were only beginning to reach physicians in western towns by the 1870s. Most residents could not grasp the concept. Many towns were filthy, with trash and garbage everywhere, but the health hazards created were not understood, any more than the importance of hand-washing and personal cleanliness generally. But town residents did object to the odor of human waste, and like people elsewhere in settled areas, they constructed outhouses or privies near their homes and businesses. Most of them probably were unaware that they were improving health conditions by doing so. They erected most outhouses 40 or 50 feet from a home, sometimes as much as 150 feet when space permitted, and these facilities were built over an open pit four feet by four feet and at least four feet deep, usually deeper. The wooden structure built over the open pit was usually three or four feet square, and about six feet high at the back and seven feet high on the front. Because there were no windows in an outhouse, the builder more often than not cut a small opening toward the top of the door.

Traditionally, the openings were in the shape of a sun for men, and a crescent moon for women. The small openings permitted light inside during daylight hours. Inside there was a wooden seat constructed with a closed front and a round hole on top where the occupant would sit to defecate. Some outhouses had two holes of different sizes in the seat, one for adults and one for children. Inside it became a common practice to have a small container of lime and a scoop. After using the facility, the user was expected to pour a scoop of lime into the hole to help control odor and absorb moisture.

For cleaning up, baskets of leaves or corncobs, discarded sheep wool, or pages torn from newspapers and magazines were kept in outhouses. After Montgomery Ward issued its first mail-order catalog in the early 1890s and Sears, Roebuck followed with its first catalog in 1894, the pages from these dream books were torn and used for this purpose, as were pages from the annual *Farmer's Almanac*, sold with a hole punched in the corner so it could be hung on a hook and the pages easily torn. Although the Chinese were apparently the first, centuries earlier, to use paper for the purpose of cleaning up, it was not until 1857 that Joseph C. Gayetty of New York produced "Gayetty's Medicated Paper," packets of premoistened flat sheets of paper medicated with aloe. But they did not sell well, because toilet paper was an unmentionable in the conservative Victorian era. The subject was taboo. Even old-timer recollections contain few references to defecation and toilet habits, perhaps because a person's sex organs are near the organs of elimination. To talk about such things was considered vulgar if not erotic. Even scholars of the time ignored the subject because of disgust for its noxiousness, and the belief that human waste had no usefulness. Rolled and perforated toilet paper was not invented until about 1880, but it took a while before it was accepted in the West. Because toilet paper was still a very sensitive subject, the inventor, the Scott Paper Company of Philadelphia, did not put its name on the product but let customers like hotels have their names printed on the rolls.[17]

CHAPTER TEN

GOING WEST FOR YOUR HEALTH

Medicine is a collection of uncertain prescriptions the result of which,
taken collectively, are more fatal than useful to mankind.

—Napoleon Bonaparte

EVEN BEFORE DR. DANIEL DRAKE of Cincinnati concluded in his 1850 classic work that there is a relationship between disease and one's environment, many people had already recognized the healthy benefits found in the western climates. Early French settlers on the upper Mississippi and Missouri rivers often sent sick family members to live in the drier climate among the trappers of the plains and mountains. When trade with Santa Fe opened in the early 1820s, traders soon realized the benefits of sunshine and the dry high plains as they traveled the Santa Fe Trail. Fur traders and mountain men also recognized the healthful benefits of the West as early as the 1820s. The frontiersman Kit Carson would later write: "I can remember that during the whole period, not a single one of them [mountain men] ever died from disease."[1] William H. Ashley, one of the founders of the Rocky Mountain Fur Company, wrote in 1825, "I have not known at any time a single instance of bilious fever among them or any other disease prevalent in the settled parts of our country, except a few instances (and but very few) of slight fevers produced by colds or rheumatic affections.... Nor have we in the whole four years lost a single man by death except those who came to their end prematurely by being either shot or drowned."[2]

When the first American immigrants settled in Texas in the early 1820s, they found the climate very healthy compared to that of the Mississippi River Valley. Stephen Austin wrote in 1828: "The climate of Texas I deem to be decidedly superior in point of health and salubrity to any portion of North America in the same parallel. The margins of our rivers in common with all rivers of the world are somewhat subject to fever, ague, and other complaints incident to similar situations but I think that the practical experience of seven years justifies me in saying that the rivers of Texas are less liable to diseases than any river of the U.S. below latitude 36. Situations back from the rivers, or near the Coast, are remarkably healthy."[3]

Austin's observations and those of other early settlers in Spanish Texas spurred the migration to Texas of people depressed about the disease-ridden Mississippi River Valley. When Matthew C. Field headed west from New Orleans, he and his companions reported that they had benefited from the dry mountain air of New Mexico. In a letter published in the *Picayune* on November 7, 1843, Field observed that their health "was fine and flourishing." He added:

> I will prove to you personally, your readers severally, panacea concoctors collectively and all the doctors unequivocally, when I get home, that consumptives must no more 'sparkle, exhale' and go to Havana, but jump into dresses of deerskin, and trot off to the mountains. We are the fattest, greasiest set of truant rogues your liveliest imagination can call up to view.[4]

Dr. Sherman Goodwin, afflicted with tuberculosis, moved his family in 1849 from Burton, Ohio, to Victoria, Texas, where he recovered and practiced medicine until his death in 1884. Texas-bound invalids, many with tuberculosis, settled in the south-central Texas towns of Boerne, Fredericksburg, and Luling Springs. San Antonio became the "Sanitarium of the West." Although no records can be found to give us numbers, in all probability a majority of the countless health-seekers like Dr. Goodwin who headed west suffered from tuberculosis, or, as it was then called, consumption. During the early nineteenth century the medical world had not yet learned that tuberculosis is a chronic bacterial infection, primarily airborne, that most often affects the lungs. In fact, over the course of the nineteenth century, tuberculosis claimed more lives in America than any other disease.

As word spread that the West was healthier, health-seekers began heading toward the setting sun. One of them was Josiah Gregg, a native of Tennessee. Born in 1806, Gregg moved west to Illinois with his family at the age of three, and to Missouri when he was six. The family finally settled in Independence, near the western border of Missouri. Gregg was a sickly child confined to his home, where he found excitement in reading books. As a young man, he tried teaching, surveying, medicine, and finally law. By 1831, as Gregg later wrote, his "health had been gradually declining under a complication of chronic diseases, which defied every plan of treatment that the sagacity and science of my medical friends could devise. This morbid condition of my system, which originated in the familiar miseries of dyspepsia and its kindred infirmities, had finally reduced me to such a state . . . so debilitated as rarely to be able to extend my walks beyond the narrow precincts of my chamber. In this hopeless condition, my physicians advised me to take a trip across the Prairies, and, in the change of air and habits which such an adventure would involve, to seek that health which their science had failed to bestow."

Gregg joined a trading expedition bound for Santa Fe to see if he could regain his health. He took along an ample supply of goods for his comfort and well-being, but, as he wrote, "I was not long upon the prairies before I discovered that most of such extra preparations were unnecessary, or at least quite dispensable. A few knick-knacks, as a little tea, rice, fruits, crackers, etc., suffice very well for the first fortnight, after which the invalid is generally able to take the fare of the hunter and teamster." Gregg observed that the "climate of most parts of the Prairies is no doubt healthy in the extreme, for a purer atmosphere is hardly to be found." He added that most of the time he slept in the open air, "for the serene sky of the Prairies affords the most agreeable and wholesome canopy. The deleterious attribute of night air and dews, so dangerous in other climates, is but little experienced upon the high plains, on the contrary, the serene evening seems to affect the health rather favorably than otherwise."

On this, his first journey west, Gregg worked as a bookkeeper for Jesse Sutton, a trader. He not only mastered the trading practices and the Spanish language but fell in love with the plains and prairies, where the warm if not hot sun and the pure, invigorating air quickly restored his strength and health. He was able to ride horseback by the time the wagon train reached the buffalo range in what is now central Kansas. When the expedition arrived in New Mexico, he described its climate as having a most interesting character. "Nowhere—not even under the much boasted Sicilian skies, can a purer or more wholesome atmosphere be found. Bilious diseases—the great scourge of the valley of the

Mississippi—are here almost unknown. . . . Persons withered almost to mummies, are to be encountered occasionally, whose extraordinary age is only to be inferred from their recollection of certain notable events which have taken place in times far remote."[5]

Gregg's observations appear in his classic *Commerce of the Prairies* (1844), published in New York. His thoughts and perceptions on climate and disease so impressed Dr. Daniel Drake in Cincinnati that they were quoted extensively in Drake's *Treatise on the Principal Diseases of the Interior Valley of North America*, published about a decade later, after the Cincinnati doctor traveled as far west as Fort Leavenworth for the purpose of studying diseases. Dr. Drake concluded that health-seekers should follow any one of three routes west—the Oregon Trail, the Santa Fe Trail, or the Missouri River. He believed that a long journey over any one of these routes would be beneficial to sufferers of tuberculosis, dyspepsia, and chronic liver, bowel, spleen, and muscular disorders, not to mention hypochondriacs.[6]

Even before Drake's book was published, missionaries who traveled to Oregon Country in the 1840s praised the healthy climate of the Willamette Valley. While some no doubt embellished their claims to attract settlers, the climate was much better than many areas in the Mississippi Valley. Dr. Elijah White observed that after nine years' residence in the Willamette Valley, he believed it had the healthiest climate he had ever known, one with fewer deaths than on any frontier since the founding of America.[7]

Francis Parkman was another easterner who traveled a portion of the Oregon Trail in part to improve his poor health. He went only as far as Fort Laramie in 1846, but spent time touring the area. Setting out one morning to go hunting in the mountains, Parkman wrote: "The morning was a glorious one, and I was in better health than I had been at any time for the last two months." However, Parkman, who did not remain long in the West, soon returned east, following the Santa Fe Trail. While there were moments when the western climate made him feel better, his journey west did not correct his nervous debilitations. They continued to affect him throughout his life.[8]

When Americans first arrived in Spanish California, they immediately recognized the healthy benefits of the climate. One of the first to praise California was Antoine Robidoux, of the prominent Robidoux family in Missouri, which established a fur-trading empire stretching from Missouri to the Rocky Mountains. In 1826, the Robidoux family built a trading post on the site of modern St. Joseph, Missouri. It was there, fourteen years later, that Antoine Robidoux spoke to a gathering of people looking to settle in the West. He described the California he had seen as being "one of perennial spring and boundless fertility." When someone asked him if there was any fever or malaria there, he supposedly replied that there was only "one man in California that had ever had a chill there, and it was a matter of so much wonderment to the people of Monterey that they went eighteen miles into the country to see him shake."[9]

One man in the audience, John Bidwell, a schoolteacher at Westport, Missouri, later wrote that Robidoux's "description of the country made it seem like paradise." Having lost his Missouri farm, Bidwell saw his future on the Pacific coast, and in May led the first wagon train of immigrants to California. The numbers of those heading west for California and Oregon gradually increased, and included the Mormons—determined to find religious freedom, with many also looking for good health—who would make their homes in modern Utah.

By the mid-nineteenth century, many guidebooks to the West were citing the healthy benefits of western climates. One such guide was *The Kanzas Region*, written by Max Greene and published in New York in 1856. Even before Kansas Territory was established in 1854, Greene had traveled through the region and observed:

As to the emigrants' bugbear of fever and ague, there is some of that; but no danger of shaking to pieces. Moreover, ague, in the Far West is like cholera in the city; You hear most of it at a distance. . . . There is a vitality in the atmosphere that is truly wonderful. As soon as you pass upon the upland swells . . . a newer life seems breathed around; and buoyancy and vigor is felt coming back to old limbs. Such was my experience; and hundreds have said to me [that] theirs was similar. Progressing westward, farther from the distressing humidity of the Mississippi region, there was to me a hopefulness, an elation in the very sense of being: an effluence which pulsed through the frame of nature, and, at times, would thrill every fibre of my body like the deep joy which penetrates the heart of a child. This is to some, the exaggerated or senseless talk of an enthusiast. And, should my reader go out from the foetid breath of the multitude, and inhale that thin, wholesome air, he might know again the elasticity of youthfulness, and be an enthusiast too.[10]

The Civil War no doubt reduced the number of health-seekers going west, but when Maurice O'Connor Morris, an Englishman visiting America, traveled west from St. Louis to Denver in 1863, he wrote: "I was greatly struck by the different appearances of the faces here from the eastern visages I had just left. There, dyspepsia or the affects of fever and ague, or consumption, were too plainly written to be ignored by any passerby, on a very large percentage of the population; here I see nothing but health visable [sic]."[11]

Following the Civil War, Samuel Bowles, editor of the *Springfield* (Massachusetts) *Republican*, made a stagecoach trip across the continent in 1865 and found several very healthful areas in the West. He was so overwhelmed with Colorado (then still a territory) that he predicted it would one day become the Switzerland of America, after the Pacific railroad was finished so that everyone could discover it. Bowles described the territory as the "fountain of health," and added that "among these hills and plains is surely to be many a summer resort for the invalid and the pleasure-seeker."[12]

A year later Albert D. Richardson, another eastern journalist, went west and was also impressed with the healthful conditions he found. He wrote: "I have seen a lady ill with typhoid fever, and barely able to sit up, travel across the plains, and reach the end of an unintermitting stage journey of seven days and nights, with the roses restored to her check and vigor in her frame. I once knew a resident of Eastern Kansas, pronounced dying with consumption, who started on the long jaunt. Too weak to sit erect, he was placed upon a featherbed in an ox-wagon, sleeping in the open air every night, and when, after fifty days, he reached the Rocky Mountains, he was enjoying comfortable health."[13]

These are only a few of the countless testimonies about the benefits of the climate in many areas of the West. Such accounts increased dramatically after the transcontinental railroad between Omaha and Sacramento was completed in 1869. Just as Samuel Bowles had predicted, the railroads made it easy for health-seekers to travel to southern California. The completion of the Kansas Pacific Railroad from Kansas City, Missouri, to Denver in 1870 made travel to Colorado simple as well. General William J. Palmer, a Philadelphian by birth, who was responsible for building the last leg of the railroad from western Kansas to Denver, was fascinated by the Rocky Mountains and traveled along the Front Range. He foresaw the possibility of creating a north–south system of railroads to cover the region. He also was impressed with the medicinal properties of iron and soda in the springs near the entrance to Ute Pass below Pikes Peak. Palmer organized the Denver and Rio Grande Railway Company, which ran from Denver south to what is now Colorado Springs, a town that was born in 1871. A few months later, on New Year's Day 1872, the Colorado Springs Hotel opened, and rapid development followed as promoters distributed pamphlets describing the healing properties of the climate and the mineral waters at Colorado Springs and at what became the nearby community of Manitou Springs.

The belief that the mineral spring waters were beneficial to health can be traced to the Ute, Arapaho, Cheyenne, and Kiowa Indians who visited Manitou Springs long before whites arrived. In fact, the area was neutral ground for these tribes, a place where they could relieve their ailments without fear of their enemies. Because the Indian diet was usually hard on their digestive tracts, the soda water in the springs was a tonic. It also improved dry skin. Whites learned of the mineral waters early in the nineteenth century, when Dr. Edwin James visited the area and wrote of the waters' health benefits. Colonel A. G. Boone, Daniel Boone's grandson, visited the spring in 1833 and may have been the first white cure-seeker. But it apparently was Dr. William A. Bell, an English adventurer traveling with General Palmer, who recognized the commercial value of the springs. When Colorado Springs was founded, the springs were first called La Fonte. It may have been William Blackmore, an English friend of Dr. Bell, who suggested the spring be given the more romantic-sounding name of Manitou, possibly borrowed from Henry Wadsworth Longfellow's poem *Hiawatha*. The name was changed to Manitou Springs about 1872.

By 1880, 30,000 invalids and tourists were visiting the area, including a large number of wealthy and educated persons hopeful of finding renewed health and seeking pleasure. The early 1880s also saw large numbers of poor people, many suffering from tuberculosis, who traveled to the region in their wagons and camped in groves of trees on the plains near Colorado Springs.

In 1883, after the Antlers Hotel was constructed in Colorado Springs, promoters widely distributed more pamphlets describing the

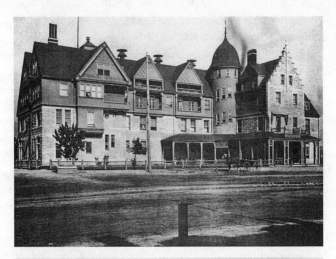

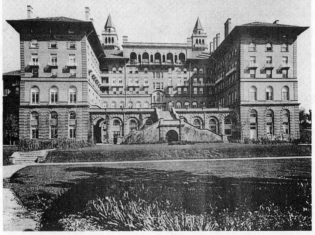

To provide health-seekers with luxury accommodations, the first Antlers Hotel (top) was built in the early 1880s in Colorado Springs. After a fire destroyed the hotel in 1898, a larger Antlers was built (bottom). In 1964 this second Antlers was razed, and a third, more modern hotel built in its place. (Courtesy Pikes Peak Library District)

health advantages of the region. It was in the Antlers Hotel in 1893 that a visiting English professor from the East, Katharine Lee Bates, wrote a poem in four stanzas after climbing to the top of Pikes Peak one day. Two years later, the poem was published and set to music as "America the Beautiful."

Of the large numbers of invalids who arrived, many were unfortunately too far gone to recover. Others never reached Colorado. Augustus A. Hayes, Jr., a native of Vermont and a chemist, toured the West, including Colorado, and wrote in 1880, "Multitudes of people in the valley of the Mississippi are slowly dying within two days' ride of perfect health. . . . Compared with other portions of the United States, the whole New West is a sanitorium."[14]

Many physicians believed this, including Denver's Dr. Charles Denison, another Vermont native, who came west seeking better health and found it. He was the first doctor to develop a formal, systematic study of climatic effects on chronic disease, including the gathering of statistics relating to all climates. Dr. Denison also proposed a "Climatic Association" made up of doctors who could advise patients which climate was best for them. The organization became a reality in 1884, eleven years after he proposed it. As it turned out, the most important climatic factor was the air. If it was pure and free of dust, pollen, and moisture, it was thought not to contain noxious vapors common in the Mississippi Valley. But, although there was a general acceptance of climatic therapeutics, many if not most physicians never took the time to understand the principles of climatology. Many doctors did not take the time to investigate carefully the benefits of one area as against another before directing their patients to this or that particular location in the West.

One physician who supported Dr. Denison's position was Dr. Samuel E. Solly, London-born and -educated, who had made Colorado Springs, Colorado, his home. He labeled those areas of Colorado between 4,500 and 8,000 feet along the east side of the Rocky Mountains as the "Invalid Belt." Dr. Solly, who served as president of the American Climatological Association in the 1880s, wrote *A Handbook of Medical Climatology* in 1899, which examined climate and its relationship to health and listed the major health resorts of the world. Solly, however, concentrated heavily on the Rocky Mountains and the Pacific slope in the United States and ignored many already estab-

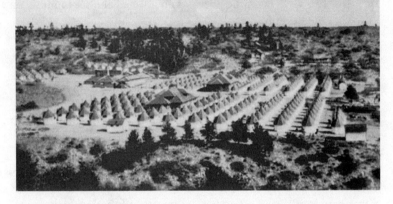

Modern Woodmen of America Sanitarium.
Twelve miles Northwest of
Colorado Springs, Colo.

In the early twentieth century, when the dry climate of Colorado was being promoted as beneficial for people with tuberculosis, the Modern Woodmen of America established this sanitarium twelve miles northwest of Colorado Springs. At the height of its operation the sanitarium employed 155 people and had 245 patients housed in Gardner tent-huts. It offered free board, lodging, treatment, medicine, dental care, and laundry to anyone who could travel to Colorado. This photo was copied from an early-twentieth-century postcard in the collection of Mark L. Gardner of Cascade, Colorado.

lished eastern health resorts such as Bedford Springs and Glen Summit in Pennsylvania.

When Dr. Solly's book was published, he was in Europe, but in 1900 he returned to Colorado Springs, then a city of 25,000, where he wrote in a letter: "Thank God we are now beginning to turn from drugs to the methods of nature for the cure of our patients. In the treatment of tuberculosis in this city the best doctors give very few drugs & do not believe in any of the specific treatments such as creasate [*sic*] & tuberculin but trust to keeping our patients when they will allow us both day & night in the open air & giving them all the nourishing food, largely meat, which they can digest. Its first & always when fever is present rest & then cautiously increasing exercise stopping short of actual fatigue."[15]

By then Saratoga Springs, New York, with its cold springs, and White Sulphur Springs, West Virginia, with its hot springs, were the

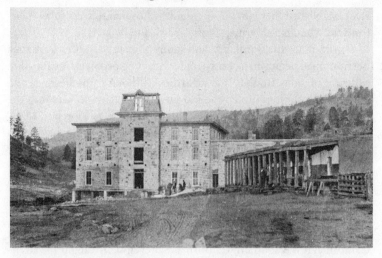

The Montezuma Hotel, built by the Atchison, Topeka and Santa Fe Railroad west of Las Vegas, New Mexico, about 1880. The hotel was located near mineral springs believed to have health-giving properties. It was destroyed by fire in 1884, but rebuilt, only to burn again in 1885; it was rebuilt yet again in 1886. The hotel remained a popular resort until it closed in 1903. (Courtesy Western History Collections, University of Oklahoma Libraries)

leading eastern resorts. In the West, Colorado was not alone in having mineral springs plus a dry climate beneficial to people with tuberculosis. After the Atchison, Topeka and Santa Fe Railroad built its line southwest across Kansas into New Mexico, it constructed the Queen Anne–style Montezuma Hotel west of Las Vegas, New Mexico, near the hot springs. But the hotel was destroyed by fire in 1884. Quickly rebuilt, it burned again in 1885, and was rebuilt once more in 1886, remaining a popular resort hotel until it closed in 1903.

Other communities in New Mexico Territory also attracted health-seekers. Albuquerque offered good hotels for them, and Silver City had a few private health resorts. Many tuberculars liked the warm, dry, and relatively sunny winter days in New Mexico, but the state never attained the reputation of the Colorado Springs area, in part because of high winds and sandstorms in late winter and early spring. In 1899, three years after the U.S. Army decommissioned Fort Stanton, New Mexico, the Marine Health Service (later the U.S. Public Health Service) established there on the site the first hospital to treat tuberculars from the Merchant Marine, Coast Guard, and Navy.*

By the 1870s the warm, dry, and sunny climate of southern Arizona Territory had begun attracting people with lung problems, asthmatics, sufferers of sinus trouble, and arthritics. Although Apache raids and poor transportation limited the movement of health-seekers into the territory to some degree, many still found their way to Florence, Maricopa Wells, and Yuma. Later, Tucson and Phoenix became major centers attracting invalids, some of whom moved to the dry and cooler portions of northern Arizona during the hot summers. By the early 1890s, physicians in the territory were claiming southern Arizona as "the finest winter climate of any section of the North American Continent."[16]

While the gold rush of 1849 attracted many people to northern California, it was southern California that eventually caught the attention of health-seekers, and by the 1870s they were being avidly welcomed there. During the next twenty years, communities like Los Angeles, Santa Barbara, San Bernardino, and San Diego were populated by countless people who had come to improve their health. The first tourist hotel in southern California was the Arlington, which opened at Santa Barbara in 1874, but few visitors stayed there until after the Southern Pacific Railroad completed its coast line in 1903 between San Francisco and Los Angeles. The same railroad, however, built the first of the great western resorts in 1880—the Hotel del Monte, located at the southern end of Monterey Bay, which opened in 1880. Next, the Santa Fe Railroad built the Raymond Hotel at Pasadena in 1886. Its proprietor was Walter Raymond, a native of New England. His hotel staff, after working the summer season in the White Mountains of New England, would move to Pasadena for the winter season, from November to May. Two years after the Raymond opened, the Hotel del Coronado at San Diego was completed, but, as

*The origin of the Public Health Service can be traced to an act in 1798 providing for the care and relief of sick and injured merchant seamen. A network of hospitals was established in 1870. Late in the nineteenth century, the Marine Hospital Service was responsible for the control of infectious diseases. Its name was changed to the Public Health and Marine Hospital Service in 1902, and was shortened to Public Health Service in 1912. The state of New Mexico took over Fort Stanton in 1952 and operated it as a sanitarium until 1967, when tuberculosis had all but disappeared in the United States.

with other large resort hotels in California, only wealthy health-seekers could afford to visit them.

By the 1880s, physicians were debating the comparative health benefits of the climates of coastal southern California and the central Rocky Mountains. Some doctors looked at the coastal areas of California as suitable only for a limited number of tubercular cases because of the often high humidity and coastal fog, which frequently blocked the warm sun. To the east in the California foothills, however, the climate was generally temperate and dry. Not surprisingly, physicians in California favored the climate in their region, while doctors in the central Rocky Mountains believed their climate was more healthful. Dr. Samuel Solly at Colorado Springs defended the elevated climate of Colorado while criticizing southern California's relative high humidity. Dr. Charles Denison of Denver also supported Colorado, and especially the state's mineral spring waters. Of Manitou Springs, Denison wrote in 1880, "These springs, with their picturesque surroundings and tonic atmosphere, yearly attracted many invalids to Manitou, which has rapidly gained favor, both as a summer and a winter resort."[17]

The medicinal benefits of the mineral spring waters in Colorado and New Mexico were analyzed. Alkaline waters were thought effective against respiratory, genito-urinary, malarial, and diabetic afflictions. Waters with a high salt content were thought beneficial in treating scrofula, syphilis, gout, malaria, and catarrhal infections. Water containing sulfur was thought helpful in treating skin, liver, and respiratory diseases, and, in combination with chalybeate (ferrous and carbonic acid) solutions, for blood deficiencies such as anemia and chlorosis. And waters containing calcic along with lime or gypsum were believed beneficial in treating dyspepsia, cystitis, and diabetes. Thermal waters, with or without chemical agents, were thought helpful to persons suffering from gout, rheumatism, paralysis, and certain skin eruptions.[18]

While physicians in the central Rocky Mountains, California, and elsewhere in the West continued into the late nineteenth century to promote the healthful benefits of their mineral waters and climate, the science of medicine was advancing. In 1896, at the annual meeting of the American Climatological Association, held that year in Philadelphia, Dr. James B. Walker presented the results of a decade-long study on climate and disease. He shattered the view that climate had a direct influence on health, and relegated therapeutic climatology to the status of a pseudo-science. Walker noted the study's conclusion that climate is not a fixed entity and that there was no way to identify elements of it that directly affect health. He added that too many physicians had failed to take sufficient time to understand what benefits existed, if any, in different geographical climates; too many patients had simply been sent west with no grounds for believing that any particular destination would be beneficial for their condition. The outcome of the study was that doctors were encouraged to give more attention to the study of microorganisms that cause specific diseases while generally stressing good hygiene, diet, and lifestyle over climate alone. Harvard professor Robert Ward, the first president of the American Meteorological Society, later wrote that the change in beliefs emphasized "pure air, good food, freedom from worry, time for rest, proper exercise, outdoor life and a congenial occupation. . . . Climate is by no means discarded as of no account . . . some climates are naturally avoided; others are sought out. The choice of a suitable climate must depend upon the disease to be dealt with and upon the individual concerned."[19]

During the latter half of the nineteenth century, many health-seekers settling in the West became merchants, teachers, clergymen, politicians, lawyers, and artists who made important contributions. In the early 1890s, Charles Schreyvogel, a New York artist, became so ill he could no longer paint. His doctors kept advising him to go west, where the air was drier. After meeting William F. "Buffalo Bill" Cody on an eastern visit, Schreyvogel began sketching cowboys, horses, and Indians. In 1893 he made his first trip west at the invitation of Dr. Thomas McDonald, post surgeon at the Ute Indian reservation in Colorado. During five months in Colorado and Arizona, he sketched, became an excellent rider, and learned Indian sign language, and his health improved. He returned to New York, where he was married in 1894. Between 1895 and 1900, the Schreyvogels made four more trips to the West, including Montana and Dakota Territory. By the early 1900s, as western art began to sell, it attracted the attention of President Theodore Roosevelt, who earlier had himself gone to Dakota Territory to improve his health. Roosevelt invited Schreyvogel to the White House for lunch in 1903. After the artist's painting titled *Custer's Demand* won the bronze medal at the St. Louis World's Fair Exposition in 1905, he was able to leave eastern city congestion and buy a farm at West Kill in upstate New York. There he lived until his death at age fifty-one in 1912.

As the twentieth century began, the myth that anyone could find perfect health in the West was being shattered. A German physician, Dr. Robert Kock, had discovered the bacterial cause of tuberculosis in 1882, and doctors in America had come to realize that social and economic factors were contributing factors in the lives of those contracting the disease, which could be spread by physical contact. Climate was no longer considered a major factor in controlling tuberculosis. New treatment methods included isolating patients in sanitariums where good sanitation and hygiene were practiced and proper diets were provided. New sanitariums were established and could be found nearer patients' homes and families.

When the operators of health resorts in the West heard that tuberculosis spread through human contact, many of them discouraged health-seekers from coming west for cures. In fact, some western states that had earlier urged invalids to visit them realized that health-seekers' dollars were no longer necessary. Local economies had grown rapidly and were now largely self-sufficient. Unfortunately, the contributions made by health-seekers who helped to populate and settle many areas of the West were forgotten. At the same time, the myth of western climate persisted in the minds of many people who either ignored or refused to believe scientific findings. During the early twentieth century countless numbers of people continued to head west, some at the recommendation of their doctors, to enjoy the watering holes and the pleasure of spending time in the dry mountain air of the Rocky Mountains or the warm climate on the Pacific coast.

CHAPTER ELEVEN

MIDWIVES AND WOMEN DOCTORS

A merry heart does good like medicine.

—Proverbs 17:22

THE SCENE IS AN American Indian camp somewhere on the southern plains in the nineteenth century. An Indian woman in labor is about to deliver her child. Tribal members have built an enclosure of bushes near a stream some distance from their lodges. Inside the temporary enclosure two stakes have been placed in the ground and a hole dug next to each stake. Soft earth fills one hole while hot stones fill the other. As the expectant mother's labor intensifies, she grabs hold of the stakes, one hand on each, and holds tightly to them as she squats over the hot stones. When she begins to discharge fluids, she shifts her body over the hole containing the soft earth that absorbs the liquids. Still squatting and holding tightly on to the stakes, she delivers her baby with the help of one or more Indian midwives.

Although Indian history was oral before the arrival of the white man, it is known that Indians used midwives long before Europeans brought the practice to North America. Midwives' duties, however, varied from tribe to tribe. Some plains tribes preferred to use family lodges for labor. Male family members left when birth was about to occur. Occasionally a man with a gun stood outside the lodge and fired a shot on signal to frighten the expectant mother. Sometimes the noise expedited delivery. Eric Stone, a doctor who spent many years researching Indian medicine, wrote in 1932 that in labor

the Utes, Navajo, Apache and Nez-Perces assumed a semi-recumbent position. The Crow and the Assiniboine knelt, resting the head against a support, while a midwife pressured in the lumbar region during the pains. The Brule-Sioux and Warm Spring Indians stood throughout labor. Delivery occurred with the woman kneeling, but she stood to deliver the placenta. In other tribes, this stage took place in bizarre fashion. The Coyotero Apache bound the woman to a tree as soon as labor began, with her hands tied to a branch above her head, and there she remained until labor was over. The Winnebago and Chippewa knelt over a bar, over which the woman was dragged belly down, in case of a difficult delivery. The Creeks lay prone with a pillow strapped to the epigastrium [the abdominal wall above the navel], as labor progressed the strap was tightened.

Dr. Stone added that as a rule Indian babies were much smaller than white or "half-breed" babies. Having small babies meant that Indian mothers were usually spared "the long train of post-partum disorders to which the white mother is prone. . . . Labor was relatively short, seldom lasting more than three hours, and was supposed to have been but slightly painful."[1]

The practice of midwifery has existed through most of the world since the beginning of recorded history. The Book of Genesis, 35:17, and the Book of Exodus, 1:20, mention midwives. The ancient Jews

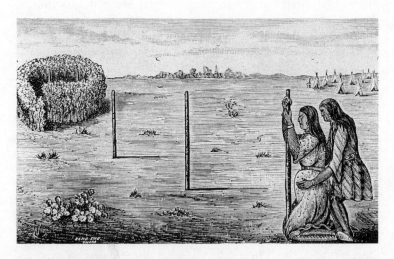

This sketch made (circa 1880) by Major W. H. Forwood, a surgeon in the U.S. Army, shows a pregnant Comanche woman in labor leaning on a post. As the time for delivery got nearer, she would move from post to post until she moved into the enclosure where she would give birth. (Courtesy National Library of Medicine)

called a midwife a "wise woman." The root meaning of the English word *midwife* is "with woman." Midwives were known for their knowledge and skill in an area of life that was a mystery to most people; sometimes they were thought to possess magical or mystical abilities. Written history suggests that many were revered, but others were feared, and sometimes tortured and killed. The first person executed in the Massachusetts Bay Colony was Margaret Jones, a midwife accused of witchcraft, in 1648. More than two decades earlier, a midwife named Brigit Lee Fuller, the twenty-year-old wife of Dr. Samuel Fuller, delivered three babies aboard the sailing ship *Anne* before it arrived in 1623 at what is now Plymouth, Massachusetts. Her husband had come to America nearly three years earlier, arriving aboard the *Mayflower* as the colony's doctor.

During the colonial period, the natural event of birthing was attended only by women, with the oversight of the midwife, who was highly respected in the community. In fact, in the colony of Massachusetts, midwives received special privileges when using ferry boats to reach expectant mothers. No one knows how many women served as midwives in colonial America and most left few records of their work, but the diary of Martha Moore Ballard provides many insights into their craft. Martha was born in the central Massachusetts town of Oxford in 1735. When she was nineteen, she married Ephraim Ballard, a millwright. Between 1756 and 1779, Ephraim and Martha had nine children. About 1777 the Ballards moved to the village of Hallowell in present-day Maine, where in 1785, at age fifty, she began keeping a diary. Although she makes no mention of abortion, she indicates that births out of wedlock were common. She describes how she cared for expectant mothers, often using home remedies. For instance, she grew coriander and chamomile in her garden and used household staples and garden vegetables medicinally. In 1810 she noted in her diary that she made a turnip poultice for a young woman named Elisa and applied it to her bowels, which soon gave relief. When an epidemic of scarlet fever struck Hallowell in 1787, Martha Ballard nursed many victims with much compassion, probably because she had lost three of her children in an earlier epidemic in 1769. Between 1785 and her death in 1812, she delivered 816 babies and lost only 5 mothers and 20 babies. Late in her life, she observed that the practice of medicine was changing. Patent medicines were plentiful and sold in most towns, and doctors were entering the field of midwifery.[2]

Before the American Revolution, childbirth was the exclusive responsibility of midwives, who were expected to offer encouragement and reassurance to women in labor. Once the baby was born, the midwife tied off the umbilical cord, made sure the placenta was expelled, and gave after-care to the mother and child. Most births were normal and uneventful, but when a birth became difficult or the labor lengthy, the midwife just did the best she could, or she might call in a more experienced midwife for help. Most midwives were unschooled, and learned their craft by observation and personal experience, because women were not permitted to receive formal medical training. That was a privilege reserved for men, but the traditions of the time barred male doctors from helping in childbirth. Ingrained notions of modesty and delicacy forbade men to enter the room where a woman was in labor.

All of this began to change about 1770. Upper-class women in colonial towns like Boston and Philadelphia began to call on medical doctors trained in midwifery (later called obstetrics) to deliver their babies. Such doctors were called *accoucheurs*, and women who used them believed these male doctors could make labor less painful and dangerous. They had received their training in Europe, since formal medical schooling was lacking in the colonies, and they were taught that childbirth should be a medically managed function handled by trained physicians and not a social activity for women to perform. The physicians, of course, were to receive compensation for such services.

One early American doctor with European training in midwifery was Walter Channing, who was born into a prominent Newport, Rhode Island, family in 1786. Channing entered Harvard College in 1805 to study medicine, but was expelled two years later for protesting against the inferior food being served to students. Determined to become a doctor, Channing apprenticed himself to Dr. James Jackson of Boston for a time and then went to Philadelphia, where he received his medical degree in 1809 at the University of Pennsylvania. Channing then studied in Edinburgh and London, where he focused on the study of midwifery. When he returned to Boston in 1811, he practiced general medicine but soon was delivering babies for upper-class women. Within a few years, Channing became professor of midwifery and medical jurisprudence at Harvard while he continued to practice medicine in Boston. When he was called to deliver a baby in the home of an expectant mother, he was, more often than not, meeting his patient for the first time. The woman would be fully clothed in loose garments, and Dr. Channing would pay strict attention to the rules of decorum by avoiding eye contact with his patient during examination and delivery. He also was very careful not to say anything that might seem indelicate.[3]

Channing and other doctors who had received midwifery training in Europe delivered babies chiefly for upper-class families of Boston and other urban areas along the East Coast. However, poor Americans, including blacks and immigrants in cities and rural areas, continued to rely on midwives as the nation was moving into the nineteenth century. Once medical schools began to appear in the new nation, the idea that only doctors (necessarily male) were qualified to deliver babies was increasingly taught. The idea gradually spread with the westward movement across the Appalachians, where doctors were practicing in larger communities. Some women did turn to male physicians to deliver their babies, but others complained that the doctor charged $10 or $20 for a normal delivery and more for difficult labors. Many women therefore ignored male doctors and continued to call upon midwives when they went into labor. Doctors in rural communities who had little training in midwifery did not object.

As medical schools grew in number by the late nineteenth century, however, more and more trained physicians sought to control the territory dominated by midwives. The medical profession worked to control if not eliminate midwives by getting lawmakers in many states to require that anyone attending a woman in labor have formal medical training and be licensed. Since women were not permitted to receive training in many medical schools, they could not qualify for licenses. Still, in many rural areas, where physicians were scarce, women ignored such laws and continued beyond World War II to answer calls to help with birthing.[4]

The names of most midwives have been lost in time, but the accounts of some exist. One revealing journal is that of Patty Bartlett Sessions, born in 1795 at Bethel, Maine. In 1847, she and her husband—both Mormons—headed for the "promised land." Between June 25 and December 13 of that year, they followed the Oregon Trail part of the way west from what is now Omaha, Nebraska, and then turned southwest at Fort Bridger to Great Salt Lake City. During this period, "Mother Sessions," as she was known, delivered 14 babies, 7 girls and 7 boys. She was then fifty-two years old. During her lifetime she reportedly delivered 3,977 babies and lost very few. She became known as the "Mother of Mormon Midwifery."[5]

When news spread in 1846 that Dr. Channing in Boston was using anesthesia in childbirth, many midwives voiced opposition to the practice and said it was not needed, that birthing should be natural. Even some doctors in eastern cities questioned the safety of anesthesia, and many members of the clergy condemned its use, calling it a transgression of God's judgment upon Eve, citing Genesis 3:16—"in pain shalt thou bring forth children." Dr. Channing, however, saw no reason why women should submit to suffering when medicine could free women from pain in childbirth.

Dr. Channing and other physicians trained in midwifery believed they were best suited to bring children into the world. Most of them also believed that the proper place to deliver babies was in a hospital. Efforts to eliminate the use of midwives grew during the nineteenth

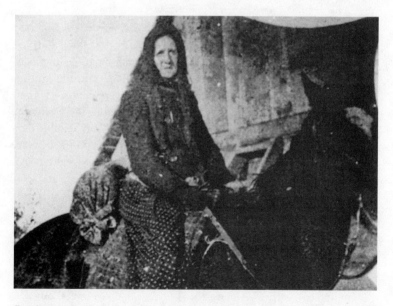

Josephine Catherine Chatterly Wood arrived in Bluff, Utah, in 1882. Since she had some nursing experience, the local Mormon bishop persuaded her to serve as a midwife. She purchased all the books she could on the subject, and became one of the leading midwives of southern Utah, known familiarly to one and all as "Aunt Judy." (Courtesy Utah State Historical Society)

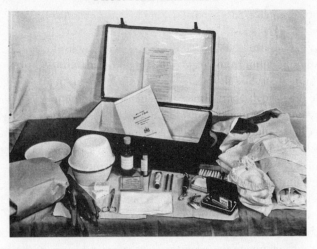

The contents of a typical midwife's kit (circa the 1920s), spread out on a table. They include bowls, apron, baby sheet, cotton, bulb syringe, sutures and needles, syringes, scissors, sanitary napkins, soap, bandages, gauze, and a thermometer. (Courtesy National Library of Medicine)

century as doctors emphasized the woman's traditional place in society. These male doctors stressed that they were trained in using innovations in technology and insisted that such things were exclusively their province. They asserted their dominance in the field by increasing the use of forceps, pioneered by the Scottish doctor William Semillie during the 1800s. Many doctors claimed that forceps aided in the delivery of the fetus by applying traction to the baby's head. Doctors also began almost routinely to use anesthesia in assisted deliveries, and episiotomy, a surgical cut made just before delivery in the muscular area between the vagina and the anus to enlarge the vaginal opening.

One Kentucky doctor clearly stated this view in 1844. Dr. John Bright of Louisville (whose life and career have already been covered in Chapter Three) wrote in his 792-page medical guide for mothers:

The forceps, vectic, perforators, and hook, as well as several other instruments are sometimes indispensably necessary in particular cases of labor, and under peculiar conditions both of mother and of child. To give a full and complete description of the case necessary for their use, and the manner of applying them, in all the circum-

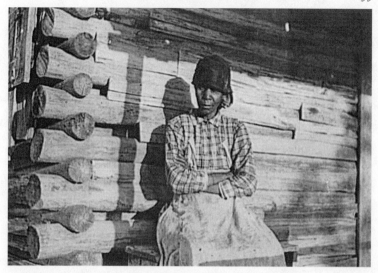

Midwives continued to deliver babies in many rural areas and small towns during the first half of the twentieth century. "Aunt Sally," shown in this 1939 photo, served not only as a midwife; for her patients in Gees Bend, Alabama, she was the only medical practitioner they ever saw. Photograph by Marion Post Wolcott. (Courtesy Library of Congress)

stances in which it would be proper to use them, would occupy a small volume; and, as no midwife in this country would be capable of using them, a doctor must necessarily be sent for when the use of instruments is required. We shall, therefore, omit that part of practical midwifery.[6]

Midwives did not relinquish control of their realm voluntarily. They pointed out that female midwives and women in general were denied medical education and thus not taught the use of new technology, especially medical instruments to ease labor or to diagnose women's problems. Without much fanfare, some women sought formal education in medicine. Oberlin College in Ohio, founded in 1835, was the first U.S. college to accept both women and black students. The first woman to graduate from a U.S. medical school, however, did not come from Oberlin but a college in upper New York State. She was Elizabeth Blackwell, who was born in England and educated by a private tutor. In 1832 she and her parents moved to America, and the family eventually settled in Cincinnati. After her father died, Elizabeth's mother opened a private school to support the family. Elizabeth became interested in medicine and determined to become a physician. She believed that women would prefer to consult with a woman and not a man about their health problems. To make a living, Elizabeth became a teacher in Kentucky and in North and South Carolina. She read medical books in her spare time. In 1847, she applied to all of the leading medical schools in the East but was rejected by every one of them. She then applied to Geneva Medical College (now Hobart College) in Geneva, New York. There the administration asked the students to decide whether to admit her. The students, apparently believing her application was a practical joke, endorsed the application.

When Elizabeth arrived in Geneva, students and townspeople were astonished to find that her application was not a joke. She was admitted but shunned by nearly everyone, and was even kept from observing

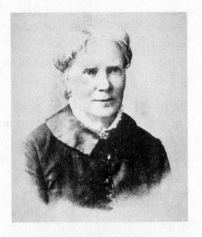

English-born Elizabeth Blackwell (1821–1910) was the first woman to graduate from a U.S. medical school. She came to America with her parents in 1832, and the family settled in Cincinnati. She first became a teacher in Kentucky before applying to Geneva Medical College (now Hobart College) in Geneva, New York. She graduated at the top of her class in January 1849. (Courtesy The Schlesinger Library, Radcliffe Institute, Harvard University)

medical demonstrations in the classroom because they were not thought appropriate for women. Her ability and persistence, however, soon impressed her fellow students, and in January 1849 she graduated at the top of her class. In ceremonies held at the Presbyterian church in Geneva, she received her Doctor of Medicine diploma, the first woman to graduate from a U.S. medical school.

With her degree in hand, Dr. Blackwell decided to study in Europe, first in England and then in Paris, where she took a course in midwifery. While there, however, she suffered a serious eye infection that left her blind in one eye. Abandoning her plans to become a surgeon, she returned to London, where she met and became friends with Florence Nightingale, a pioneer of nursing and a reformer in hospital sanitation methods. Dr. Blackwell returned to New York in 1851 and tried to set up a medical practice. But she was refused office space, and hospitals and dispensaries denied her privileges. To start her private prac-

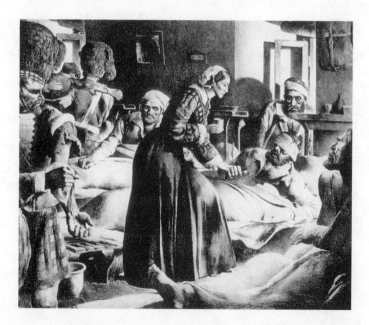

Florence Nightingale (1820–1910) was a pioneer in nursing and a reformer of sanitary conditions in English hospitals. Her achievements in Victorian times inspired many American women to enter nursing. (Courtesy National Library of Medicine)

tice, she purchased the house where she lived and set up an office there where she saw women and children. Two years later she opened a dispensary in the New York slums, where she was joined in her work by her sister Emily Blackwell after Emily had earned her medical degree. When not practicing medicine, Elizabeth lectured and wrote articles that enhanced her reputation as a female physician. She made a one-year lecture tour of England and in 1859, before returning to America, became the first woman to have her name on the British medical register. During the Civil War she and her sister helped to organize the Women's Central Association of Relief, which selected and trained nurses for the war. Their organization inspired the creation of the United States Sanitary Commission. Following the war, they opened the Women's Medical College at their New York City infirmary, which operated for thirty-one years. Toward the end of her life Elizabeth was appointed professor of gynecology at the London School of Medicine for Children. She died in England in 1910 from a serious fall.[7]

Elizabeth Blackwell received her medical degree at Geneva Medical College one year after the New England Female Medical College opened in Boston in 1848. The small school began to attract faculty and students, and between 1850 and 1874 it trained more than 280 students and granted ninety-eight medical degrees. One of the recipients was Rebecca Lee, the first black female doctor to receive a medical degree in the United States. In 1850, two years after the New England Female Medical College opened its doors, the Female Medical College of Pennsylvania (later the Women's Medical College of Pennsylvania) was founded in Philadelphia with six male professors. In 1870, the University of Michigan became the first state medical school to accept females. On the West Coast in 1876, the San Francisco Medical College of the Pacific accepted its first female student, Alice Boyle Higgins, who graduated in 1877 and went east for additional study at the Women's Medical College of Pennsylvania. In 1882, she returned to California to practice medicine. Married and with three children, she did not begin her medical training until age forty.

By 1880, there were 100 medical schools in the nation, with 11,826 students. The number of schools increased to 160 by 1903, with 27,615 students. By 1905, there were 8,201 female doctors practicing in the United States. Most were located in urban areas and most still experienced problems obtaining clinical experience because most hospitals, ambulances, and dissection rooms were not considered proper places for women. Many of these women doctors had no choice but to restrict their practices to caring for women and children. Rejected by most local medical societies, they were prevented from entering the mainstream of medicine. In many rural areas, however, they seem to have been more generally accepted by other physicians. Local history books contain countless biographies and stories about women doctors who made significant contributions to their communities without ever gaining national attention.

One such woman was Susan LaFlesche, the daughter of an Omaha Indian chief. Born in 1865 on the Omaha reservation in Nebraska, she spent her first fourteen years there before attending an institute for young ladies in New Jersey for three years. She returned to Nebraska and worked for two years on the Omaha reservation in a mission school. She then returned east to Virginia for more studies. The Women's National Indian Association then gave her funds to attend the Women's Medical College in Philadelphia. She graduated in 1889 at the top of her class and became the first female Indian physician to graduate from a medical school. In 1894, she married Henry Picotte and moved to Bancroft, Nebraska, where she established a private medical practice treating Indians and whites alike. After her husband died in 1905, she moved to Walthill on the Omaha reservation. There she became the county health officer and helped to organize a medical association. She next raised private money to establish the first hospital on the Omaha reservation, which opened in 1913. After her death in 1915, the hospital was named in her honor.[8]

Another little-known female doctor was Susan Anderson, known as "Doc Susie," born in Indiana in 1870. After graduating from the University of Michigan Medical College in 1897, she joined her family in Cripple Creek, Colorado, where she established a medical practice. Her father, however, thought a mining town was no place for a lady and encouraged her to move to Denver. She did, but was unable to overcome the local prejudice there against female doctors. The same was true when she moved to Greeley and later to Eaton, Colorado. She turned to nursing to make a living, only to contract tuberculosis. Moving to the mountain community of Fraser, Colorado, to cure the disease, she realized that the isolated community needed a doctor, and that the need for medical care in Fraser outweighed any local prejudice against women doctors. Anderson renewed her medical practice. Most of her patients were poor, but she treated anyone needing her services.

Her financial situation improved when she became a railroad doctor and coroner of Grand County, which gave her a regular income. She never became wealthy, nor did she own a horse or auto. Patients provided her transportation. She left her mark on Fraser and inspired many young girls to pursue goals higher than their mothers'. She died in a Denver rest home in 1960 at the age of ninety, and is buried at Cripple Creek.[9]

Another woman doctor of note in Colorado was Justina Laurena Carter Ford, the first black woman licensed to practice medicine in Denver. Born in 1871 near Galesburg, Illinois, she became interested in medicine at an early age. In 1899, she graduated from Herring Medical College in Chicago and first practiced in Normal, Alabama, before moving to Denver. Because Denver's hospitals denied her privileges, she specialized in women and children of all races, including those who were poor. During a career of fifty years she delivered more than 7,000 babies and was affectionately known as the "Lady Doctor" until her death in 1952.[10]

In Texas, another female doctor, Sofie Dalia, made her mark. She was born in 1846 in Austria, where her father was a doctor. At age fourteen, Sofie Dalia married another physician in Vienna, Dr. August Herzog, and they had fifteen children, including three sets of twins. Eight of the children died in infancy. In 1886, Sofie Herzog's husband accepted a position at the United States Naval Hospital in New York City, and the family moved to the United States. Sofie began to study medicine in New York and then returned to Austria to earn a medical degree from the University of Graz. Returning to the United States, she opened an office in Hoboken, New Jersey, and enjoyed a successful practice for nine years. After her husband died in 1895, she moved herself and her practice to Brazoria, Texas, where one of her daughters had married a merchant a year earlier. At first, residents were not quite sure what to think of a woman doctor, especially one whose hair was cut short, who wore a man's hat, and who wore a split skirt so she could ride horseback astride. But when residents realized her medical skills and dedication to her patients, she was soon accepted as a physician and called "Dr. Sofie." She established her office in a drugstore she purchased, where she made many of her own medicines, and across the street she had a hotel constructed which she called The Southern. It operated for many years. She became wealthy from real estate investments. Because shootings were common in the area, she became very skillful at removing bullets from patients. In time, she took twenty-four bullets she had removed from victims to a Houston jeweler and had them strung between gold links as a necklace. She wore the necklace as a good-luck charm for the rest of her life and had it placed in her coffin when she died.

When the St. Louis, Brownsville and Mexico Railway began laying track in South Texas early in the 1900s, Dr. Sofie was frequently called to treat ill and injured railway workers. She used any mode of transportation, including trains, handcars, and whatever else. When the job of chief surgeon for the railroad opened, she was hired, but when eastern officials of the line learned a woman had been given the job, they asked her to resign. She refused and told them that if she did not perform her tasks to their satisfaction, they could fire her. They never did. She remained with the railroad and continued her medical practice in Brazoria until a few months before her death at age seventy-nine in 1925.[11]

Nevada had its share of female doctors. There was Ruth E. Newland, who practiced in Virginia City in 1882. She received a degree from the Medical Eclectic College in Cincinnati. Another woman doctor was Hattie F. Atwater, who received her degree from Wooster Medical College in Cleveland before practicing in Carson City, also in 1882. The medical schools both women graduated from were not viewed by the medical profession at large as being very strong, requiring as they did only minimum training of one or two years. Catherine Nicholas Post, who practiced in Virginia City during the early 1880s, received her degree from the University of the Pacific Medical Department (later the Cooper Medical School) in 1879, a truly pioneering medical school with a professional faculty.[12]

The story of Lucy Hobbs Taylor is different. The seventh of ten children, she was born in Ellenburg, New York, in 1833. Orphaned at the age of twelve, she worked as a seamstress to support herself through school. By the time she graduated at age sixteen from Franklin Academy in Malone, New York, in 1849, she knew she wanted to be a doctor, but women were not admitted to medical schools. She turned to school teaching and found a job in Michigan, where she taught for ten years. She then moved to Cincinnati, Ohio, and sought admittance to the Eclectic College of Medicine. She was turned down, but even though she was now twenty-six she did not give up. She found a professor at the college who agreed to let her study medicine with him.

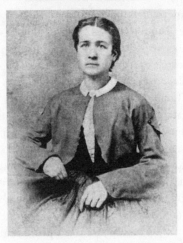

Lucy Hobbs Taylor (1833–1910) was born in Ellenburg, New York. She was a schoolteacher when she sought to enter a school of medicine in Cincinnati. Turned down, she began studying with a professor, who suggested she enter the field of dentistry, which she did. She opened her own practice at Cincinnati in 1861. A year later she moved to Iowa, where her male colleagues admired her work and helped her to enter the Ohio College of Dental Surgery. In 1866, she became the first woman in the United States to earn a doctorate in dentistry. She later married and spent the remainder of her life practicing dentistry in Lawrence, Kansas. (Courtesy Kansas State Historical Society)

Early in her studies, the professor suggested that Lucy consider dentistry and sought a dentist with whom she could apprentice. At the time prospective dentists had to serve an apprenticeship before applying to the handful of dental schools that existed. Unable to locate a dentist who would accept her as an apprentice, she again became a private pupil and studied under the dean of the Ohio College of Dental Surgery, and later apprenticed herself to a graduate of the college.

At age twenty-eight, she then opened her own practice in Cincinnati in 1861. The following year she moved her practice to Bellevue, Iowa, for a year and then to McGregor, Iowa, where she remained until 1865. There she became known as "the woman who pulls teeth." By then she had proven she was a worthy equal to any male dentist. The Iowa State Dental Society accepted her as a member and sent her as a delegate to the American Dental Association convention in Chicago. Her fellow Iowa delegates made a formal appeal at the convention for Lucy to be accepted into a dental college. They even threatened to boycott any college that refused to admit her. The Ohio College of Dental Surgery, where she had first been denied admittance, accepted her as a student. She was admitted to the senior class and because of her professional experience, she earned her degree within a few months and graduated in February 1866, becoming the first woman in the United States to earn a doctorate in dentistry.

She soon moved her practice to Chicago and there met and married, in 1867, a Civil War veteran and railroad maintenance worker, James M. Taylor. Under his wife's guidance, he also became a dentist. Late in 1867 the couple moved to Lawrence, Kansas, where they established a successful practice treating many women and children, who came to call her "Dr. Lucy." Following her husband's death in 1886, she retired from dentistry but remained active in civic and women's causes, including the suffrage movement. She gained recognition as a pioneer who had opened dentistry to women. By 1900, nearly a thousand women had entered dentistry. Lucy Hobbs Taylor died in 1910 at the age of seventy-seven. Years later the American Association of Women Dentists established the Lucy Hobbs Taylor Award, the organization's highest honor, recognizing women dentists who have contributed to the advancement, enrichment, and betterment of the role of women in the field of dentistry through their achievements in civic, cultural, humanitarian, and academic areas.[13]

Not all of the female doctors of the late nineteenth century had medical degrees. For instance, Amy M. Loucks was born in 1843 in Pennsylvania, where she received a good education and studied medicine and surgery with a brother who was a physician. After she married William P. Loucks in 1866, they moved to western Kansas in 1879 and settled in the tiny town of Lakin in ranching country. Lakin, located on the Santa Fe Railroad line, had no school, churches, or other trappings of civilization aside from the railroad depot, a restaurant, a saloon, and a general store operated by John O'Laughlin, which supplied ranchers, buffalo hunters, and travelers. The nearest doctor was located in Dodge City, seventy-five miles away. She came to know everyone in the area and gradually people came to her when they were sick or injured. One day a man who had been scalped by Indians and left on the prairie for dead was found and brought to Lakin. Amy Loucks was called. She found that the scalp had not been entirely removed but had been pulled down over the man's eyes. She replaced the scalp and re-attached it to the man's head using a fiddle string and common needle. She nursed him back to health, contacted his relatives in the East, and sent him to them. The man lived for many years, though he never fully regained his sanity. Another time a posse of lawmen asked her to treat a prisoner who had been shot. Using a small vial of carbolic acid as an antiseptic, a knitting needle as a probe, and a pair of common pincers, she removed the bullet and saved the man's life. Another time she was called by the railroad to deliver a baby. There was not enough time to take the expectant mother to her home, so Amy Loucks brought the baby into the world on a freight truck at the depot. When a train wreck near Lakin killed several people and injured many other passengers, she treated the injured until a special train carrying the railroad sur-geon arrived from Dodge City. The doctor was so impressed with her work that he got the railroad to give her a permanent pass on the line.[14]

Another woman doctor without a medical degree was Lillian Hath, who dressed like a man and carried pistols while she studied medicine with the only other doctor in Rawlins, Wyoming. She became the town's first obstetrician in 1893. In Palo Alto County, Iowa, where doctors were scarce during the late nineteenth century, Etta May Lacey Crowder learned medicine from a medical book brought from the East. It described treatments for numerous illnesses and injuries, as well as homemade medicines. Following instructions in the book, she made medicines from many wild plants, most of which were steeped in hot water and drunk as tea. Her tonics were made from the butterfly weed, sweet flag root, sassafras bark, and boneset. She used the dande-lion, both as extract and as wine, to help the liver. She insisted that everyone take sulfur and molasses each spring. To treat colds she made use of pennyroyal, prairie balm, and horse mint, and mullen was used externally for pleurisy. Smartweed was employed externally for boils, while cubeb berries were smoked to treat catarrh.

For more than thirty years, her neighbors counted on her for help. When an expectant mother was about to give birth, a neighbor would drive by and tell her when they wanted her, and she was always there. She never charged for her services, saying she was just trying to be a good neighbor. Neighbors, however, would sometimes give her things. One neighbor gave her a cream ladle and another a calico dress.[15]

WHILE, AS DISCUSSED ABOVE, some pioneering women gained admittance to some medical schools, proved their academic merit, and earned their medical degrees, in the late nineteenth century they constituted only about 5 percent of the more than 7,000 physicians then practicing in the nation. Many among that 5 percent found little support and experienced discrimination in urban areas especially. In rural areas, women doctors, because they often filled an urgent need, tended to enjoy a more favorable reception. During the early years of the twentieth century, there was a decline in women seeking to become doctors because of new positions for them in allied health fields such as nursing, public health, and social work. The closing or consolidation of medical colleges that had earlier accepted women, and high entrance requirements, may also have been partly responsible. Medicine itself was changing, becoming more scientific and less humanistic.

CHAPTER TWELVE

PATENT MEDICINES

*Folks with their wits about them knew that advertisements were just
a pack of lies—you had only to look at the claims of patent medicines!*

—Frances Parkinson Keyes

W HEN I WAS A BOY, my grandmother regularly gave me a dollar bill
to walk to a drugstore near my home in Manhattan, Kansas, to
purchase a bottle of "white medicine." When I got there and told the
pharmacist, a family friend, what she wanted, he would smile and go to
his back room. There it took the pharmacist about three minutes to
mix and bottle a chalky white liquid. He would then use his old manual
typewriter to prepare the drugstore's label, with the words *White Medicine* and the simple instructions—"Shake well. Take one teaspoon as
needed and then drink one full glass of water." Years later, I learned
that my grandmother's physician had arranged with the pharmacist to
mix for her this compound that was similar to milk of magnesia, a
saline-type laxative also recommended for heartburn or indigestion.
The doctor knew it was cheaper to have the pharmacist do this than for
her to buy the commercially produced Phillips' Milk of Magnesia—a
patent medicine first concocted by an English pharmacist, Charles
Henry Phillips (1820–1882), and still sold over the counter.

Patent medicines first appeared in England in the late 1600s when
the Crown issued letters patent for Anderson's Scots Pills. A letters
patent is a legal document, an open letter issued by a monarch granting
a right, title, monopoly, or status to someone or some entity. Anderson's Scots Pills, already mentioned in Chapter Two, were concocted
by a Scottish doctor, Patrick Anderson, who claimed he had obtained
the recipe in Venice. Anderson passed the formula to his daughter
Katherine, who in turn passed it to a doctor named Thomas Weir in
1686. Weir obtained letters patent on its contents from King James II
in 1687 and began manufacturing and selling it as a laxative. Because

Weir held the patent, no one else could duplicate his formula and sell it as a medicine. The patent holder, however, did not have to show proof of its effectiveness, but he did have to reveal the ingredients. Twenty-four years later, in 1711, Timothy Byfield patented the first compound medicine in England, *sal oleosum volatile*. It contained spirits of Hartshorne. Byfield claimed it cured gout. The recommended dosage was one teaspoon mixed in a glass of wine and taken at bedtime.[1]

In the history of medicine, patenting is significant. Before medicines were patented, people used home remedies, Indian cures, or medicines prepared by doctors who knew their patients. Patent or proprietary medicines, however, were concocted by individuals with little medical education and no knowledge of the people buying and using them. To sell them, however, the manufacturers had to promote them. They used newspaper advertisements, handbills, posters, pamphlets, and endorsements from those who had used the medicines. The more prominent the user, the better. The medicine makers also relied upon cash sales instead of the longtime practice of bartering for goods and services. While some manufacturers of pills, powders, cordials, and elixirs did patent them, others sought to keep the ingredients of their medicines secret and only registered their trademarks or the name of the creators.[2]

Elixirs were among the earliest medicines patented and endorsed by the Crown. Elixirs originated in the mysticism of ancient Greece. It was believed that they prolonged life, but the ingredients of many early elixirs were nothing more than sweetened aromatic water and alcohol. An early English elixir, mentioned in Chapter Two, was "Elixir Salutis: The Choise [*sic*] Drink of Health or, Health-bringing Drink, Being a Famous Cordial Drink." It was concocted by Anthony Daffy, an English clergyman, who had a pamphlet printed and distributed to promote his product. Daffy said it could be taken for gout, kidney and bladder stones, languishing and melancholy, shortness of breath, tuberculosis, scurvy, dropsy, rickets, pestilence, ague, and the "king's evil," a tubercular infection of the lymph glands in the throat. Daffy added that his elixir was a "pleasant inoffensive Drink" that he believed safe to give to his wife when she was expecting a child, and to their newborn baby. It contained aniseed (anise), fennel seed, parsley seed, Spanish liquorice, senna, rhubarb, elecampane, jalap, saffron, manna, raisins, cochineal, and alcohol (usually gin). It was among the first English patent medicines shipped across the Atlantic to the American colonies in the mid-eighteenth century. By then most people were simply calling it "Daffy's Elixir." Daffy branded his product with his name.[3]

Daffy's Elixir was advertised in colonial newspapers and sold by physicians, apothecaries, grocers, tailors, goldsmiths, postmasters, and just about anyone in business, including the post riders carrying the mail between Williamsburg and Philadelphia. In addition to Daffy's Elixir and Anderson's Scots Pills, another popular patent medicine in pill form was concocted by a London physician, Lionel Lockyer. He labeled it "Pillulae Radiis Solis Extractae" and claimed the pills were extracted from the "rays of the sun." Lockyer appeared before King Charles II to demonstrate how they were manufactured, but kept the ingredients secret. A London chemist, however, tested the pills and found the chief ingredient was antimony, a metallic element having four allotropic forms, the most common of which is a hard, extremely brittle, lustrous, silver-white, crystalline material. Like other medicines with long names, it soon became known simply by its inventor's name, in this case as Lockyer's Pills. Lockyer printed and distributed 200,000 copies of a pamphlet promoting his pills. Selling them at 16 shillings per ounce, he became wealthy. When he died, he left the current equivalent of more than $200,000, leases on four properties, and a quarter-share in the ship *Batchelour*, which sailed out of London.[4]

The patent medicine business grew, and many other products appeared on the market, including Dr. Hooper's Female Pills, Dr. Batemen's Pectoral Drops, and Robert Turlington's Balsam of Life. Turlington's Balsam first appeared in England in 1770, a few years before the American Revolution. It was the concoction of Dr. John Hill, who claimed that "the medicine was made from American plants which had been taken to the king and queen some years before by an American botanist named William Young, Jr.," who really existed. Hill reported that the medicine would cure everything from whooping cough to the "hypochondriacal disease," an individual's exaggerated fear or belief that he or she had a serious disease. Hill noted that since the medicine was compounded from American plants, it was "no wonder" that "it must have the best effect in that country," an obvious pitch for Americans to buy it. Unlike many patent medicines, Turlington's Balsam of Life did have genuinely beneficial properties and is still listed in the American *Pharmacopoeia* as "Compound tincture of benzoin." Its principal ingredient comes from the tropical benzoin tree, and it is used as an antiseptic for dry, cracked skin and as an expectorant for respiratory conditions such as severe bronchitis.[5]

When English imports, including medicines, ceased during the American Revolution, apothecaries along the East Coast filled customers' empty medicine bottles with English recipes. If the apothecaries did not have all of the ingredients necessary, they substituted their own. Many customers were unaware of what was in their refilled medicine bottles. When the war ended, American apothecaries imported empty bottles in all shapes and sizes and began filling them with their own medical compounds and selling them for less than the English imports. This marked the start of the American patent medicine industry and resulted in a decline in sales of English patent medicines that lasted until after the War of 1812.

As the new nation was taking shape, the framers of the U.S. Constitution borrowed the English concept of patents and included it in Article 1, Section 8. It grants Congress the power to regulate such protections. Thomas Jefferson then had a hand in helping to draft the Patent Act of 1790 (H.R. 41), which was passed on March 10, 1790, and included the establishment of a patent office. The first American to patent a medicine in the United States was Samuel Lee in 1796. His medicine was called "Bilious Pills." Although the original government patent records were lost in a fire, a copy of Lee's recipe was later located, and it listed the ingredients of "Bilious Pills" as gamboges, aloe, soap, and nitrate of potassa. Lee, who lived in Windham, Connecticut, claimed his pills would battle bilious and yellow fevers, jaundice, dysentery, dropsy, worms, and female complaints. Then another Samuel Lee—Dr. Samuel H. P. Lee, of New London, Connecticut—secured a patent for *his* "Bilious Pills," containing ingredients that were partly the same as those in the first Lee's concoction—aloes, scammony (tropical American morning glory), gamboge, jalap, soap, syrup of buckthorn, and calomel. The first Samuel Lee could do nothing, since his patent applied only to the contents and not the name of his product. Soon two other men named Lee, in Baltimore—Richard and Michael—introduced their own bilious pills to the public. Serious competition in the American patent medicine business was under way as the new nation experienced a wave of cultural nationalism and citizens sought American products.

Thomas W. Dyott became the first American to build a patent medicine empire. Born in the British Isles in 1777, he came to America about 1804, settling in Philadelphia, and made bootblack. Soon, however, he produced a series of patent medicines in bottles blown in his own mold and embossed "Dr. Robertson's Family Medicine Prepared by T. W. Dyott." They included Robertson's Infallible Worm Destroying Lozenges, Robertson's Vegetable Nervous Cordial, and other compounds credited to a Dr. Robertson of Edinburgh who Dyott claimed was his grandfather. The editor of a Philadelphia medical journal did some checking and found there had not been a Dr. Robertson in Edinburgh for two hundred years. Dyott ignored the editor and continued producing his medicines, often bartering them for produce, tobacco, brandy, rum, candles, and castor oil.

In a few years, Dyott's business grew considerably. He was manufacturing his medicines in a large building at the corner of Second and Race streets in Philadelphia. Outside there was a large sign across the front that read "Philadelphia Cheap Drug, Medicine, Chemical, Colour [meaning dyes] & Glass Warehouse." About 1810, Dyott gave

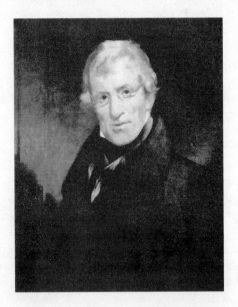

Thomas W. Dyott (1777–1861) was the first American to build a patent medicine empire. He was born in England and came to America about 1804, settling in Philadelphia. (Courtesy Pennsylvania Historical Society)

himself the honorary title of doctor, perhaps to lend more credibility to his medicines. He had forty-one agents in thirty-six towns in twelve states, and by 1814 he had added agents in fourteen towns in New York State, including New York City. He purchased an interest in a New Jersey glassworks to produce the bottles he needed and later, about 1824, he bought a glassworks on Gunner's Run along the Delaware River near Philadelphia. Around his glass factory, Dyott created a quasi-utopian community known as Dyottsville, consisting of dormitories, a bank, a school, an infirmary, and a chapel for his workers. His business grew because Dyott realized the importance of branding his products through their packaging, which included custom-made bottles, and of good marketing, with much advertising. He called his products "family medicines" and advertised extensively in daily and weekly newspapers across the growing young nation. Dyott eventually, however, fell victim to the financial panic of 1837. His creditors took him to court and won, and Dyott was sent to jail, though he was released early. He lived until he was ninety years old and died in 1861.[6]

While the feeling of nationalism in the new nation contributed to the sale of American patent medicines, most Americans apparently used them because of their low cost or manufacturers' claims or both. Few Americans sought curative treatments from doctors, toward whom there was a deep-rooted mistrust because many Americans sensed that most had limited medical knowledge and little training in pharmacology. Many people also refused to submit themselves to the heroic medicine still being practiced by most doctors, with its purging and bleeding. So it was that Americans continued to rely on home remedies and turned to an increasing number of patent medicines even though the more popular ones increased in cost. Many manufacturers of patent medicines took advantage of the public's distrust of doctors and stressed that their products contained no harsh mercury or other harmful ingredients. Some buyers prized the patent medicines for their alcoholic content or solutions fortified with opium, morphine, or cocaine. When the age of the common man emerged with the presidency of Andrew Jackson, the popularity of patent medicines increased even more. This was the era when highly emotional popular religion put doctors in a bad light, especially, as already noted, those physicians who wanted to deliver babies. Many Americans, especially those in rural areas, considered childbirth a natural act that needed no professional intervention.

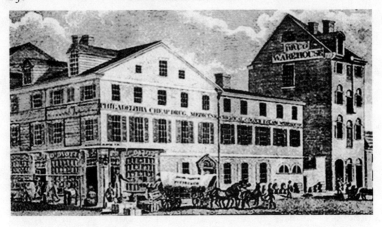

During the early nineteenth century, Thomas W. Dyott manufactured medicines in this building at the corner of Second and Race streets in Philadelphia. He also manufactured glass bottles to hold his medicines in a nearby glass factory. (Courtesy American Institute of the History of Pharmacy)

As the patent medicine industry grew during the first half of the nineteenth century, eastern apothecaries realized the need to institute reliable standards for drugs and to produce qualified pharmacists (*pharmacist* being the modern term that now began to replace the older word *apothecary*). Pharmacy was becoming a profession in its own right. Sixty-eight apothecaries held a meeting at Carpenters Hall in Philadelphia in 1821 to consider higher standards for drugs to protect the public. A few years later they organized and incorporated the Philadelphia College of Pharmacy, the nation's first such college. It was during this period that pharmacists gradually began to take over the task of preparing medicines, something that till then doctors had done.

Pharmacists were well aware of the growing number of patent medicines. One New York wholesale drug catalog in 1804 listed about ninety by name, but in the 1850s, a Boston catalog listed about six hundred. The expanding patent medicine market owed a great deal to the nation's growth, and especially the growth of newspapers (from 200 in 1800 to nearly 4,000 by 1860). Then, too, the development of daily newspapers in cities—including the penny papers in the East, directed at a mass audience—fit perfectly with the sensational nature of the papers' treatment of news. The patent medicine makers were the first

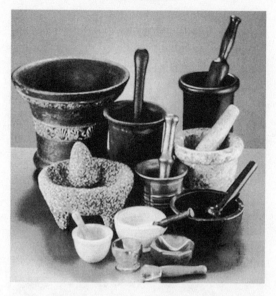

A collection of antique mortars and pestles. In the compounding of medicines a handheld club-shaped pestle was used for grinding or mashing substances. (Courtesy American Institute of the History of Pharmacy and the Smithsonian Institution)

businesses in America to seek a national audience for their products, and they spent thousands of dollars to promote them.

The concern for higher standards expressed by the apothecaries who met in Philadelphia in 1821 was some years later enacted at least partially into law: A change in the patent law in 1836 made it more difficult to patent a medicine. Anyone seeking such a patent now had to divulge the medicine's ingredients and provide evidence that it would not cause injury to those who used it. If a compound was substantially the same as one already known to practicing physicians, moreover, it could not be patented. Yet, while these stricter regulations reduced the number of medicines patented, they did not in the end hamper the patent medicine makers, who simply patented the design of their bottles and secured copyrights for their labels. They could still put anything they wanted into their bottles. For instance, one manufacturer created what he called "Vital Sparks" and claimed it could enhance masculine virility. It was nothing more than rock candy rolled in powdered aloe. A cure-all balm called "Tiger Fat" was supposedly made

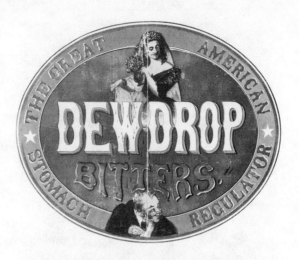

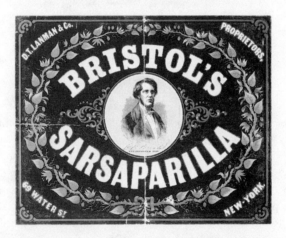

Popular patent medicines in the nineteenth century included Dewdrop Bitters, recommended as a "stomach regulator"; Bristol's Sarsaparilla, described as a healthy beverage; Cherokee Liniment, which supposedly had healing powers; and The Lone Star Liniment, which was recommended "for man or beast." (Courtesy Library of Congress)

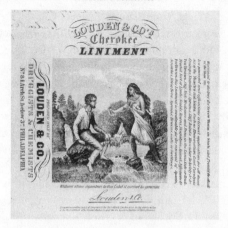

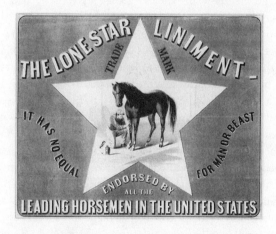

from the backbones of Royal Bengal tigers. In truth it contained turpentine, camphor, petroleum jelly, wintergreen oil, eucalyptus oil, and paraffin. Red pepper was the principal ingredient of "Liver Pad," an alleged cure for liver diseases. The pads were simply small swatches of cheap cloth onto which the manufacturer put a dab of glue on which he placed red pepper. When body heat melted the glue, users thought the sting of the red pepper was a healing sensation.

Another manufacturer was James Cook Ayer (1818–1878), who decided to enter the patent medicine business in 1843. He owned a drugstore in Lowell, Massachusetts, and began concocting medicines in the back room. He soon offered to the public "Ayer's Cherry Pectoral," claiming it would treat pulmonary troubles. It contained sweet spirits of nitre (natron), spirits of bitter almonds, and syrup of squills (made from bulbous plants of the genus *Scilla*). Sold first as sugar-coated pills in small boxes, the concoction was bottled in liquid form beginning about 1865. By 1870, Ayer was advertising in nearly 2,000 periodicals, both magazines and daily and weekly newspapers, across the country. Soon he was marketing other products, including an extract of sarsaparilla in 1855, an ague cure in 1857, and Ayer's Hair Vigor in 1869.

Ayer claimed to have a medical degree, but it is questionable whether he did. As he became increasingly wealthy, he claimed to be as well a member of the Society of Arts and Sciences, the Chemical Institute, the College of Pharmacology, the U.S. Medical Association, and the College of Physicians and Surgeons. By then he had helped to finance a railroad from Boston to Lowell, Massachusetts, and donated $10,000 to the town of Lowell to build a town hall. In the 1870s he turned over the management of his company to A. G. Cook, who continued to build the business. When James Ayer died in 1878 at the age of sixty, his brother Frederick assumed control. The company continued to manufacture medicines in Lowell well into the twentieth century.[7]

By the mid-nineteenth century, Ayer fit perfectly into one of two categories of patent medicine makers that had emerged. One was the individual or family honestly seeking to produce a beneficial medicine. These people genuinely wanted to relieve pain, improve health, and prolong life. Making money was secondary. For members of the second group, which included Ayer, however, making money was the primary motive. They sought to capitalize on people's weaknesses, lack of education, and gullibility so they would uncritically accept claims about these medicines. Some of the individuals in this second category produced what became known as "snake oil" medicines, which were sold by roaming "snake oil peddlers" who put on "medicine shows." The roots of such shows go back to medieval Europe, where mountebanks peddled pills, potions, and herbal tonics after their assistants—called zanies—attracted an audience by clowning, juggling, tumbling, performing magic tricks, or the like.

Exactly when the first medicine show appeared in America is not clear, but some were staged in the colonies well before the American Revolution. Records indicate that the colonial assembly in 1773 outlawed mountebanks because they produced "harmful social results" and "the corruption of manners, promoting of idleness, and the detriment of the good order and religion." After the Revolution, however, medicine shows again emerged in the East and spread westward, especially after the Civil War. The typical show followed a simple pattern. A peddler moved into a town, set up a platform, a table, or a tent and began to pitch the medicine and its cures with a pitch that was something similar to a fire-and-brimstone sermon. To attract a crowd many medicine shows provided entertainment that might include musicians, a small theatrical show, magicians, jugglers, or anything else that might fascinate the public. Members of the audience got caught up in the entertainment and ended up buying the "medicine." The peddler and his associates then left town quickly before the claims about their potions were found to be false and traveled to another town, where the process was repeated. These medicine shows were a forerunner of Wild West shows.

In time, medicine shows developed more sophisticated promotional techniques to sell their concoctions. Some manufacturers used the word *Indian* in the name of their medicines to suggest they were long-lost native cures. They no doubt recalled the nation's early years when Indian remedies were popular, sold widely to the public, and used by many doctors. Early in the nineteenth century, however, Indian medicine fell out of favor because Indians were thought to be uncivilized and inferior. Many doctors, sensing a change in national attitudes, began rejecting Indian remedies and treatments. Peddlers of patent medicines, however, knew that many Americans distrusted white doctors and still thought kindly toward Indian remedies because they had become family remedies. Thus, when peddlers began selling what they labeled as Indian cures, many Americans sensed truth in the pitch and bought them.

One of the better-known "Indian snake oil" firms was the Kickapoo Indian Medicine Company, started in the East in 1881 by John E. Healy, a New York patent medicine manufacturer; Charles F. Bigelow, a farmer called "Texas Charley"; and N. T. Oliva, known as "Nevada Ned." Their major product was "Kickapoo Indian Sagwa," a tonic reportedly first made from stale beer and aloe. By the early twentieth century, the company identified its ingredients as bicarbonate of soda, gentian root, mandrake root, cubebs, rhubarb root, senna leaves, aniseed, red cinchona bark, yellow dockroot, dandelion root, burdock root, sacred bark, licorice root, aloe, alcohol, glycerin, and water. To sell "Kickapoo Indian Sagwa," the company hired many Indians (tradition says none of them was a Kickapoo) to accompany the pitchmen in traveling medicine shows. The Indians demonstrated Indian ways and customs and the pitchmen sold the medicine. Members of each touring show would mix the contents and bottle them backstage for about 7 cents and sell each bottle for a dollar.

The business was so successful that within a few years, and through the 1890s, the company had nearly eighty troupes touring the nation. (Cartoonist Al Capp later incorporated "Kickapoo Joy Juice," as he called it, into his twentieth-century comic strip *Li'l Abner*.) The company also began adding other medicines under the Kickapoo label, including a cough cure, a worm killer, a salve, liver pills, and an oil that was highly successful as a remedy for rheumatism, earache, cholera, toothache, and diarrhea, bellyache, cramps, sore throat, and as a mouthwash. It was first offered in only one size, but became such a best seller that about 1908 it was offered in three sizes.

From all indications, some of the Kickapoo troupes sold medicines prepared for one distinct region of the country. William D. Naylor traveled with one Kickapoo Indian Medicine Company troupe in southern Missouri, Arkansas, and Indian Territory. In 1938, at the age of seventy-two, Naylor recalled that what he used to sell when he was with the medicine show was

'Chill and Ague Eliminator.' It was put up in a square pint bottle and guaranteed that two bottles would drive out the worst case of chills on the market. Whether it would or not I don't know. But, I do know it was mighty potent and bitter. I think it was probably a straight 'emulsion' of quinine and whiskey and the directions told the 'patient' to take enough of it before his chill started to make him go to sleep . . . theory was, no doubt, that if a person about to have a chill could be gotten drunk enough to go to sleep he'd never know he had it when he waked up and naturally think he had missed it entirely and was cured!

[The] . . . medicine was strong but it wouldn't have worked on the kind of chills people got down in the Ozark country of Arkansas, South Missouri, and over in the Indian Territory where I spent a lot of time. . . . Down in that country people didn't call chills and ague, 'chills and ague'; they called it the 'shakes.' And that was the right

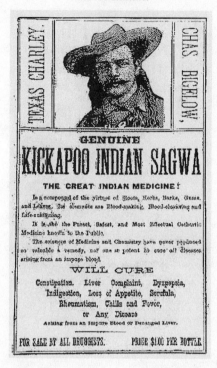

A newspaper advertisement for Kickapoo Indian Sagwa, sold by the Kickapoo Indian Medicine Company, started in New York in 1881 by John E. Healy; Charles F. Bigelow, known as "Texas Charley"; and N. T. Oliva, called "Nevada Ned." Bigelow's likeness appeared often in advertisements for the product. (Author's collection)

name. For when a man with the 'shakes' started to shake, he shook! He couldn't stop shaking till the chill was over.

There were two kinds, the 'every-other-day shakes,' and the 'every-day shakes.' I had both kinds. They started on me as the every-other-day kind and after a week or two turned into the every-day kind, then switched back and forth that way, first one sort and then the other till I finally got rid of them. The 'shakes' were so common in the Ozark country along back in the 1890's . . . that practically everybody would have them some time or other.

And people would talk about their 'shakes' with a sort of pride,

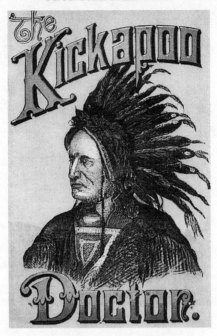

The cover of The Kickapoo Doctor, *a thirty-two-page pamphlet distributed by the Kickapoo Indian Medicine Company in 1890. It was designed to sell the company's medicines to the public. (Author's collection)*

something like a lot of people like to talk in these later days of their 'operations' after they've been to the hospital and had something cut out. The harder a man shook when he had the shakes the prouder he seemed to be![8]

Another patent medicine company not only used the Indian theme to sell its products but capitalized on the mystique of Oregon, the destination of thousands of immigrants seeking better lives, beginning in the 1840s. The Oregon Indian Medicine Company was founded by Thomas Augustus Edwards in 1876. Edwards, who was born in Saugerties, New York, in 1832, entered the patent medicine business when he was about forty after years of adventure. He left home at seventeen and worked in the whaling industry and as a grocer until he met

John Robinson, a circus showman. Edwards became business manager of the Spaulding and Rogers' Circus. In 1857, he left the circus and went west with General Albert Johnston's campaign against the Mormons in Utah. He returned east a year later and found work in Memphis, Tennessee, until the Civil War began. Edwards then joined the U.S. Secret Service and was a spy behind enemy lines. He was captured but managed to escape and spent the rest of the war scouting for General Frederick Steele in Arkansas. By then Thomas Edwards reportedly held the rank of colonel. The Secret Service in 1866 then sent Edwards to the Pacific Northwest during the Snake Indian War.

It was in Oregon that Edwards learned about Indian medicine through Dr. William C. McKay, one of four sons of Alexander McKay, who had been a partner in John Jacob Astor's Pacific Fur Company. Dr. McKay was a physician to the Indians. His brother, Donald McKay, was a prominent scout and Indian fighter. Both men had Indian wives. Both McKays returned east with Colonel Edwards about 1874, taking with them a party of Warm Springs Indians. Edwards and the Indians toured Europe and then New England demonstrating Indian skills and customs. In 1876 he took the Indian show to the Centennial Exposition in Philadelphia. It was there that he began selling Indian medicines.

In the fall of 1876, Thomas Edwards and his brother Alfred organized the Oregon Indian Medicine Company, with its headquarters in Pittsburgh. Dr. William C. McKay and Donald McKay also were part owners. At first, the company sold its medicine to the public in raw form, as supposedly gathered by Indians in the Pacific Northwest. Buyers would then mix the herbs and berries in their own homes. Thomas Edwards, however, complained that buyers mixed the ingredients carelessly, and he found a chemist who showed him how to prepare the medicines so they could be bottled. Edwards next purchased land in Corry, Pennsylvania, and constructed a factory that covered nearly a city block. As the factory was being built, Edwards asked his old friend John Robinson, the veteran circus showman, how he would sell the medicine. Robinson told him the then popular medicine show format was best. By 1885, the medicine factory was in full production and the Oregon Medicine Company used Donald McKay's name and image in advertising its products. While the operation was not as extensive as that of the Kickapoo Indian Medicine Company, the Oregon Indian Medicine Company at its height had several shows touring much of the nation simultaneously. Thomas Edwards had a promotional flyer printed called *The Ka-Ton-Ka Story*, along with a booklet, *The Last War Trail of the Modocs* (1885). Thomas Edwards left the business in 1901 and died in 1904. His daughter continued to operate the company until it was sold about 1912.[9]

Medicine shows using Indian themes continued to tour the country well into the twentieth century. Shows with an Indian theme had the most success because Americans believed strongly that Indians had a deep and secret knowledge of medicine. A rare glimpse of what it was like to work for an Indian medicine show company was offered by Grace McCune in 1939. Her husband was employed by such a company headquartered in a large old house in Athens, Georgia. Soon after she married McCune, she, too, was hired by the company. Here is her story in her own words:

"The first thing I did was label bottles. At first, this was done by hand, but business grew so that we had to have a machine to label as well as fill the bottles and it wasn't long until I could label more bottles than anyone else. I was paid more. I think I was raised to ten dollars a week. It wasn't long then until I was taken in the laboratory where the medicine was made, and the doctor in charge of this department taught me how to make the medicine up. I really enjoyed this work for it was really interesting and you know it was really a good medicine. We used it ourselves as you know it was good. I could soon make it as good as the doctor. When we had a good supply made, we were ready for the road work. I was looking forward to this for I didn't realize what it meant and thought it would be fun.

"But I soon learned better than that. As I said the medicine was really good and was in demand. It was sold all over the United States. Why, one man that run a chain of drugstores bought about one hundred carloads at one time. We had salesmen on the road to make the sales and then we did the advertising also giving our circulars and coupons and for this my husband carried several crew managers with him. But the others were hired to work under them in the towns where we were working.

"As it was an Indian medicine, all the people that advertised [it] were made up as Indians. The crew managers went on a day ahead. Yes, they had enough of them so that they could do this. They carried a supply of the Indian suits for the men giving out the circulars. The medicine sold for a dollar a bottle and the coupons that we gave away was good for thirty-five cents on a bottle of medicine.

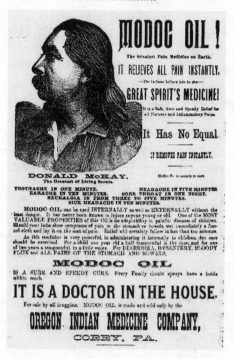

This newspaper advertisement for "Modoc Oil" appeared often during the 1890s. The Oregon Indian Medicine Company was started in Pennsylvania by Thomas and Alfred Edwards in 1876. Dr. William C. McKay and Donald McKay, an Indian fighter, were part-owners of the company. To give the product credibility, Donald McKay's likeness was featured in the advertising. (Author's collection)

"My job was to advertise at the drugstores while the crew managers and their men canvassed the town. My husband saw that it was all done and the first day or so it was alright. I thought it was fun. I was dressed in a soft leather suit, all trimmed up in beads and fringes, leather moccasin shoes with beads, my face and hands were stained and I wore a wig with coarse black hair and feathers in my hair, and hanging down over my shoulders. You know how it all looked for I know you have seen pictures of them. I stood at the door of the drugstore and gave away coupons.

"Yes, I made good money for when I went on the road I was paid twenty-five dollars a week. My husband made fifty dollars. The crew managers were paid fifteen dollars. Of course all our expenses were paid by the company. The men or boys that he hired in the towns were paid twelve dollars a week or two dollars a day for it was a large town if they stayed there for a week. My husband and I only stayed one day at the town and then we went on to the next town.

"We didn't travel in cars but went on the trains. I soon grew tired of it for standing all day and then getting the make-up off and rushing to catch trains sometimes didn't have time to eat and very little sleep and very often we could not get a good place to stay.

"Sometimes we almost froze to death in the winter time. Maybe we would get in about light and have to get ready for the day's work, probably have to get on the job before we had time to eat and we had to be on the job for that was in the company rules for those doing all the advertising. I was the only woman on the road, but my husband saw that I did my part.

"We didn't go to the small towns where there were no trains. The salesmen and crew managers took care of them. But hard as the work was I would want to laugh sometimes especially at the kids. They would get off and look at me and just knew they were looking at an honest to goodness Indian woman, but then some of the grown-ups were as bad as the children and have asked me all kinds of questions. I was not supposed to be able to talk any English and I even had one to pinch me one day to see if I was real." She laughed and said, "That is one time I could hardly keep still. . . .

"We would stay on the road until the medicine gave out and then we had to come back in and help get another supply made up. We had to keep up with all those Indian suits that were used by the crew managers for their boys that distributed circulars. This was not as easy as one might think for they [were] sent in from many different towns at times to [be] laundered and we had to send out fresh ones. There was always something to keep you on the move. I did not get very much in the evenings for any pastime or pleasure for when we were on the road I was really too tired to think of it and too I had no time for it since I had to catch a train and was off so I could be at another town by morning.

"I was young and grew tired of all this. I realized then what I had done and every day it grew worse but I didn't know what to do and I just stood it for three years and we separated."[10]

Of all the medicine shows that toured America into the twentieth century, only a few came close to matching the success of the Kickapoo Indian Medicine Company. One successful company was organized by John Austen Hamlin, a professional magician. Following the Civil War he sent troupes from his headquarters in Chicago touring towns across America to sell "Hamlin's Wizard Oil." Hamlin, however, used music and not magic to attract audiences. Each of Hamlin's troupes had a special wagon equipped with parlor organs pulled by a four- or six-horse team. Each consisted of a lecturer, a driver, and a male quartet. At night the wagon became the stage where the lecturer—the pitchman—told of the wonders of Hamlin's Wizard Oil, and the quartet entertained with popular songs of the day. The performers were usually dressed in formal wear, including silk top hats, frock coats, and pinstriped trousers. They distributed countless pamphlets containing songs that the audiences were invited to sing along with the quartet. Each troupe spent several days in a town. During the day, the lecturer tried to place Hamlin's Wizard Oil in local drugstores while the quartet performed for church groups and any organization that asked them to perform. At night they presented their show from atop their wagon.[11]

The history of patent medicines suggests that just about anyone could concoct something and sell it. E. W. Grove, who owned and operated a small drugstore in Paris, Tennessee, following the Civil War, came up with many concoctions. One was "Grove's Chill Tonic," first marketed in 1878. Another was "Grove's Bromo Quinine Cold Tablets." As his modest business grew, Grove established the Paris Medicine Company in 1889, and two years later moved the business to St. Louis. After he died in 1927, his son operated the company until 1934, when he died. The company then became Grove Laboratories.

The popularity of patent medicines during the late nineteenth century also gave rise to many solo peddlers who simply went from town to town selling their cures without the fanfare of the medicine show. Clement Flynn was one such traveling salesman. He spent forty-five years selling one medicine, and only in Colorado and Nebraska. Born in Stone Quarry, Michigan, in 1862, he and a brother moved to Harvard, Nebraska, in 1877, and operated a small general store for two years. Not having much business success, they moved to Yuma, Colorado, in 1879 to file homestead claims. In Yuma, Flynn obtained a recipe for a medicine which he began to make and sell, called "The

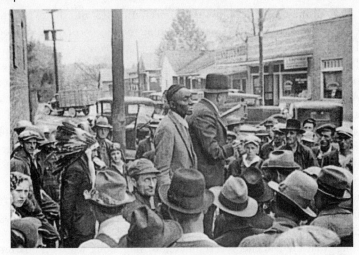

Although medicine shows declined during the first half of the twentieth century, some continued to tour small towns in rural areas into the 1940s. This 1935 photo taken in Huntington, Tennessee, shows a pitchman (right of center wearing hat) pitching some medicine. The black man standing next to him provided entertainment to attract an audience. Farther back (left of utility pole) another member of the medicine show, wearing an Indian head bonnet, is apparently waiting his turn to give his spiel. This photo was taken by Ben Shahn. (Courtesy Library of Congress)

Great Remedy." Late in 1938, when Flynn was seventy-six and retired, he recalled his life and his patent medicine days selling The Great Remedy, which contained

> Garden Sage, Lobelia, Gum of Myrtle and Peppermint. A chemist at Topeka, Kansas, analyzed it. He said it was as good as any medicine in the world. It cures anything. Pains, Colds, Cough, Pneumonia, Rhumethism [sic], Arthritis, Burns, etc. When you don't feel well just take a spoonful twice a day and it will do the work. One lady over 80 yrs old here in Hastings [Nebraska] claims that this medicine restored her sight. It does miracles. I never tried to make money by selling this medicine. I would work a while then lay around during the winter or until I needed money again, then I would sell my medicine again.[12]

The label on bottles of The Great Remedy contained specific instructions for using the medicine to provide relief for fourteen ailments. There were no claims of its curing anything. The label read:

For Neuralgia and Toothache, use it warm, bathe the face and the gums until pain is gone.

For Earache use it warm, moisten a piece of cotton with the remedy, place it in the ear and pain stops.

Burns will not blister if you apply cloths instantly and keep them wet with the remedy.

For coughs, mix the remedy with an equal amount of molasses, boil it, and take a teaspoonful every half hour.

For Dyspepsia, Liver Complaint, Palpitation of the Heart, take inward one tablespoon morning and night until relieved.

For Nervous and Sick Headache, bathe the head and temples with the remedy and take a teaspoon diluted with two of water internally.

For Fev[e]r of all kinds, bathe the head and chest and lay on cloths with remedy.

For Corns, Bunions, Chilblains, Frosted Feet, rub on with hand.

For Sour Stomach, Indigestion, Hart [*sic*] Burn, take a tablespoon night and morning for several days.

For Ulcerated Eyes, with four parts of water use it in the eye several times daily.

For Flesh Wounds, Burns, Cuts and Bruises, wash the wound with the remedy several times a day, applying bandages wet with it till well.

For Piles, Dilute it with an equal amount of water, and saturate a piece of cotton and apply to parts frequently.

For Hay Fever and Colds, sniff up the nostrils every morning four times with water.

For Rheumatism, bathe the parts frequently with the remedy hot and pour a tablespoonful of the remedy into a tumbler of hot water sweetened with sugar and take, repeat this dose every three hours until you are relieved.

Flynn's Great Remedy never became well known outside the areas where he sold it.

Probably the best-known patent medicine of the late nineteenth and early twentieth centuries was a vegetable compound concocted in the early 1870s as a home remedy, chiefly for women, in the Lynn, Massachusetts, kitchen of Lydia Pinkham. When a batch brought positive results to Pinkham, she shared it with her neighbors, who also found it helpful. After her husband's real estate business collapsed in 1875, she decided to sell her medicine to the public to produce income for the family. She put her compound in 14½-ounce bottles, and because she believed so strongly that her medicine would help women who used it, she loaned her own name to it, calling it "Lydia E. Pinkham's Vegetable Compound" and included her picture in the advertising. She claimed it would cure any "female complaint," from nervous prostration to a prolapsed uterus. Although its ingredients were not listed on the bottle's label when it was first introduced, it was later found to contain unicorn roots (*Aletris farinos*), life root (*Senecio viscosus*), black cohosh (*Cimicifuga racemosa*), pleurisy root (*Asclepias tuberose*), fenugreek seed (*Trigonella foenum-gracecum*), and alcohol.

The medicine quickly gained wide acceptance. With her name and picture used extensively in advertising, Pinkham herself became known around the world. She was the first woman in America to experience wide business success. Her company grossed $300,000 in 1883, the year she died. She and her medicine became so popular that they were subjects of drinking songs. The words of one traditional song are, in part:

> *Here's a story, a little bit gory.*
> *A little bit happy, a little bit sad.*
> *Of Lily the Pink and her medicinal compound,*
> *And how it slowly drove her to the bad.*
> ....
> *Meet Ebenezer, thought he was Julius Caesar,*
> *So they put him in a home.*
> *And then they gave him medicinal compound,*
> *And now he's Emperor of Rome.*
> *We'll drink a drink a drink*
> *To Lily the pink the pink the pink*
> *The savior of, the savior of, the human race.*
> *She invented medicinal compound*
> *Most efficacious in every case.*

Her family took over the company's operations after her death. During Prohibition in the 1920s, Lydia Pinkham's medicine enjoyed especially great success because it gave respectable women a legal pretext for drinking alcohol. The company reportedly earned $3.8 million in 1925. Her family continued to manufacture the product until the 1960s, when the company was sold.[13]

William Radam, another patent medicine maker, never became as

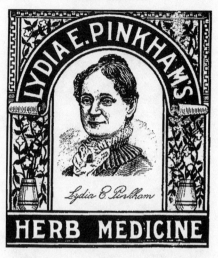

Lydia Pinkham (1819–1883) invented and man-ufactured one of the most popular patent medicines of the late nineteenth century. Although it was a vegetable compound for women, it contained 20 percent alcohol. Pinkham had her likeness printed on every bottle and became well known herself. The product supposedly provided relief to women from the symptoms of menopause. (Courtesy National Library of Medicine)

well known as Lydia Pinkham but he became wealthy relying on pseudo-science in developing and marketing his remedy. Radam came from Germany and settled in Austin, Texas, where he ran a feed store and a successful plant nursery. When he contracted malaria, doctors and their medicines did not help him. Radam then decided to cure himself and began to experiment with different compounds. After many months he produced "Microbe Killer," as he called it, and took doses of the liquid for six months. He claimed that it worked, and then began to sell it in the late 1880s.

Radam exploited what became a popular belief once germs were found to be the cause of some diseases—that they caused them all. He claimed Microbe Killer would cure them all. "I treated all my patients with the same medicine, just as in my garden I would treat all weeds alike." Radam was soon making money selling his medicine. He had bottles manufactured embossed with the words "Cure All Diseases."

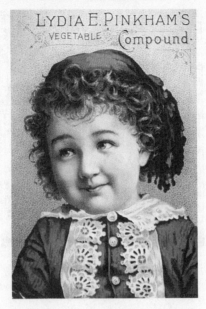

This illustration appears on a trade card distributed by Lydia Pinkham's company.
(Courtesy National Library of Medicine)

By 1890, Radam had factories from coast to coast producing his potion. It cost him 5 cents to make one gallon, which he sold for 53 cents in small jugs. No lot was ever exactly the same as another. An analyst found one batch to be 99 percent water, with a little red wine and tiny amounts of hydrochloric and sulfuric acids. Some batches contained larger amounts of these acids, which if taken in large quantities would be poisonous. Radam made so much money with his medicine that in the 1890s he moved from Austin to New York City and bought a mansion overlooking Central Park. There he died in 1902. He is buried in Austin's Oakwood Cemetery.[14]

Another patent medicine manufacturer who became wealthy was Asa Soule. He was the eleventh child of a Quaker family who became a farmer and fruit grower and then worked in banking and hotel management before making patent medicines. Perhaps his first concoction, about 1870, was "Soule's Hop Cure for Colds and Coughs." Next came "Dr. Soule's Balm Syrup." He bought out the New York City firm of

Doyles Bitters and moved the plant to Rochester, New York, where he strengthened the formula and changed the name to Hop Bitters. Its sales increased rapidly and he became wealthy, because bottled bitters were essentially alcohol disguised as medicine. Even after the temperance movement grew, there was a popular belief that a dose of bitters each day was respectable as a supposed means of maintaining good health. By the early 1880s, Soule was known worldwide as the Hops Bitter King.

When Soule learned in 1882 that two promoters from Spearville, Kansas, had decided to make drought-stricken southwest Kansas a garden spot by building a vast irrigation system, Soule invested in the scheme. He founded the town of Ingalls, Kansas, named for then U.S. senator John J. Ingalls of Kansas, on the line of the Santa Fe Railroad. Soule dreamed of building a canal from Ingalls to Spearville, located east of Dodge City, to carry water from the Arkansas River for irrigation use. But while a portion of the canal did open in 1886, the whole scheme soon collapsed. Soule made a hasty exit from Kansas and returned to Rochester and his patent medicine business.[15]

By the late nineteenth century, thousands of patent medicines were on the market. Among bitters alone, there were nearly five hundred different brands competing for public attention. Even more physicians and pharmacists were producing their own concoctions on a small scale, using tablet machines or ointment mills, and experimenting with different compounds. And, like the established patent medicine manufacturers, these doctors and pharmacists could make any claim they wished about their products, because there was no outside control. Pharmacists sold their concoctions in their drugstores. Doctors would sell theirs to their patients and get local drugstores to carry them.

John Bull, a prescription clerk in Louisville, Kentucky, produced several patent medicines, including a "Balsam of Wild Cherry." He also made a sarsaparilla remedy after the Civil War that became very popular and made him a wealthy man. The sarsaparilla root was first found in Mexico and was taken to Europe in 1536, where it was thought useful as a cure for syphilis and rheumatism. From the sarsaparilla root grows a tropical vine distantly related to the lily. In time, the root gained a reputation as a blood purifier and a general tonic. Exactly how John Bull used sarsaparilla as a remedy is not known, but it may have been produced as a tea or a beer.

While John Bull was at work in Louisville, Charles Hires, a Philadelphia pharmacist, discovered a recipe for a delicious herbal tea while on his honeymoon. First, he sold a dry version of the tea mixture and then began developing a liquid version that consisted of more than twenty-five herbs, berries, and roots which were used to flavor carbonated soda water. He introduced his "Root Beer" to people attending the 1876 Philadelphia Centennial celebration. The beverage was a hit. In 1893, the Hires family began to bottle the root beer and sell it.

Root beer, in various forms, can actually be traced back to colonial times, when people produced what were called "small beers" in their homes. Some contained alcohol, others did not. They had various names depending upon the ingredients—"birch beer," "sarsaparilla beer," "ginger beer," and "root beer." A wide range of ingredients was used, including allspice, birch bark, coriander, juniper, ginger, wintergreen, hops, burdock root, dandelion root, spikenard, pipsissewa (a low evergreen plant), guaiacum chips, sarsaparilla, spice wood, wild cherry bark, yellow dock, prickly ash bark, sassafras root, vanilla bean, hops, dog grass, molasses, and licorice. No two recipes were alike. One well-known brand, A&W Root Beer, did not come on the market until 1919 and is credited to Roy Allen.

In 1885, Charles Courtice Alderton, a pharmacist in Wade B. Morrison's drugstore at Waco, Texas, set out to concoct a new medical tonic without using alcohol. He began by combining carbonated water with fruit extracts and sweeteners. Those who tried it liked the drink but did not view it as medicine—it was simply a refreshing beverage that local residents called a "Waco." As it became popular, townspeople urged Alderton's boss, Wade Morrison, to name the drink. He did. Legend has it that he named the drink after a friend, Dr. Pepper of Christianburg, Virginia (not a Dr. Charles T. Pepper of Rural Retreat, Virginia, as is sometimes reported), because Morrison was in love with the doctor's daughter. The demand for Dr Pepper became so great that Morrison could not produce enough in his Waco drugstore. The making of Dr Pepper moved to a separate facility, and the distribution spread throughout Texas and the Southwest. In 1898 the Southwestern Soda Fountain Company of Dallas purchased the rights to produce and sell Dr Pepper fountain syrups to drugstores, and so drugstore soda fountains became the primary place where the public could buy what is considered the first popular soft drink in America.[16]

Three years after Dr Pepper was born in Waco, Texas, Dr. John Pemberton, a physician in Atlanta, Georgia, concocted Coca-Cola in

1885, in a three-legged brass kettle in the backyard of his home. Pemberton intended the drink as a tonic, and it was his bookkeeper, Frank Robinson, who suggested the name *Coca-Cola*, since it contained extracts of cocaine as well as the caffeine-rich kola nut. It was first sold at the soda fountain in Jacob's Pharmacy in Atlanta in May 1886, where sales averaged only nine servings of the drink each day—Pemberton actually lost money on the tonic during its first year. In 1887, another Atlanta pharmacist and businessman, Asa Candler, paid Pemberton $2,300 for the drink's formula. Applying good business practices, Candler aggressively marketed Coca-Cola syrup, and sales increased by 4,000 percent between 1890 and 1900. Candler not only sold to soda fountains but began selling syrup to independent bottling companies licensed to sell the drink. Coca-Cola became the second major soft drink to be created in America.[17]

Coca-Cola had to end its use of cocaine in its drink, and most patent medicine manufacturers, including doctors and pharmacists, had to make changes in the ingredients of their products when Congress passed the Pure Food and Drug Act in 1906 and it was signed into law by President Theodore Roosevelt. The act prohibited interstate commerce in misbranded and adulterated foods, drinks, and drugs.

The legislation was long in coming. It was approved after decades of campaigning by government agencies, the growing medical establishment, and journalists in many newspapers and magazines. Perhaps the most effective journalist in calling the problem to the attention of the American people was Samuel Hopkins Adams, whose series "The Great American Fraud" was published by the weekly magazine *Colliers* beginning late in 1905. Adams exposed 264 fraudulent firms and hucksters, and when Congress finally acted, patent medicine empires began to crumble.

With regard specifically to medicines and drugs, the 1906 law required their manufacturers to list the presence and amount of selected dangerous or addictive substances such as heroin, alcohol, morphine, and cocaine on the product's label. The law, however, fell short of what lawmakers had intended. While it required a label on each medicine, the misbranding provision in the law did not compel a full listing of ingredients, or include directions for use, or provide warnings. Drug manufacturers therefore could and often did simply omit such information from their labels. Congress amended the Food and Drug Act in 1912 and required that the government prove fraudulent intent on the part of anyone who made false statements on the label. This still missed the mark and was difficult to enforce. It was not until 1938 that further amendments to the act eliminated all such shortcomings by mandating a complete list of ingredients and directions for safe use on the label. By then the government had also decided that some drugs were too dangerous to give the consumer free access to even with directions on the label. From that point on, such drugs were labeled for prescription distribution only.

By then America was changing. There were better roads, and motion pictures and radio provided new forms of entertainment. Medicine shows faded and were all but gone by the middle of the twentieth century. In the meantime, the language of medicine also changed, as manufacturers who had formerly promoted their products as a *cure* dropped that term also, in favor of the more cautious and honest word *remedy*. What had been called "pills" became "tablets," sometimes "capsules." The changes did not occur overnight, but manufacturers were required to prove at least the safety of their drugs even if not yet their effectiveness. By the mid-twentieth century, manufacturers, however, were indeed required to show both safety and effectiveness.

Many of today's major pharmaceutical companies got their start with patent medicines.

CHAPTER THIRTEEN

QUACKS

We have not lost faith, but we have transferred it
from God to the medical profession.

—George Bernard Shaw

THERE IS AN OLD STORY about a city doctor who moved his practice to a rural area. One day he was called to treat a sick farmer. But after making a few house calls, the doctor stopped coming to the farm. The farmer called the doctor and asked him where he had been. The doctor replied, "I do not like your ducks. Every time I walk up to your house, they verbally insult me."

Quacks claim to have medical knowledge but usually peddle unproven and sometimes dangerous medicines, cures, or treatments. They have been around for centuries. They existed in Europe long before Columbus arrived in the New World in 1492. They existed in the colonies and then in the new United States. It was not, however, until the middle of the nineteenth century that they gradually became a problem in the eyes of physicians trying to make medicine a respectable profession whose practitioners were fully trained, educated, and certified. The more educated physicians sought ways to identify quacks, but it was difficult because there were no commonly or universally accepted standards by which to distinguish the quack from the qualified professional. And this question remains even now difficult to answer.

It is not surprising that when most Americans are searching for a physician, they ask their friends and neighbors whom they would recommend. It all boils down to a physician's reputation. If a person is satisfied with what he or she hears, he or she usually seeks out the doctor in question. From the mid-1850s on, however, some doctors began advertising. They promised to cure patients by using some secret formula or new medicine or a treatment that would work overnight. As medicine became more impersonal, many people responding favorably to these medical pied pipers learned by experience that the so-called cures did not work. An old adage applied—"If it sounds too good to be true, it probably is." The quacks survived and prospered because people were ignorant and susceptible to their claims.

Probably the first popular quack to gain national attention was Samuel Thomson (1769–1843), who realized Americans were increasingly displeased with conventional heroic medicine, which still included the bloodletting and purging practiced by heroic doctors. Thomson, a self-taught botanical irregular, opposed mineral purgatives like calomel in favor of distillates of native American plants. In 1813, he received a patent for "Thomsonian Materia Medica," which became known as the Thomsonian system. He stressed safe herbs and plants in the treatment of illnesses and for maintaining good health. In 1822, he published a book, *New Guide to Health; or the Botanic Family Physician*, and then sold patents to people who wanted to use his system. In 1840 alone, Thomson sold more than 100,000 patents. Thom-

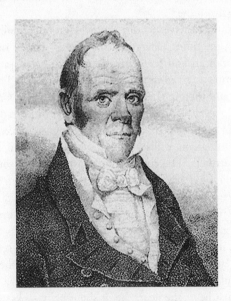

This portrait of Samuel Thomson (1769–1843) appears in his 1835 book New Guide to Health; or, Botanic Family Physician. *(Courtesy National Library of Medicine)*

son's system was popular because doctors were not needed and every man could treat himself. Buying a patent to use the system cost $20 and enabled the buyers to obtain a manual and guide to the system; it also gave him or her the right to prepare and use the remedies described. Thomson required buyers of his patents to purchase the basic botanical ingredients from him. Patent holders also automatically became members of their local chapter of Thomson's Friendly Botanic Society, which held regular meetings where members could share experiences and seek counsel; members, however, were forbidden to reveal secrets to nonmembers.

Although Thomson was very critical of formal medical training for physicians, he opened his own Botanic Medical College in Columbus, Ohio, in 1840, which provided him with the trappings of traditional medicine to give his system more credibility. In the end, however, the freedom that Thomson had in establishing his system also worked against him. Although the system was patented, Thomson lacked control. His medical manual was pirated. Some of his agents set out on their own. These "mongrel Thomsonians," as they were called, even

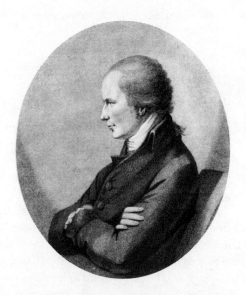

Franz Joseph Gall (1758–1828), anatomist, physiologist, and founder of phrenology. (Courtesy National Library of Medicine)

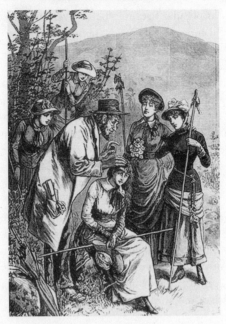

This nineteenth-century illustration from an unidentified newsweekly shows a practitioner of phrenology at work somewhere in America. Phrenologists spread into rural America offering their services to anyone they met. (Courtesy National Library of Medicine)

compounded his botanicals. As a result, Thomson did not gain much profit from his enterprise, although his system spread over wide rural areas of the West, South, and New England.[1]

Phrenology was another form of quackery that became popular during the first half of the nineteenth century. It was a theory claiming that a person's personality could be determined by the bumps on his head. Although founded in 1796 in Vienna by Franz Joseph Gall (1758–1828), it was not promoted in the United States until the early 1830s by Orson Squire Fowler, a native of Steuben County, New York. Fowler, born in 1809, attended Amherst College and became friends with Henry Ward Beecher. In college both young men became interested in Gall's phrenology. After they graduated in 1834, Beecher went into the ministry but Fowler remained devoted to phrenology. He began lecturing on the subject, claiming that a person's character was made up of thirty-seven faculties that could be "read" on the cranium at the site where each was located. He believed that the size of the bump in a given location would reveal the strength of that particular faculty. Phrenology was even adopted by artists, including sculptors and painters who did phrenological profiles of their subjects to make sure their portrayal would accurately reflect the traits of their subjects.

During an early lecture tour, Fowler visited southeastern Colorado and had a vision. He leased 5,000 acres of land thirty miles east of Pueblo on the Arkansas River and filed a plat (town layout) under the name of Fowler Town and Development. He wanted to build an irrigation ditch and import a colony of fruit growers. Land improvements were started, and a mile of the ditch had been completed when Fowler became ill and returned to his New York home, where he died on his large estate near Amenia, New York, in August 1889. He did not live to see the Fowler Colony become a reality, but the town of Fowler, Colorado, still exists as do copies of the books he published on phrenology.

Fowler promoted phrenology as a science. Americans enthusiastically adopted the system because it was the era of Jacksonian democracy and citizens believed society benefited from science. They viewed phrenology as based upon common sense and reason, two traits of

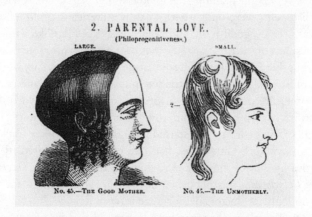

The New Illustrated Self-Instructor in Phrenology and Physiology *by Orson and Lorenzo Fowler was published in 1875. This how-to-do-it book included more than one hundred engravings similar to the one above. (Author's collection)*

Jacksonian democracy. Phrenology also mixed well with the religious revivalism and social reform of the period. By the 1850s, however, phrenology began to lose its appeal because the common man began to question its validity.[2]

Hydrotherapy, the intensive application of water internally and externally (later it was referred to as hydropathy), was another form of quackery. Formulated by an Austrian farmer, Vincent Preissnitz, in 1829, it was introduced in England about 1840. Preissnitz claimed to have, as a young man, healed his own broken ribs by applying cold cloths to the affected area. He preached that the "water cure," as it became known, would improve personal hygiene when combined with preventive medicine. He believe in three types of treatments: applying water by bath, applying water to a particular part of the body, and cleaning the body internally by drinking lots of water or by injecting it.

Dr. Joel Shew (1816–1855) introduced the system in America in 1844. Shew later adopted the Hygeio-Therapy dietary and exercise plan with its emphasis on fresh air and sunlight. In 1853, he founded the New York College of Hygeio-Therapy. Another early practitioner of hydropathy was George H. Taylor, who in 1853 established a water cure practice in New York.

To many Americans, the water cure seemed logical and sensible, and they took to it avidly. It spread mostly by word of mouth, and became very popular among the middle and upper classes. A few fancy establishments were built where wealthy Americans could lounge in hot tubs, enjoy good food, and receive massages. Unlike with other new systems of the time, few societies originated to promote the water cure, but there was a water cure "institute" in New York City where for a fee of $50 individuals were trained in its fundamentals and qualified as "water cure doctors." The institute sought to make hydro theory scientifically respectable to improve its credibility. About 1841 promoters of the hydro theory started a magazine, *The Water-Cure Journal*, in New York City, which had one of the largest circulations in America by mid-century. In 1843, Russell T. Trall's book *The Hydropathic Encyclopedia* was published in New York, explaining the water cure not only for doctors but for the curious public.

Mark Twain's mother may have learned of the cure from reading Trall's book, or else heard of it by word of mouth. Regardless, Twain later recalled his personal experience with the cure when it reached Missouri in the early 1840s: "I can remember well when the cold water

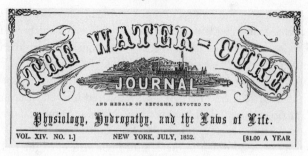

THE WATER-CURE JOURNAL

AND HERALD OF REFORMS, DEVOTED TO

Physiology, Hydropathy, and the Laws of Life.

VOL. XIV. NO. 1.] NEW YORK, JULY, 1852. [$1.00 A YEAR

The masthead of The Water-Cure Journal, *which had a wide circulation in the United States during the mid-nineteenth century. (Author's collection)*

cure was first talked about. I was then about nine years old, and I remember how my mother used to stand me up naked in the back yard every morning and throw buckets of cold water on me, just to see what effect it would have. Personally, I had no curiosity upon the subject. And then, when the dousing was over, she would wrap me up in a sheet wet with ice water and then wrap blankets around that and put me into bed. I never realized that the treatment was doing me any particular good physically. But it purified me spiritually. For pretty soon after I was put into bed I would get up a perspiration that was something worth seeing."[3]

During the first half of the nineteenth century, most Americans were caught up in the romantic philosophy then spreading across the country. It was spurred by the notion of Manifest Destiny, a belief in expansionism and other popular ideas such as everyone being entitled to health and happiness. Many Americans, however, were not well educated—many, in fact, were quite ignorant. Then, too, they believed in the supernatural. Medical historian Fielding H. Garrison has observed that many Americans have a "fetichistic instinct, a craving for the supernatural which is ever latent in man." Rabbits' feet, for example, supposedly bring good luck to the owner, and there are love potions, voodoo bags, charms, and many other such things. The selling of such items was and is big business. This craving for something positive in itself was prevalent in primitive medicine and has always been capitalized on by quacks.[4]

Conditions in nineteenth-century America were perfect for quackery. Francis J. Shepherd, writing on quacks and quackery in *Popular*

Science Monthly in June 1883, noted: " 'Ailment plus medicine equals cure' is an equation widely cherished as true. But the algebra is not so simple. Countless times, of course, the true equation is 'Ailment plus Nature equals cure,' and if any drug is added its value is zero. Why, a physician once asked, was quackery more prevalent in medicine than in other areas of science? 'Because,' he answered himself, 'the medical quack attributes to himself what is due to Nature. Nature cannot build a railway, but she can very often cure disease.' "[5]

Quacks secretly relied on natural healing instead of their claimed remedies to treat patients. Sometimes, however, quacks were not concerned with the process of natural healing as a way to fleece their patients. In one western state, two fast-talking men and a woman plied their quackery in a different way. One man claiming to be a doctor would arrive in a town and spend several days searching out and visiting with residents who complained of chronic illnesses, whether real or imagined. No one questioned the "doctor's" credentials because he simply talked to them about their symptoms, learned how long they had been suffering, and determined their ability to pay. Residents found the "doctor" likeable since he was friendly and did not try to force any medications on them. Having completed his research, the man would leave town and meet his partners in some nearby spot. A week or two later the second man and the woman would come to the town, calling themselves a doctor and his nurse. The "doctor" would set up an office and advertise his presence in the local newspaper. When a patient visited the office to see the new doctor, the nurse would take the patient's name and give it to the doctor. He would look up the patient's history in the notes prepared by the first man. The patient would then be ushered into the doctor's office, where he would rattle off the person's symptoms, giving an impression of extraordinary medical ability. The patient would be amazed at the doctor's brilliance and when a guaranteed cure was offered—payable in advance—the response was immediate. When the quack had exhausted the patients interviewed by the first man, he would quickly leave town with the woman and join the other "doctor" in another town to start the process all over again. Their quackery apparently escaped detection until the second doctor left town. By then their patients were too embarrassed to discuss the traveling medical men.

As medicine was becoming more oriented to scientific rigor during the latter half of the nineteenth century, Thomas Edison, Alexander

Graham Bell, Guglielmo Marconi, Madame Curie, and others were making discoveries and advances that would change the world. With each such advance, quacks sought to use it to cheat an unsophisticated public that was awed by scientific developments. For example, most Americans did not fully understand electricity, which seemed magical and powerful. Quacks jumped on the discovery and created what they called "electropathy." Unlike many magical quack cures, electricity could be felt, and when patients felt it they believed the claimed cure was working. One of the earliest contraptions in the United States based on electricity's supposed healing powers was the Davis Kidder Magneto, patented in 1854. It was a simple device that generated electricity using a magnet. A hand-turned crank operated the gears that spun a velvet-covered armature that generated a flow of electricity conducted over cloth-insulated wires to two brass electrodes about two inches in size. The patient was hooked up to these electrodes, and the low-voltage current generated by cranking the machine usually caused involuntary muscle contractions that were not unpleasant. Quacks promised patients using the device cures for most diseases and conditions, including mental illness. The device was manufactured by the Jerome Kidder Manufacturing Company in New York City.

Numerous other electrical devices appeared late in the nineteenth century, including electric belts. Sears, Roebuck and Company advertised Heidelberg Alternating Current Electric Belts. There was no alternating current; the belt contained nothing more than a copper disk in front and two to four chrome-plated nickel disks toward the back. The manufacturer claimed interaction between the copper and nickel was what created electricity. Dr. James J. Walsh, in his book *The Story of Cures That Fail* (1923), observed that such devices multiplied once Americans became hooked on electricity as possessing a potent force for good on the human system. There also were belts designed as shoulder straps, and electrical chest protectors and hairbrushes. Some devices sold for as much as $25—a substantial sum at the time.

The public's interest in electropathy took off after Thomas Edison introduced in 1879 incandescent lighting and three years later created the electric industry with the first commercial power station in lower Manhattan that provided light and electrical power to customers in a one-square-mile area. While Edison was certainly no quack, his son Thomas A. Edison, Jr., who tried to follow his father's example as an inventor, was. He found his greatest success in the Magno-Electric

Vitalizer, a "miracle" machine that claimed to cure everything from rheumatism to deafness and paralysis, using a combination of magnets and batteries. The machine, of course, had no medical value, and the federal government closed his company for fraud in 1904. In court, young Edison's father entered an affidavit noting that his son "has never shown any ability as an inventor or electrical expert, and that deponent believes his said son is incapable of making any invention or discovery of merit."

Another electrical device called for a patient to hold a metal cylinder, a hand electrode, and for the "doctor" to attach a second electrode to the ailing part of the body. The electrodes were connected to an electrical source such as a magneto, chemical battery, or box battery. As with the Davis Kidder Magneto, a low-voltage current was generated that could be felt by the patient and could cause involuntary muscle contractions. Medically speaking, of course, it was worthless.

Still another device making use of electricity was the Violet Ray, invented and first sold by Nikola Tesla in the early 1900s. Quack doctors purchased many of the devices and claimed they would cure circulation problems, falling hair, germ infections, aches and pains, deafness, constipation, and just about any other problem in the human body. Violet Ray machines produced a very high voltage by increasing the voltage from a wall socket with a step-up transformer. The high voltage was impressed on the end of a glass tube filled with a gas that lighted up with a violet color when the voltage was applied. The lighted tube looked very impressive to a patient and became even more impressive as the "doctor" described how it was "curing" the patient. The device was something like a magic wand to cure illness, but about the only thing it cured was head lice: The Violet Ray killed them.[6]

Dr. Albert Abrams created another form of quackery in his native California. Born in San Francisco in 1873, Abrams became a physician with good credentials. He reportedly earned a medical degree from the University of Heidelberg, and worked at the Cooper Medical Institute and later at Stanford Medical School. In 1893 he served as president of the San Francisco Medical Surgical Society and was highly regarded by his colleagues. He published a number of articles in prominent medical journals. During World War I, however, Abrams suddenly changed his focus and came up with the theory that electrons were the basic element of all life and that all matter contains certain vibrations and harmonics that can be manipulated. He described his theory as

"Electronic Reactions of Abrams," or ERA. Soon Abrams introduced machines that he claimed operated on the principles of ERA. Probably the most important one was called the Dynomizer, a machine that looked something like a radio. Abrams claimed it could diagnose every known disease from a single drop of blood. The blood sample was first "polarized" by a magnet before being inserted into the machine, which would then sense the frequencies of the vibrations. The blood did not have to be fresh. In fact, Abrams claimed his machine would work with dried blood samples sent to him through the mail, and therefore that he could conduct his medical practice over the telephone using his machine to determine a patient's personality characteristics and medical problems. Radio was in its infancy in America and was on everyone's mind. Abrams implied that his Dynomizer could detect disease just as a good radio receiver could bring in distant stations. His invention sounded marvelous. Interestingly, in 1918, when his Dynomizer was at the height of its success, a silent film was released that dramatized Mary Shelley's early-nineteenth-century novel *Frankenstein* and portrayed Dr. Frankenstein's monster brought to life by electricity.

Abrams became wealthy with his machine, even though he earned only one fee when using it to diagnose patients. Deciding he needed a machine that patients would turn to and use repeatedly, he came up with the Oscilloclast (sometimes called the Radioclast). His new machine also looked like a radio and came with lists of frequencies. Each frequency would attack a different disease. His machine supposedly could diagnose health problems including syphilis, cancer, and diabetes. A specific frequency would then be set on the machine to treat the disease. Patients using the Oscilloclast usually had to receive and pay for several treatments. Abrams even came up with a disease he called bovine syphilis. Orthodox physicians had never heard of it, but Abrams claimed that most of the time his machine could detect and treat it. Of course, he added, the Oscilloclast was a machine, and no machine is perfect.

As Abrams's reputation grew, students from across the nation came to his San Francisco clinic to enroll in his training course. Each student paid $200. Abrams then leased machines to his students to take home and use in their practices. Before leaving, each student had to agree not to open his machine, because to do so might disrupt its delicate adjustments. Abrams was so successful that by 1921 about 3,500 "doctors" were using Electronic Reactions of Abrams (ERA) and cutting into the business of orthodox physicians. Abrams's downfall began about 1924, when the Mayo Clinic in Minnesota diagnosed an old man as having inoperable stomach cancer. As a last resort, the man went to an ERA practitioner for treatment and afterward was told he was completely cured. A month later he died. This case led to a battle between Abrams and his supporters, who included writers Upton Sinclair and Sir Arthur Conan Doyle, and the American Medical Association.

In hopes of learning the truth about Abrams's ERA, the highly respected magazine *Scientific American* entered the conflict. The magazine's investigators developed a series of tests and even invited readers to suggest their own tests. Next the magazine gave a leading practitioner of Abrams's system, whom it called "Doctor X," six vials containing pathogens unknown to him and asked him to determine what they were. The doctor gave the magazine permission to witness his tests, but he failed to correctly identify the contents of even one of the six vials. The doctor concluded that the labels in red ink confused his machine. The investigators gave the doctor vials with new labels, but he still failed to identify any of the contents.

The magazine published the results and received many letters from both sides. Abrams offered to cooperate but begged off when investigators stipulated conditions he did not like. He never participated in any of the tests and actually claimed he was the victim of unjust persecution. This conspiracy claim was a typical tactic of quacks seeking to gain sympathy from their supporters and others when confronted by orthodox medicine. Meantime, however, a member of the AMA sent a blood sample to another practitioner of the Abrams system and received a diagnosis that the patient in question had malaria, diabetes, cancer, and syphilis. It turned out that the blood sample came from a chicken. Similar tricks were played on other Abrams practitioners, and some were charged with fraud in courts. In one 1924 case at Jonesboro, Arkansas, Abrams himself was called as a witness. He replied that he could not attend because he was dying of pneumonia. He was sixty-two and he did die. People, including many of his supporters, began to wonder why his machines had not been able to cure him.

Soon after Abrams's death, officials of the American Medical Association publicly opened one of his ERA machines and found nothing but wires connected to lights and a buzzer. The so-called machine was nothing more than a fancy prop, and it proved Abrams was a deliberate fraud. In its *Journal*, the AMA later described Dr. Abrams as "the dean of twentieth-century charlatans." In the meantime, however, other quacks moved into the vacuum he left and created similar devices and new theories in their ceaseless efforts to make money.[7]

Hundreds if not thousands of quack devices came and went during the first half of the twentieth century. Perhaps as many as fifty sought to copy Abrams's techniques. One such doctor was Heil Eugene Crum, a native of Indiana, who after graduating from high school enrolled in a diploma mill called the College of Drugless Physicians in Indianapolis, and in one year received degrees of Doctor of Naturopathy, Doctor of Electro-Therapeutics, Doctor of Chiropractic, and Doctor of Herbal Materia. He was licensed in 1927, without examination, and began a practice in Indianapolis. Some years later, in 1936, he patented his Co-Etherator machine. The government's granting of a patent, however, does not imply that the device will accomplish what the patent holder claims it will do or that it has any merit at all. But Crum apparently believed that telling the public a device was patented gave it and him more credibility. His device was nothing more than a small wooden box with twenty-six holes in the front. Tissue paper printed with letters of the alphabet in various colors was pasted over the holes, one letter per hole. Inside the box was an ordinary lightbulb with a cord. The bulb could be moved around inside to shine through one or another of the paper-covered holes. Crum also placed in the box a tangle of disconnected wire apparently representing an antenna, and there was a glass vial filled with tap water. On the outside was a pedal and a dial that were not connected to anything inside the box. The patient was asked to moisten a slip of paper with saliva and then insert the paper into the box through a slot. The machine operator then rubbed the pedal with his thumb and talked to the machine, reciting a list of common diseases. The light would then shine through one of the holes and the letter supposedly indicated the patient's disease.

Crum claimed his Co-Etherator could diagnose and cure anything from an amputated finger to cancer. Interestingly, the doctor's patient did not have to be with the doctor to be diagnosed and cured. Crum also said his machine could help a patient's financial situation by fertilizing his farmland within a distance of seventy miles, killing dandelions, and treating golf course greens. Crum's claims were too much for orthodox physicians in Indiana. The Indiana State Board of Medical Registration and Examination took Crum to court, accusing him of using a device of no possible therapeutic value under any recognized system of treatment, and that he knowingly made false and fraudulent claims about it for profit and to the injury of others. In November 1941, the Indiana Supreme Court revoked Crum's medical license and upheld a trial court ruling that found him "guilty of gross immorality."[8]

Another form of quackery evolved from Madame Curie's discovery of radium. Born Maria Sklodowska in Warsaw, Poland, in 1867, she also discovered that radium could kill diseased human cells, and she sought ways to isolate radium to use in killing tumors. The public did not fully understand what radium was. When they learned that many of the popular hot springs contained radon, a gas emitted by radioactive material in the earth's crust, many concluded that if radon was in the water it was good for you and radium itself was even more effective. Even though Madame Curie's fingers fell off before her death from radiation, the gullible public looked with awe at the radioactive products that appeared on the market during the 1920s and 1930s. It was then possible to buy an array of radium-containing products, including beauty creams, earplugs, toothpaste, soap, and even chocolate bars. Manufacturers claimed their products could cure tuberculosis, high blood pressure, arthritis, cancer, epilepsy, and kidney problems, among other ailments.

One pioneer radium quack was Dr. William J. A. Bailey, who was born in Boston in 1884. Although from a poor family, Bailey graduated from Boston Public Grammar School and entered Harvard in 1903. After two years he had to drop out of college because he had no money. He never graduated but later claimed to have a bachelor's degree from Harvard and a doctorate from the University of Vienna. Evidence that he was an accomplished con man surfaced about 1915, when he and two other associates established the Carnegie Engineering Corporation, a name that falsely implied a relationship with the Carnegie Steel Corporation. Bailey's company sold automobiles by mail for $600, requiring a $50 advance deposit on each. The company accepted 1,500 advance deposits but could not deliver. In the fall of 1915, the government issued an injunction for fraud against Bailey's company, and he was convicted of swindling and given thirty days in jail.

Bailey surfaced again in 1918, when he was fined $200 for selling Las-I-Go, an impotence "cure" that contained strychnine. Meantime, he had latched on to sex cells, the human sperm and egg that have only half the number of chromosomes that other body cells have. By the early 1920s, Bailey was combining sex with the nation's interest in radium. He started Associated Radium Chemists, Inc., in New York City and began promoting several radium cures, one for coughs and flu, a radioactive liniment, and Arium, a radioactive aphrodisiac in tablet form. Bailey claimed Arium would bring renewed happiness and youthful thrills into the lives of older couples. Bailey even guaranteed that radium was used in Arium's preparation. The U.S. Agricultural Department investigated the claim and found it to be false and fraudulent and ordered Arium off the market. Bailey did not give up. He began selling Thorone, which he claimed was 250 times more active than radium, and would cure impotence.

By the late 1920s Bailey had entered into partnership with Ward Leathers and started the American Foundation Laboratories in New York City. Two other quacks—Dr. C. Everett Field and Dr. Herman H. Rubin—joined the company, which soon was selling Radiendocrimator, a device promoted as something like the fountain of youth. It was nothing more than two pads, two inches long by three inches wide and three-eighths of an inch thick, attached to the body by a belt called an "adaptor." The pads were "charged with pure radium, carefully and perfectly screened to avoid every possible alpha or burning ray. The gamma ray is amplified by the use of mesotharium and actinium, elements rarer and in some cases much more expensive than radium." The pads of the Radiendocrimator were worn over the thyroid, adrenals, ovaries, pituitary, and prostate glands. Treatments of ten to thirty minutes were sometimes recommended as often as three or four times a day. Overnight treatment of the "gonads" was also suggested. Bailey's advertising said the device worked by causing ionization of the endocrine system, thereby increasing hormone production. In simple words, the pads were effective at "lighting up dark recesses of the body." The result, according to the advertising, was rejuvenation, with results guaranteed in thirty days. The Radiendocrimator first sold for $1,000, but soon after the stock market crash of 1929 it was priced at $500. When the American Medical Association attacked radium cures during the 1930s, the price was reduced to $250. At their peak, Bailey's laboratory sales of the device reached $200,000 annually with a net profit of $50,000.

In 1925, while still enjoying much success with his Radiendocrimator, Bailey was already producing another quack cure using radium called Radithor, probably his best-known piece of quackery. It was premixed radium water packaged in a small brown bottle with a cork. Each bottle sold for $1, but a minimum order was thirty bottles, or a month's supply. The contents were actually triple-distilled water containing at a minimum one microcurie each of the radium 226 and 228 isotopes, as well as one microcurie of isothiouronium, a less expensive radioactive compound. Bailey advertised Radithor as "A Cure for the Living Dead" and as "Perpetual Sunshine." The true nature of this "cure" became clear with the eventual death in 1931 of a steel tycoon from Pittsburgh, and of a onetime U.S. Amateur Golf champion, Eben M. Byers, from Radithor consumption and the associated radiation poisoning. Byers reportedly drank more than 1,400 bottles, until portions of his mouth and jaw had to be surgically removed. He died of radium poisoning in April 1932. The cause of Byers's death was widely publicized and led to the strengthening of the Food and Drug Administration's powers and the demise of most radiation quack cures. As for William Bailey, he died of bladder cancer in Massachusetts in 1949.[9]

Since the middle of the nineteenth century, countless other devices have been produced by quacks to cure just about everything, including failing eyesight. The roots of one quack who exploited this last concern, Urbane Barrett, go back to 1906, when his brother Wesley M. Barrett founded the Barrett Institute in Los Angeles. After reading Dr. William Horatio Bates's book *The Cure of Imperfect Eyesight by Treatment Without Glasses*, published in 1920, which put forth the theory that failing eyesight could be corrected by exercising the eyes, Urbane Barrett bought out his brother's mail-order business and changed the name to National Eyesight Institute. A lawyer, Urbane Barrett developed his own "system," created a device for the eyes, and wrote advertising copy to promote what he called the Natural Eye Normalizer. It was a metal instrument finished in chrome, with rubber gaskets fitting over the eyes. The device shut out all light. A handle on the side, however, permitted the patient to rotate the gaskets slightly to massage the eyelids. He claimed the device relaxed the eyes and by doing so corrected any and all vision problems. In truth, Barrett's instrument corrected nothing. He was convicted of mail fraud in 1937, following a hearing where experts testified that his Natural Eye Normalizer was useless.[10] As for Dr. Bates's theory that eye relaxation can solve visual problems, it is considered useless and his theories unscientific by most experts, except that relaxing the eye may help correct lazy eye or crossed eyes.

Bates was something of a mystery. Born in 1860, he received his medical degree in 1885 from the College of Physicians and Surgeons at Cornell University. He soon practiced and later taught medicine in New York City medical schools. But he disappeared twice during his lifetime. His obituary in the July 11, 1931, issue of the *New York Times* relates how he first vanished seven years after receiving his medical degree. His wife found him later in London in a state of nervous exhaustion, with no recollection of recent events. She took him to a hotel, but two days later, Bates disappeared again. His wife looked for him throughout Europe, but she died before locating him. A friend found him in 1910 living in Grand Forks, North Dakota. He could not remember how he got there. The friend persuaded him to return to New York City, where he practiced medicine until 1922. It was there that he wrote his book containing his theory on how to correct failing eyesight through eye exercises.

John Harvey Kellogg was another physician with impressive credentials. He never was a true quack, but his beliefs were often questioned by orthodox doctors. He was born in 1852 at Tyrone, Michigan. His family, devout Seventh-Day Adventists, moved to Battle Creek, Michigan, when John was four years old. As a boy, he came to believe in the tenets of healthy living, including a rejection of meat, advocated by the Adventist religion. Ellen and James White, the church's founders, opened a Health Reform Institute in 1866 and practiced the water cure. The Whites needed someone to be the institute's full-time medical director and they helped finance John Kellogg's medical studies at the Bellevue Medical College in New York City. When he graduated in 1875, the twenty-three-year-old Kellogg returned to Battle Creek and became HRI's medical superintendent. His brother, Will Keith Kellogg, a former traveling broom salesman, became its bookkeeper and business manager. Soon thereafter, John coined the term *sanitarium* and changed the institute's name to Battle Creek Sanitarium. He also changed its focus from hydrotherapy to medical and surgical treatment.

During the years that followed, he studied medicine, surgery, and physiology in Europe with leading doctors and became a fellow in several leading medical societies, including the American College of Surgeons, the American Association for the Advancement of Science, and the American Medical Association. Dr. Kellogg introduced several new techniques in surgery and during his career had an extraordinarily low mortality rate in the thousands of operations he performed. Long before medicine looked at smoking and cancer, Dr. Kellogg warned that smoking caused lung cancer. He was also a pioneer in advocating exercise and "biologic living."

The Kellogg brothers worked to develop more grain-based foods for their vegetarian patients. They also devised a coffee substitute—and, by accident, wheat flakes. They discovered the flakes in 1894 as they were preparing wheat meal by running boiled wheat through rollers to create a very thin cracker-type sheet. They would then roast the wheat and grind it into meal. One night, however, they left a batch of boiled wheat out and forgot about it. The next morning they found it and ran it through the roller to see if the stale wheat was salvageable once it was ground. But instead of emerging as a unified flat sheet, the wheat came out in flakes, one for each wheat berry. They roasted the flakes and served them to their patients. They were a hit. Soon former patients at the sanitarium were requesting the cereal flakes by mail. Within two years the Kellogg brothers were in the cereal business, manufacturing what they called "Granose" for patients and church members. Later, Will Kellogg created corn flakes and tried to persuade his brother John that they should sell their discoveries in grocery stores. But John opposed the idea, believing such a commercial venture might compromise his integrity as a physician.

Realizing the potential of their discoveries, Will Kellogg bought out his brother's portion of the cereal patents, created the Kellogg Company, and introduced their cereals in grocery stores. A good businessman who believed in advertising, Will Kellogg was responsible for the 1907 advertising slogan "Wink at your grocer and get a free box of Corn Flakes." In three years, the company's sales reached a million cases of Kellogg's Corn Flakes.

Although Will's doctor brother John had outstanding medical credentials, he became involved in questionable medical practices during the years that followed. The Battle Creek Sanitarium offered water cures, electropathy, mechanotherapy (medical treatment by mechanical methods such as massage), and radium cures. For a time he even believed in "Fletcherizing," the chewing of food until it slithered down the throat. He then decided that excessive chewing destroyed the fiber content of the food. He even opposed sexual activity and claimed he never made love to his wife. His favorite medical subject was the bowel, and he claimed that 90 percent of all illness originated in the stomach and bowel. He soon made the bowel, till then a subject avoided in polite conversation, something of a national obsession. People came to believe their bowels were full of harmful substances, and Kellogg's solution was to clean out the bowels, starting with every patient at the sanitarium. A favorite device was an enema machine that could run fifteen gallons of water through a patient's bowel in seconds. Next, he had each patient eat half a pint of yogurt. The other half was administered by enema. Dr. Kellogg believed the yogurt replaced the intestinal flora of the bowel, making it clean. If the treatment did not work and left a portion of the intestine dirty, he removed it. On some days, he performed nearly two dozen operations on patients to accomplish this. Dr. Kellogg claimed that his approach had cured ulcers, cancer of the stomach, schizophrenia, diabetes, acne, migraine headaches, and neurasthenia, and even stopped premature aging. He continued to run the sanitarium, despite increasing financial problems. By the end of the 1930s it was clear it could not survive at its current size. In 1942, he sold the main building to the federal government and moved the treatment center to another structure up the street. Kellogg's former sanitarium was soon converted into the Percy Jones General and Convalescent Hospital, an orthopedic hospital that served the nation's veterans through World War II and the Korean conflict. In 1954 it was the U.S. Army's largest medical installation.

While Will Keith Kellogg died in 1898, his brother Dr. John Harvey Kellogg lived until December 1943, when he died at the age of ninety-one. Today his medical contributions are often overshadowed by the Kellogg name and the breakfast cereal empire it represents.[11]

I STILL REMEMBER my parents talking during my Kansas boyhood about the radio broadcasts of Dr. John R. Brinkley, the "goat gland doctor." His radio station was located next to his hospital at Milford, about thirty miles west of my home in Manhattan, Kansas. The Federal Radio Commission refused to renew his station's license in 1930 and his station was taken off the air a year or two before I was born. Later, my parents told how he used his station to pitch goat gland transplants, claiming men would be rejuvenated. I was not sure what all of this meant, but my parents enjoyed some of the station's informational programs on farming and recipes, and musical programs featuring concerts by high school music groups and the U.S. Army Ninth

Cavalry band from nearby Fort Riley. Individual entertainers like Uncle Bob Larkin and his fiddle and Dutch, the boy blues singer, entertained between Brinkley's medical pitches. Brinkley even broadcast lectures and correspondence courses from nearby Kansas State College (now Kansas State University) in Manhattan.

Putting a radio station on the air was easy in 1923 when Brinkley built his five-hundred-watt station at Milford. Broadcasting was just beginning. It was a novelty. The AM radio broadcast band was expanded that year by the Department of Commerce in Washington, D.C. Brinkley simply filled out a government form and sent it to Washington. Call letters of his choice were assigned as a way to identify the station, and Brinkley selected the call letters KFKB, an acronym for "Kansas First, Kansas Best," "Kansas Farmers Know Best," and "Kansas Folks Know Best."

When a young girl, a crippled shut-in, supposedly called KFKB "the Sunshine Station in the Heart of the Nation," Brinkley used this as the station's slogan for his predominately rural audience in Kansas and surrounding states. When legal rulings caused federal regulation to break down in July 1926 and stations became free to use any power they wanted, Brinkley raised his station's power to 1,000 watts. At night his station could be heard over much of the nation and in Canada.

"Doc" Brinkley was born John Romulus Brinkley near Beta, Jackson County, North Carolina, on July 8, 1885. (He later changed his middle name to Richard.) Orphaned at an early age, he was raised by an aunt. Between 1907 through 1915, he attended Bennett Medical College in Chicago but lacked the money to earn his degree. Later he received a degree from the Eclectic Medical University in Kansas City, Missouri. Even though his credentials were dubious, Brinkley was granted a license to practice by the state of Arkansas, and in 1916 in Kansas, after he answered a newspaper advertisement that said Milford, Kansas, needed a doctor. He thought Milford had a population of 2,000 until he arrived and found only 200 residents. Brinkley and his second wife, Minnie, rented the Milford drugstore, which had two rooms plus the store. They lived in one of the rooms while Brinkley set up his office in the other. His wife operated the drugstore, which had a soda fountain and carried patent medicines, cosmetics, and knick-knacks.

One day, Milford businessman William Stittsworth came by to see

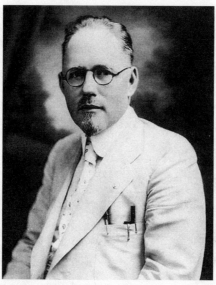

Dr. John Romulus Brinkley (1885–1942) was born in North Carolina. He earned a medical degree from a questionable institution in Kansas City, Missouri. In 1916, he moved to Milford, Kansas, rented a drugstore, and opened a medical practice. He achieved fame for his claim that he could restore male sexual potency by transplanting glands from goats into men. (Courtesy Kansas State Historical Society)

the doctor about his impotence, a condition he claimed he had suffered for sixteen years. Brinkley told him he had been studying a theory according to which goat glands could be transplanted into men to make them virile. Stittsworth agreed to the surgery, which was performed on November 22, 1917. When Stittsworth's wife produced a child less than a year later, Brinkley claimed this as proof that the operation worked. The news spread by word of mouth, and within weeks another Milford businessman came to Brinkley wanting the same operation. Brinkley knew he had found a good way to make money and announced a fee of $750 for the goat gland operation.

On the advice of a consultant from Kansas City, Missouri, Brinkley began to advertise his operation in newspapers and by direct mail. His

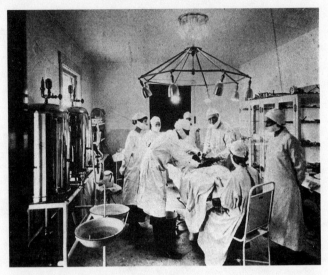

Dr. John Brinkley's operating room at Milford, Kansas, about 1919. (Courtesy National Library of Medicine)

business grew, and in 1918 he constructed a 2½-story, sixteen-room hospital in Milford to accommodate more patients. Five years later, he built a radio station to publicize his business and to attract customers. He soon added a program called *The Question Box* to the station's schedule. Brinkley answered listeners' questions on the air twice daily, offering advice and prescriptions from his Milford Drug Company. He prescribed common drugs such as castor oil and aspirin, but he gave each a number instead of its name. Listeners could order the prescription by asking for the number recommended. The listener who received advice on the air would then send in his payment and the specific prescriptions were sent back postage paid. The business was so successful Brinkley hired up to fifty girls to open the mail, which at its peak reached 50,000 letters a day.

Brinkley's business attracted the attention of other druggists around the country because it was cutting into their sales. A delegation of druggists visited Brinkley in Milford to complain. After a meeting of about an hour the Brinkley Pharmaceutical Association was formed, each member of which had access to Brinkley's numbering system. As

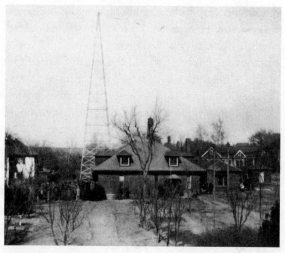

John Brinkley's hospital (left), home, and radio station in Milford, Kansas, in the 1920s. The antenna tower for his station, KFKB, is faintly visible in the center. (Courtesy Kansas State Historical Society)

Brinkley prescribed drugs on the air, he would tell listeners they could get it from their local druggist if he was a member of the Brinkley Pharmaceutical Association. The local member druggists charged $3 per prescription, sent $1 of it to Brinkley, and increased their own profit for common drugs. Brinkley reportedly earned about $750,000 annually through this scheme.

In 1927, Brinkley successfully applied to the Federal Radio Commission to increase KFKB's power from 1,000 watts to 5,000 watts, winning out over WDAF, a competing station owned by the *Kansas City* (Missouri) *Star*. KFKB became one of the most powerful stations in the nation. The newspaper sent one of its best reporters, A. B. MacDonald, to investigate Brinkley, and a series of articles was published alleging that he was a quack. About the same time Dr. Morris Fishbein, the vocal executive secretary of the American Medical Association, began attacking Brinkley for diagnosing illnesses and then prescribing medicines on the air. In 1928, Brinkley began using his station to attack Fishbein and the AMA. This went on for more than a year. At last, in 1930, the Kansas State Medical Board revoked Brinkley's medical license, and the Federal Radio Commission refused to renew KFKB's broadcasting license. His station, however, remained on the air until early 1931 while Brinkley appealed the ruling.

In February 1931, however, the U.S. Court of Appeals upheld the Federal Radio Commission's decision to cancel Brinkley's station license. Brinkley's response was to enter the Kansas governor's race against Alf Landon. Brinkley hoped to win so that he could appoint new members to the state medical board. He ran as an independent write-in candidate, and came close to winning; he lost only because thousands of votes were tossed out on technicalities. Two subsequent bids for the governorship, in 1932 and 1934, also failed.

Meantime, Doc Brinkley obtained permission from Mexican officials to build a powerful 75,000-watt radio station at Villa Acuña, Mexico, across the Rio Grande from Del Rio, Texas. It went on the air in the fall of 1931 and station XER blanketed the nation with its broadcast signal. Brinkley remained in Milford and broadcast by telephone

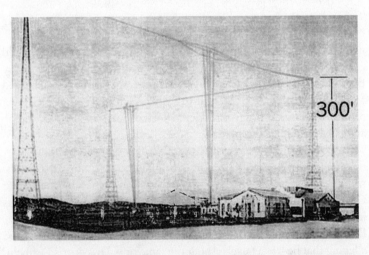

Dr. Brinkley received permission in 1931 from the Mexican government to build radio station XER in Villa Acuña, Mexico, just across the Rio Grande from Del Rio, Texas. At first, it had a 75,000-watt transmitter, and the station could be heard across the United States. In 1934, he received permission to increase the station's power to 500,000 watts. The station then not only blanketed the United States but could be heard in Canada and Europe. This photo, showing the station and its huge antenna system, appeared on postcards Brinkley mailed to his listeners who sent in reception reports. (Author's collection)

to the XER transmitter at a cost of thousands of dollars. By then he had moved his medical staff and facilities to the Roswell Hotel in Del Rio. XER, however, was easily heard at night in Kansas, where he was running for governor. In 1934, after his final electoral defeat, Brinkley moved to Texas, where he got permission to increase the power of his Mexican station to 500,000 watts. His new call letters were XERA.

At night, XERA was heard not only in Kansas, but also throughout the United States and in Canada. Its signal was so powerful that it went over the North Pole, and XERA could be heard in the Soviet Union, where his broadcasts were reportedly used to teach English in the NKVD spy school. In the meantime, Brinkley was getting richer. He enticed listeners to visit his clinic in Del Rio, and he also sold an array of gimmicks by mail, including ampoules of colored water at a price of six for $100. In Del Rio, he rarely implanted goat glands, but began offering Mercurochrome shots and pills to help restore youthful vigor in men with prostate trouble. During the Depression, from 1933 to 1938, Brinkley lived in a lavish mansion built overlooking his Mexican radio station. He accumulated expensive autos, planes, diamonds, and yachts, including his last, the huge *John R. Brinkley III* requiring a crew of twenty-two and costing Brinkley $1,000 a day to operate.

During this time, the U.S. government seems to have tolerated him. But that changed when Brinkley in his broadcasts from XERA expressed open sympathy for Hitler and the Nazis in Germany. This was too much for President Franklin Roosevelt, who was trying to persuade Americans to back the Allies before the U.S. entered World War II. Under pressure from the United States, on the grounds of Brinkley's Nazi sympathies, the Mexican government silenced XERA late in 1939. The government in Washington also passed what was called "the Brinkley Act" under the Communications Act of 1934, banning any cross-border studio transmitter links originating in the United States, including telephone lines like those that Brinkley had used from Kansas to his Mexican radio station.

In 1938, he moved his medical activities to Little Rock, Arkansas, but maintained his residence in Del Rio. About this time, he lost a libel suit against Fishbein, fought numerous malpractice suits, and battled the Internal Revenue Service over back taxes. All these things together forced Brinkley into bankruptcy in 1941. The following year he experienced circulatory problems, and one of his legs was amputated. On

May 26, 1942, he died of heart failure in San Antonio, Texas, and was buried in a Memphis, Tennessee, cemetery.[12]

IF JOHN BRINKLEY was a spectacular quack, a small-town Iowa boy named Norman Baker would turn out to outdo him. Born in Muscatine, Iowa, three years before Brinkley was born in North Carolina, Baker was the youngest of ten. In 1898, at the age of sixteen, he quit high school and took a job as a machinist. He wandered about the region for a few years, earning his living as a tool-and-die man. One evening Baker attended a show put on by a magician who claimed to be a mentalist. Fascinated, Baker soon read up on the subject and appeared himself as a mentalist. By 1904, Baker had established a successful show using a "mind reader" he called Madame Pearl Tangley. Soon Baker's outfit was on the vaudeville circuit. When the mind reader quit in 1909, Baker hired a college girl named Theresa Pinder to be the new Madame Tangley. About a year later Baker and Pinder were married and the mentalist show continued until 1914, when the couple went to Muscatine for a break.

The Bakers had intended to take their show back on the road in the fall of 1914, but while tinkering in his brother's machine shop, Baker invented a new kind of pipe organ, which used air instead of steam. He called it the Air Calliaphone. Baker sold the first one for $500. He built and sold two more Air Calliaphones and decided to quit vaudeville and turn to the full-time manufacture of his organ, calling his enterprise the Tangley Company after the stage name of his mind reader in vaudeville. The year was 1915. He divorced his wife and devoted himself full-time to manufacturing air organs; within a few years he had earned $200,000 from his enterprise. Then in 1920, Baker opened an art correspondence school that he called the Tangley School. Baker admitted that he could not draw himself, but he reportedly earned $75,000 in three years ostensibly teaching people who signed up for his correspondence course in learning how to draw and paint.

In the meantime, he became very active in civic affairs in Muscatine, enhancing his local reputation. In 1925, he proposed building a radio station that would call attention to this town of a few thousand people located on the Mississippi River in eastern Iowa. He told the Muscatine Chamber of Commerce and the city fathers that he would build the station if they would provide free electricity and water, and not tax the station. They agreed, and Baker then asked for and obtained a government license to establish a five-hundred-watt radio station on a high hill overlooking the Mississippi River. Its call letters were KTNT. Just as John Brinkley had done in Kansas, Baker sought to attract small-town folks, farmers, and laborers. KTNT went on the air on Thanksgiving Day 1925, with Baker telling his listeners that his little station was fighting big business for freedom of the airwaves.

Using the airwaves and a magazine he started, Baker became a crusader seemingly for the common man by attacking the moneyed establishment, including large newspapers, the emerging radio networks, Wall Street, the Aluminum Trust, and the American Medical Association. He soon gained listeners and realized radio was a highly effective way to promote Norman Baker and his opinions and to sell products. Three years after KTNT went on the air, Baker received permission to raise the station's power to 10,000 watts. The increased power meant his station could reach more than a million homes in the Middle West. Its call letters supposedly stood for "Know the Naked Truth." Baker soon started *TNT* magazine to expound on his populist views, with the slogan "The Naked Truth." He also started a gasoline service station and opened the TNT Café. As his popularity grew, he became more vocal and personal in attacking those he considered the enemies of the people. Baker's attacks, however, began to turn people against him, and KTNT received many letters of complaint.

In 1929, Baker decided to branch out into medicine, claiming that aluminum, especially in the form of cooking utensils, caused cancer and that radium, X-rays, and operations could not cure cancer. When he learned that a Dr. Charles Ozias was operating a cancer sanitarium in Kansas City, Baker told listeners that in the public interest Dr. Ozias should be investigated to see if his cure worked. Baker asked for five volunteers to go to Kansas City for treatment, promising to pay their expenses. He got his volunteers and sent them off. Although all five patients died between November 1929 and May 1930, Baker reported in his magazine that all of them had been cured. He proclaimed in *TNT* magazine, "Cancer is Cured," and announced that he had acquired the Ozias cure and was opening the Baker Institute in Muscatine. He claimed the patients, who were actually dead, had been cured by a liquid solution containing carbolic acid, glycerin, and alcohol that was mixed with tea brewed from watermelon seed, clover leaves, and brown cornsilk. Baker advertised his new hospital on KTNT and hired

Harry Hoxsey, a quack with an alleged cancer cure. Why Baker hired Hoxsey is something of a mystery, since he claimed to have already acquired Dr. Ozias's cure. Regardless, in 1930, Baker made more than $440,000 from cancer patients.

In April 1930, however, Morris Fishbein and the American Medical Association began a campaign to expose quackery in the association's journal, of which Fishbein was editor. He realized that Baker's attacks on the AMA were undermining the trust Americans had in the ortho-dox medical establishment, and he set out to put Baker out of business through articles in the journal. In the April 12, 1930, edition, Fishbein reported:

> In Iowa at Muscatine, over KTNT, broadcasts a business man named Norman Baker who is selling a cancer cure, with cigars and cheap magazines as side lines. His cancer cure includes the old Hoxsey fake, originally promoted in Illinois, and apparently now resident also in Iowa. This nostrum for cancer is boomed by Mr. Baker over his radio station KTNT, which can be heard almost anywhere after 11 o'clock at night. This is exceedingly proper since it is the time of night when many devious and doubtful ventures are promoted. . . .
>
> Baker has even claimed that the American Medical Association offered him one million dollars for his cancer cure with the intent of forcing it from the market so that patients might be compelled to resort to surgery for the saving of their lives. The lie is so obviously false to any person of intelligence above that of a moron that it needs little thought to convince his hearers of its fallacy. . . .
>
> The viciousness of Mr. Baker's broadcasting lies not in what he says about the American Medical Association but in the fact that he induces sufferers from cancer who might have some chance for their lives, if seen early and properly treated, to resort to his nostrum. The method can result in Muscatine, Iowa, as it did in Taylorville, Illinois, merely in death certificates signed by the physicians who have been so poor in finances and in morals as to sell their birthrights to Mr. Baker for his mess of garbage.

Meantime, the *Des Moines Register*, the state's leading newspaper, investigated Baker and established that his radio talk claims were false. The AMA journal soon called for the revocation of Baker's medical license and for the Federal Radio Commission to put KTNT off the air. Baker soon went on the offensive, filing a half-million-dollar law-suit against the AMA for libel and defamation. He even claimed the AMA had sent three assassins to KTNT to kill him. In hopes of gaining public support he announced he would hold a public demonstration of his cure in Muscatine. Perhaps forty thousand people went to Musca-tine to watch it. With his theater experience, Baker knew how to manipulate a crowd, and he first had former patients stand up and tell about their miraculous healing from the cure. Baker next drank an enormous dose of his purported cancer cure to show there were no harmful effects. Next, one of Baker's doctors ostensibly opened the skull of a sixty-eight-year-old man who was still conscious and applied the cure to what was supposedly cancerous brain tissue. Baker then dra-matically told everyone, "Cancer is cured." Having gained the support of the audience, Baker then began a verbal attack against the "medical trust," accusing them of concern for profits over patients. Baker told the audience that the initials *M.D.* really stood for "More Dough." He assured everyone present that he would not give up his fight for them.

As more patients came to Muscatine, the AMA published new arti-cles calling Baker's public operation a hoax and continued to lobby the Federal Radio Commission to revoke Baker's radio license. In May 1931 the FRC refused to renew the license, forcing Baker off the air. He then lost his suit against the AMA as relatives and former patients began to testify in court against him. A court found Baker guilty of practicing medicine without a license, but before an arrest warrant could be served, Baker fled to Nuevo Laredo, Mexico. There he built a new 100,000-watt radio station, XENT. The station went on the air in 1933 with programs similar in content to Baker's broadcasts on KTNT, including anti-Jewish, pro-Hitler commentary, and attacks on the American Medical Association. Baker remained in Mexico, broad-casting from his station. He also established a small cancer hospital at Nuevo Laredo. In 1937, however, he decided to return to Muscatine. He pleaded guilty to practicing medicine without a license, and served a one-day sentence in jail. He ran as a candidate for governor of Iowa in 1932 but lost and then left the state.

Baker then moved to Arkansas and purchased a Victorian hotel called the Crescent in the Ozarks town of Eureka Springs. The hotel sat on a hill above the town and Baker christened it the "Castle in the Air." He turned the hotel into the Baker Hospital and resumed the same medical frauds that had made him wealthy in Iowa. Two years later, however, federal authorities arrested him on a charge of using the U.S. mails to defraud. He was found guilty and his appeal was denied. He was fined $4,000 and sentenced to four years in prison at the federal penitentiary at Leavenworth, Kansas. He was released from prison in the summer of 1945. Baker retired to Florida, where he lived a comfortable life from his quackery earnings until his death from cirrhosis of the liver at age seventy-five in 1958. Norman Baker was buried in the cemetery at Muscatine, Iowa, not far from the hill where his radio station had once stood.[13]

LIKE MODERN SCIENTIFIC MEDICINE, medical quackery continues and is constantly evolving with technology. Quackery persists in spite of legislation and self-policing by medical associations and public groups. With each generation, new scoundrels seek to take advantage of people's ignorance about conventional medical treatments. People are attracted to them by their claims and promises. Quacks often appear to be caring individuals whose medicines and treatments may or may not be harmless. Sometimes the patients say they work. More often than not, this is caused by the placebo effect of mind over matter. People who go to quacks usually do so because they mistrust orthodox medicine and government regulation. Others go because conventional medicines may be costly and the quacks provide cheaper alternatives. Others who have terminal or untreatable illnesses turn to quacks in desperation. They ignore scientific medicine and the fact that some common ailments are often cured naturally in the course of time. With no exact standard for what constitutes quackery, quacks survive because too few people ask, "What is the acceptable evidence for the efficacy and safety of the medicines and treatment proposed?" Unfortunately, there remains some level of uncertainty with all medical treatments. It is also often difficult to distinguish between those who knowingly promote unproven medical therapies and those who are honestly mistaken about the effectiveness of their treatments and misrepresent their benefits and risks. Responsible physicians follow the common ethical practice—which is in some cases a legal requirement—of stating the promise, risks, and limitations of a medical choice. The same is true of pharmaceutical companies. Quacks do not. The late Marlene Dietrich perhaps summed it up when she said, "Not everyone called a quack is a quack—except quacks and ducks."

CHAPTER FOURTEEN

INTO THE TWENTIETH CENTURY

The physician's is the highest and worthiest of all occupations, or would be if human nature did not make superstitions and priests necessary.

—Mark Twain

Humorist samuel langhorne clemens, who used the pen name Mark Twain, wrote much satire about health, medicine, and doctors. Growing up in Missouri, Clemens remembered that "doctors were not called in cases of ordinary illness, the family grandmother attended to those. Every old woman was a doctor and gathered her own medicines in the woods and knew how to compound doses that would stir the vitals of a cast-iron dog."[1]

Clemens's life spanned the nineteenth and early-twentieth centuries, and he witnessed many changes in medicine. Clemens had great creative genius; he was a philosopher and a keen observer. He came to understand the difference between disease and illness, concluding that diseases arise in the physical body, and have biological origins, while illnesses arise in the soul, are less often biological in origin, and are shaped by the patient's own attitudes, beliefs, and expectations, as well as those of society. He realized that anyone can have both a disease and an illness at the same time, and even that some illnesses can be described as the way a person experiences a disease. He also realized that the treatments for illnesses and diseases differ.

While Clemens respected and trusted individual doctors, he was cynical about the profession overall. A recurring theme in his writings was what he saw as the ineffectiveness of medical treatment. In 1883, in his book *Life on the Mississippi*, a memoir of his early years, he wrote: "There is something fascinating about science. One gets such wholesome returns of conjecture out of such a trifling investment of fact." As Americans became fascinated by science, Clemens's satire reflected the truth as he saw it, and his views were fresh and humanistic. By the late nineteenth century, he concluded that the education of physicians was not what it should be. In one of his notebooks, found after his death, Clemens had written, "A half-educated physician is not valuable. He thinks he can cure everything."

When scientific medicine began to label illnesses, Clemens expressed his views in a letter to Dr. W. W. Baldwin, dated June 15, 1904: "I was born with an incurable disease, so was everybody—the same one that every machine has—and the knowledge of the fact frightens nobody, damages nobody; but the moment a name is given the disease, the whole thing is changed: fright ensues, and horrible depression, and the life that has learned its sentence is not worth the living. Medicine has its office, it does its share and does it well; but without hope back of it, its forces are crippled and only the physician's verdict can create that hope when the facts refuse to create it."

Clemens died at the age of seventy-five in 1910, a year when Amer-

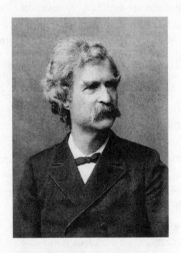

Samuel Langhorne Clemens (1835– 1910) used the pen name Mark Twain. The great American humorist, satirist, writer, and lecturer made many comments, often satirical in nature, about doctors and medicine. This photo was taken in Berlin in 1892, when Clemens was fifty-six years old. (Courtesy Bancroft Library, Berkeley)

ican medicine was trying to find order and struggling to improve in an atmosphere where quackery was rampant. The American Medical Association, founded sixty-three years earlier, was on the verge of bankruptcy. Few doctors belonged, and those who did paid little attention to the organization. Four years earlier, the AMA had created a committee to examine medical education. They made little progress because of differences among the committee members and a lack of funding. It was then that the recently funded Carnegie Foundation offered financial assistance, put Abraham Flexner in charge, and quietly worked with the AMA to complete the project. In 1910, Flexner's *Medical Education in the United States and Canada* was published in New York.

Flexner (1866–1959) was not a medical doctor. He was a former secondary school teacher and principal for nineteen years in Louisville, Kentucky. He then took graduate work at Harvard and the University of Berlin and became a consultant to the Carnegie Foundation's advancement-of-teaching project in New York, where he wrote his report that sought to standardize the medical profession. He surveyed medical training across the nation with help from the AMA and made specific recommendations for improving it. Flexner failed to acknowledge in his report that some medical schools and associations were already working to improve standards in medical education. In his report, however, he condemned medical schools including the proprietary operations run for profit. Of medical education for women, he wrote, "It is clear that [women] show a decreasing inclination" to become doctors. Of the seven black medical schools, Flexner described five of them as "ineffectual." He concluded that American medical schools should follow the German model, providing a comprehensive grounding in the biomedical sciences together with hands-on clinical training. Flexner concluded that there has been an "enormous over-production of uneducated and ill-trained medical practitioners . . . in absolute disregard of the public welfare."[2]

Flexner's report was widely circulated, and the public soon joined him in calling for improved medical education. His report shook medical education, and with the resulting publicity many medical schools closed. From 160 in 1900, the number of medical schools dropped to 85 by 1920 and to 80 by 1927. Most of the schools that remained open adopted the reforms Flexner proposed because the Carnegie and Rockefeller foundations offered grants to study and teach drug therapy

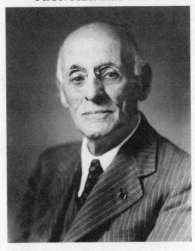

Abraham Flexner (1866–1959) was an educator whose 1910 report for the Carnegie Foundation shook the foundations of medical education and emphasized the need for scientific training in medicine. His report had far-reaching effects on the practice of medicine. (Courtesy National Library of Medicine)

and chemical research. Through these grants medical education in America slowly began to change. Flexner made clear in his report his view that medicine should be taught only as a laboratory science. Medical schools, he stressed, needed teachers trained as researchers in laboratory work. Not being a medical doctor and not conversant with the day-to-day demands of medicine as actually practiced, Flexner downplayed the importance of studying clinical medicine—the treatment of patients. Some practicing physicians who had taught part-time in medical schools were replaced by full-time research-oriented faculty to intensify the focus on scientific medicine. This created a culture in many schools dominated by salaried medical faculty trained only in laboratory science teaching students who were destined to spend their lives caring for patients. This pattern, however, was gradually reversed, and by the late 1930s many schools of medicine were going back to some clinical training taught by practicing doctors.

William Osler, former head of medicine at Johns Hopkins in Baltimore and perhaps the greatest internist of his generation, had a worldwide reputation for teaching based on his bedside study of patients. He related his views in a highly respected textbook, *The Principles and Practices of Medicine* (1892). The combination, in his book, of historical perspective, detailed discussion of disease pathology, and exhaustive clinical experience set it apart from other medical texts of the day. In 1911, after Osler became chair of medicine at Oxford University in England, he wrote to Ira Remsen, president of Johns Hopkins: "I cannot imagine anything more subversive to the highest ideal of the clinical school than to hand over our young men who are to be our best practitioners to a group of teachers who are ex-officio out of touch with the conditions under which these young men live."[3]

While Flexner's report, and subsequent grants from the Carnegie and Rockefeller foundations, did impact medical schools and in turn medical education in America, so did the fact that many American physicians had studied in Germany and were trained in the research-oriented approach to medicine and the ability to think critically, solve problems, and acquire new information. At the time the teaching of such things in American medical schools was marginal. But, whereas German schools would shortly drop this concept of medical education, it took on new life in America because of Flexner's report, which gave strength to the struggling American Medical Association. The AMA began projecting allopathic or scientific medicine as the best form.

As medical education was undergoing changes in America, so was the pharmaceutical industry. Before the Flexner report, most drug companies were still producing patent medicines. Pharmacologists, who studied drugs and their origin, nature, properties, and effects on living organisms, first organized in 1908, when eighteen of them formed the American Society of Pharmacology and Experimental Therapeutics in Baltimore. The society, however, excluded from membership anyone employed by a drug company. As for the pharmacists, who compounded and dispensed drugs, they had organized in 1852. Then, in 1906, the New York State legislature passed legislation requiring a college degree for pharmacists seeking a license, the first state to do so. Still, Flexner in his 1910 report criticized the pharmaceutical industry and called for better scientific training of people in that industry because many of the nation's drug companies were still producing patent medicines containing plant-based treatments. As the pharmaceutical industry shifted toward scientific medicine, the drug industry gradually moved away from plants and herbs toward synthetic drugs that could be patented. They needed patented drugs that could make more money with which to conduct more research and to conduct clinical studies required by the government before new drugs could be approved. The shift to synthetic drugs, packaged by drug companies, directly affected pharmacists. During the 1920s, for instance, about 80 percent of the prescriptions filled by pharmacists in drugstores and elsewhere required knowledge of compounding. By the early 1940s, only about 55 percent of doctors' prescriptions did so, because of the move toward synthetic drugs.

Across the nation, however, many practicing physicians, especially in rural areas, viewed with caution the use of synthetic drugs, the changes in medical education, and the increasing power of the American Medical Association. Many small-town doctors had either been trained by other physicians or attended one of many medical schools that operated for profit. The quality of their training and understanding of medicine was dependent upon their teachers. As medical education changed, most of these practicing physicians followed the changes that were reported in medical journals. Many physicians, however, chose not to become involved in the politics and kept their views to themselves. Most were in any case too busy practicing medicine using proven medical treatments that included plant and herbal preparations to treat common illnesses and ailments. Why not? American doctors had used them since colonial times. In addition, their medical reference books still characterized plant drugs, herbs, and spices as proven-by-use prescription medicines.

Such reference books originated about 1820, when a few persons from colleges of medicine, state medical associations, pharmacists, and the U.S. surgeon general got together to select those drugs thought to have the greatest therapeutic value. The list was distributed to selected pharmacists and pharmaceutical chemists, who then formulated the standards of quality and potency. They compiled a book titled *Pharmacopeia*, which was first published in 1820, one year before the first U.S. school of pharmacy was established at Philadelphia. As pharmacists organized, they founded the American Pharmaceutical Association in 1852, and in 1888 the association took over the compiling of the *National Formulary*. These volumes contained hundreds of medically useful references on leaves, resins, berries, barks, roots, twigs, and flowers. Many of these medical books containing such information continued to be published until about 1940.

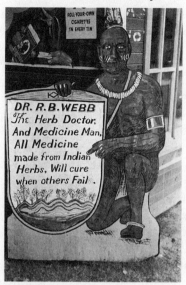

Many doctors continued to treat illnesses with herbs and plants during the first half of the twentieth century. This sign outside the office of Dr. R. B. Webb in Pine Bluff, Arkansas, advertised his medicines in the fall of 1938. (Courtesy Library of Congress)

Even during the first four decades of the twentieth century, many long-practicing doctors continued to use plant and herbal preparations in treatments. One such doctor was this writer's paternal grandfather, Gilbert Dary, M.D. Like most doctors of his day, he was a general practitioner who had developed many medical and pharmaceutical skills as a country doctor in Kansas. Born Gilbert Derry on July 17, 1858, at Madoc, Hastings County, in Ontario, Canada, he moved to Kansas with his parents when his father, Thomas Derry, homesteaded south of Abilene in 1873. Thomas later changed the spelling of the family's last name to Dary when he proved up on his claim. (He thought the *Derry* spelling looked too foreign.) Gilbert married Sarah Douglas Russell in 1881, farmed, and started a family. In the mid-1890s, at age thirty-eight, he decided to become a doctor and in 1896 entered the Wisconsin Eclectic Medical College at Milwaukee, Wisconsin. He graduated that year in the college's only graduation class.

After his return to Kansas, he learned that the dean of his college in Milwaukee had been arrested for selling diplomas to some students, though not Gilbert. But Gilbert realized his medical education was not the best, and he began reading medical books. He and Sarah had four children to feed, and he had to make a living.

Gilbert opened his practice at Strong City, a small town in the ranching country of the Flint Hills. He did not need a license to practice. Kansas did not begin licensing physicians until 1901. Having practiced medicine since 1896, Gilbert received his Kansas license to practice medicine and surgery in 1901.

After Gilbert's father was killed in an accident at Strong City, Dr. Dary moved his family and practice to Strawn, another small Kansas town, where he remained until early 1918. Realizing that medicine was becoming more scientific and that he needed more training, he left his family in Kansas and went to Chicago, where he enrolled in the Post Graduate Medical School and Hospital. He graduated in June of 1918 and returned to his practice in Strawn. There he remained until early 1919, when he again left his family and traveled to Indianapolis, Indiana, and enrolled in The National College of Electro-Therapeutics, graduating in May 1919. After returning once again to Kansas, he soon moved his family and practice to Hartford, a small town east of Emporia. There he spent the rest of his life working as a country doctor and helping his wife Sarah raise eight children—five boys and three girls.

When I was a small boy, it was always a treat to visit my grandfather Dary in Hartford because he raised chickens in the backyard of his home. Looking for eggs in the chicken coop was always fun. Gilbert and Sarah lived in a large two-story white frame house about a block east of Main Street. He also maintained his office and pharmacy in their home. My older cousin, Leonard J. Dary, was born in the house, delivered into the world by his grandfather, Dr. Dary. As Leonard recalled, "With such good prenatal care, I weighed thirteen pounds at birth." At the time, Leonard's parents were living with Sarah and Gilbert. Leonard's earliest memory was "the sound of a Model A Ford, of which Dr. Dary had two, going out of the garage and down the gravel driveway in the middle of the night for a run to help someone in need. . . . I remember the room at the end of the hall in his farm-style home that served as his pharmacy. There were many large brown medical bottles on the shelves with strange-sounding names that I couldn't begin to read or understand. It was in this room that he would mix for his patients the amounts of medicine needed and fill the small brown bottles that he had. The main medical item that Dr. Dary would mix in this room that I used and benefited from was a pink salve. It worked great on all types of skin irritations, scratches, skinned knees, and rashes. I never knew what ingredients he mixed together to create the salve; however, I can remember we called the medication the 'Pink Salve,' and indeed it was a dark pink color. Believe it or not, and to my amazement, today I can purchase a similar salve in my local drugstore. It looks the same, it smells the same, and it does the same job; however, it is known as Resinol.

"The medication I disliked the most from his pharmaceutical room was castor oil. The doctor would always take a dosage with me and he liked it or maybe he just acted like he did! Sometimes I would see different persons come to the office looking for what they called medicine, but I learned later they were after illegal drugs. Dr. Dary, not being sympathetic to their cause, would send them on their way," recalled Leonard. "In the winter, the doctor and I would spend many evenings playing checkers. He was an excellent player and he wasn't one to 'let me win.' Occasionally we would go to a silent movie together. In the summer, he would relax by sitting on a green park-like bench that was under a big cedar tree in his front yard.

"There was a radio in the dining room. It was a rectangular box with a big speaker on the top. Dr. Dary enjoyed listening to Dr. Brinkley broadcasting from Mexico. He was a kind, gentle, soft-spoken person who was totally unmaterialistic. His payment for services was seldom in cash. If he was paid at all, it was very common for the payment to be in apples, potatoes, or some other produce that could be stored in the cellar."[4]

Gilbert died in 1938 and his wife Sarah passed on in 1942. Dr. Dary never publicly claimed affiliation with any of the various medical sects, although he seems to have leaned toward eclectic medicine, the practice of treating patients with whatever was found to be beneficial. He learned of the discovery of vitamins and increasing knowledge of hormones and body chemistry and the 1921 discovery by Canadian physician Frederick Banting of insulin, the first effective treatment for diabetes. Dr. Dary read of the discovery of the antibiotic penicillin in London by Dr. Alexander Fleming in 1928, but Dr. Dary did not live to see it mass-produced in the early 1940s. Just before his death in 1938, he learned of the discovery of sulfa drugs, a class of synthetic

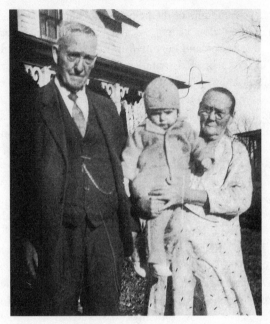

Dr. Gilbert Dary and his wife, Sarah, pose for this photo outside of their Hartford, Kansas, home in 1936. Dr. Dary had his office and pharmacy in his home. Sarah Dary is holding the author, her grandson, who was then two years old. (Author's collection)

chemical substances, developed in Germany, that was effective in treating some bacterial infections. Had he lived longer, he probably would have used the new medical discoveries in treating patients. He never joined the American Medical Association. Like many other small-town doctors across the nation, he sought to avoid the controversy that arose in the aftermath of the Flexner report. Dr. Dary continued to practice medicine as he had learned it helping his patients in and around Hartford, Kansas. Until his death, he had a great deal of autonomy, as did countless other practicing physicians across the nation, because the full impact of scientific medicine was not felt until after World War II.

Dr. Dary might have read *Book on the Physician Himself and Things That Concern His Reputation and Success* by Daniel Webster Cathell, M.D., of Baltimore, Maryland, and published in 1882 by F. A. Davis

Company, a medical publishing house in Philadelphia. The book, which sold for $2, was so popular that it went through twelve revised editions between 1892 and 1931. Dr. Cathell frequently revised his book, which he had written to help new physicians in America prosper in a period before the reforms driven by the Flexner report occurred in medical education. In the book, Cathell noted that in the court of public opinion the doctor had to behave with dignity, look the part, and show himself properly to his hoped-for patients. In 1890, when home visits were at the center of most medical practices, the doctor either walked or went by horse to see his patients. In the 1890 edition, Cathell wrote, "If you unfortunately have a bony horse and a seedy looking buggy, do not let them stand in front of your office for hours at a time, as if to advertise your poverty, lack of taste or paucity of practice." Later, in the 1922 edition, Cathell recommended that doctors use cars, which, unlike buggy horses, did not get tired going uphill.

Dr. Cathell added, "Clean hands, well-shaved face or neatly trimmed beard, unsoiled shirt and collar, unimpeachable hat, polished boots, spotless cuffs, well-fitting gloves, fashionable, well made clothing of fine texture, cane, sun-umbrella, neat office jacket . . . indicate gentility and self respect."

In the last printing of the book, in 1931, Cathell wrote: "The majority of people will employ a well-dressed medical man with clean genteel appearance and manners, always neat but never gaudy. They will accord him more confidence, and willingly pay to him larger bills, even though he may have a homely figure and a baboon face." He added that "a knowledge of Latin to a limited extent is of inestimable value. Employ some scholar to teach you at least as much of the elements of Latin as you need in writing prescriptions, etc. You can get one [a scholar] at a small cost by advertising anonymously in any daily paper."

Cathell urged doctors to follow good business practices and ask to be paid in cash, not credit, which would be paid promptly by grateful patients who could easily seek care elsewhere. He said the measured outcomes of professional tact and business sagacity were freedom from debt and money in the bank. He also urged doctors to attend to their own personal health by not working to the point of exhaustion. As for their offices, Cathell suggested diplomas and "modest size busts or statues of our great medical heroes are in excellent taste," as was a nice bookcase with medical books in it. Cathell warned doctors not to display a miniature museum in their offices, with "sharks' heads, stuffed alligators, tortoise-shells, impaled butterflies, miniature ships, mummies, snakes, tape worms, devil-fish or any thing else that will advertise you in any light other than that of an educated and cultivated physician."

A doctor, Cathell said, is a public figure about town. He should not be seen "loitering around drug-stores, hotel-lobbies, saloons, club-rooms, cigar-stores, billiard-parlors, barber-shops, corner-groceries, moving pictures etc. with 'splendid fellows' who love doing nothing." He also advised: "Never ask the age of a patient more than once during attendance on his case. Take care also neither to ask any questions twice at the same time nor to do anything else that would indicate lack of memory, lack of interest or incompetence."

Other advice offered by Dr. Cathell:

It is very pleasing to the sick to be allowed to tell in their own way whatever they deem important for you to know. Allow every one a fair hearing, and, even though their long statements are tedious, do not abruptly cut them short, but endure them and listen to them with respectful attention.

Never write a prescription carelessly. Legibility is the first requirement, neatness the second. Cultivate the habit of scrutinizing every thing you write after it is written, to assure yourself that there is neither omission nor mistake and sign your name or initials to every prescription, but not until you have satisfied yourself that it is as intended. Mistakes are seldom discovered unless at the moment of their occurrence.

There are two kinds of reputation a physician may acquire—a popular one with the people and a purely professional one with his brethren. These are often based on entirely different grounds and are usually no measure of each other. Try to possess both.

Bear, therefore, the greatness of your trust and the responsibility and glory of your almost divine mission, ever in your mind. Remember at all times that every phase of your conduct, every word you utter, every look, every nod of your head, tremble of your tongue, quiver of your lips, wink of your eye, and shrug of your shoulders, will be observed and considered. Therefore, strive to make your manner and your methods as faultless as possible ... observe punctuality and system in attending all who place themselves under your care, and strive to do the greatest absolute good for each and every one of your patients that you may merit to be called A MODEL PHYSICIAN.

In the tenth edition of Dr. Cathell's book, published in 1895, he urged doctors not to send patients far away to the crowded wards of hospitals mostly populated by sailors, soldiers, and paupers, unless they "feel assured that the management is kind, humane, and skillful, for while hospitals and almshouses are an unspeakable blessing to sick wanderers, to the castaways, the forgotten, and the homeless ...," it was far better to let patients stay at home with families and friends and "all the little endearing sympathies and solaces of domestic life."[5]

This view of hospitals changed early in the twentieth century, when American hospitals changed. No longer were they primarily places for long-term care for the sick, especially for the poor. Hospitals began to become places where patients could be diagnosed, tested, treated, and then released as fast as possible. To cover the added costs for such services, such hospitals turned to cost accounting—fees for services. As modern hospitals gradually emerged, they gave physicians a new partner. Physicians in turn helped to safeguard hospitals from intrusion by government and other external agencies through self-regulation. Fueled in the 1920s by the growing publicity given to modern surgery, especially safer childbirth, tonsillectomies, appendectomies, hernia repairs, and other such operations, hospitals created a growing demand for their services during the 1920s and 1930s.

The Great Depression of the 1930s, however, slowed the expansion of hospitals and personnel. Many Americans now had trouble paying for the medical care they needed. Doctors tried to make allowances for patients in financial straits, but hospitals with higher fixed costs had much less flexibility. In 1929, just before the stock market crash, the cost of a hospital stay averaged about $200; once the Depression began, that figure dropped to about $60. Hospitals then began to turn to insurance plans to guarantee steady cash flow by spreading the financial risk. Baylor University Hospital in Dallas, Texas, introduced the first insurance plan in 1929. A group of 1,500 schoolteachers contracted with the hospital to provide care should it be needed. Each teacher paid a fee whether or not he or she ever used the services. Such a health insurance plan was acceptable to the medical community, since the hospital benefited.

Another prepaid medical plan was started at a clinic in 1929 in Los Angeles, California, by two doctors under contract with the city's Department of Water and Power to provide medical services to the department's employees. That year another plan was established in western Oklahoma by Lebanese-born Michael Shadid (1882–1966), who came to America late in the nineteenth century and earned his medical degree from the School of Medicine at Washington University in St. Louis. Dr. Shadid practiced in Elk City, a town of six thousand residents in the farming region of western Oklahoma. When the Depression began, medical costs were rising. Dr. Shadid, opposed to the expensive fee-for-services medical system supported by the American Medical Association, organized the Farmers Union Hospital Association Cooperative in Elk City. It was the nation's first cooperatively owned and managed comprehensive prepaid medical care program. Farmers in a ten-county area contributed a one-time fee of $50 to become shareholders in the cooperative association, whose first goal was to build a hospital. The plan then called for members to pay $25 a year to receive comprehensive medical and hospital care. By May 1930, the association had seven hundred shareholders and was making plans to construct its hospital. However, three other doctors in the Elk City area publicly opposed the plan and ran a notice in the *Elk City News* calling it "unethical" and declaring that they would never send any of their patients to the hospital.

The two-story brick hospital building was completed by October 1931 and named Community Hospital. It was then that opposition to the association increased. The county medical society reorganized, thereby compelling all its members to reapply for admission. Since membership in the AMA required the signatures of two other physicians in the local medical society, and no one would support Dr. Shadid for membership, he was no longer a member and could not receive the AMA journal. He fought back and gained the support of the Oklahoma Farmers Union and Oklahoma governor Bill Murray. Later, when he sought accreditation for the hospital and was turned down by the AMA, he threatened to sue the American Medical Association's Council on Medical Education and Hospitals for violating antitrust laws. The AMA then dropped its opposition and the hospital gained accreditation. The cooperative continued to be successful in spite of continued opposition from the medical profession, including local doctors in Elk City. Peace finally came in the early 1950s, when country doctors sought and received permission to have their patients use the hospital.[6]

Another physician in the West who gained national prominence in medicine early in the twentieth century was Dr. Samuel J. Crumbine. Born in Pennsylvania in 1862, he worked as a pharmacist's apprentice before enrolling in the Cincinnati College of Medicine and Surgery. During summer vacations he traveled to the town of Spearville near Dodge City in western Kansas to work in a drugstore. After graduation from the Cincinnati medical school in 1885, he married, moved to Dodge City, and established his practice. Dodge City was then in its last years as a roaring cattle town, and soon Dr. Crumbine gained a good reputation as a physician. He remained there for nineteen years. In 1904 he was offered the position of executive secretary, or director, of the Kansas State Board of Health. After giving the offer much thought, he accepted the position and moved his family to Topeka, the state capital.

For nearly two years, the Board of Health had had no executive director. The agency was in turmoil. There had been no leadership in organizing responses to disease outbreaks or complaints. Dr. Crumbine faced the problem of reorganizing the operation. He improved the organization of health officers in the state's 105 counties. Next, he initiated major campaigns to eliminate common towels and drinking cups from public places, reduce public expectoration, and "swat the fly." These were all things he had preached about in Dodge City. By making public health education a focus for public and professional audiences across Kansas and the nation, he was able to have a widespread impact on public health.

Dr. Crumbine had learned in Dodge City that "an ounce of prevention is worth a pound of cure." In Dodge City, he had convinced the Fred Harvey diner chain on the Santa Fe Railroad to stop selling milk out of open jugs and pitchers and use bottles instead. He used the germ theory as the reason to get the chain to employ methods that would reduce the transmission of contagious diseases caused by bacteria, parasites, and unknown agents later identified as viruses. Dr. Crumbine was a pioneer in the practice of taking new scientific knowledge about disease to the physicians and citizens he served. He knew he had to change people's behaviors and he was successful. In fact, his work helped to shape the national movement to change society's attitudes about cleanliness, germs, and health.

In Topeka, he expanded his efforts of educating everyone in Kansas by issuing statewide bulletins and establishing statewide campaigns designed to convince everyone that reform was needed in personal behavior and in state laws. Even before Congress passed the Food and Drug Act in 1906, Dr. Crumbine was able to get the Kansas legislature to pass laws on pure food and drug purity, knowing they would help cut down on contamination by reducing bacteria and foreign substances in such ingested items. The public supported his efforts.

It was after military researchers reported that flies carried disease-causing bacteria onto food that Dr. Crumbine started his "swat the fly" campaign, which spread not only across the nation but around the world. A Kansas schoolteacher gave Dr. Crumbine a yardstick with a square piece of wire screen attached to kill flies. He called it the "fly swatter" and it became the model for commercially produced swatters using wire screen. Some citizens also worked to outlaw manure piles that attracted flies.

His continuing campaign to ban expectoration was tied to the fight against tuberculosis. He convinced a Kansas brick-maker to print his slogan "Don't spit on the sidewalk" on every third brick manufactured. Other brick manufacturers soon joined the campaign. Many such bricks can still be seen today in towns and cities in Kansas and elsewhere in the West.

By 1913, Dr. Crumbine had gained a worldwide reputation in public health. He was asked to become dean of the University of Kansas School of Medicine while continuing to serve as executive director of the Kansas State Board of Health. This was just after Abraham Flexner's report was issued and the school needed to improve its reputation in medical education. He worked to improve the school and continue his health crusades in Kansas. In 1914, he started a crusade to "save the baby," focusing attention on clean milk, clean mothers, visiting nurses, and child welfare. When a new governor took office in Topeka and tried to replace his Board of Health staff with political appointees, Crumbine fought back and the public supported him. The following year he resigned as dean of the University of Kansas Medical School to devote himself full-time to his work at the Board of Health.

In 1923, at the urging of then secretary of commerce Herbert

Hoover, Dr. Crumbine resigned from the Kansas State Board of Health to become head of the American Child Health Association in New York. After his retirement he lived on Long Island, New York, but frequently returned to Kansas for speaking engagements before his death at the age of ninety-two in 1954.[7]

Another Kansas doctor became nationally known for his best-selling book *The Horse and Buggy Doctor* (1939). Born in 1870, Arthur E. Hertzler graduated from Southwest Kansas College at Winfield and then entered Chicago's Northwestern University Medical School, where he earned his medical degree. He returned to Kansas and set up his practice at Moundridge. When a tornado struck the farming community of Halstead, fourteen miles north of Moundridge, Dr. Hertzler rushed there to treat the injured. He liked the town and moved his practice there and soon opened a clinic and a hospital. He visited his patients in rural areas around the town by horse and buggy or on horseback. He often practiced surgery using a patient's kitchen table or delivered babies in less-than-desirable settings. He was known for sometimes recommending home remedies and gained a fine reputation as a country doctor. He found time to write and began producing books on medicine, including a two-volume set on abdominal surgery (1919) and books on his case studies. He was asked to teach at the University Medical College in Kansas City (now the University of Kansas School of Medicine) about 185 miles northeast of Halstead. His teaching methods were considered unconventional but effective, and he earned the affection and respect of countless students.

Dr. Hertzler approved of changes in medical education and wrote: "The advance in medical education is a source of pride to medical men, because it has come from within the profession. The public has not demanded it. The standards of medical practice, for that matter, always have been higher than the public has required or was willing to accept. In fact, when the public has become articulate it has been to criticize the actions of the medical profession or obstruct its advancements. There has been a constant conflict between the medical profession, the press and the clergy but the contest is drawing to a close. This progress is due to the public. We are helpless to lessen the opposition, except as we acquire the help of the laity."

Dr. Hertzler noted that medicine "in large measure is able to protect the public from infectious disease whether it [the public] wishes it or not. The cure of individual disease is much more difficult to force

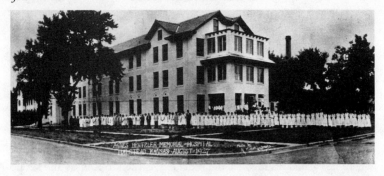

The Hertzler Hospital in Halstead, Kansas, in 1927. Standing in front of the structure are the members of the hospital staff (faintly visible). (Courtesy Kansas State Historical Society)

on the patient. The difficulty, therefore, lies not in the availability of adequate medical service but in the intelligence of the patient to use it. The term intelligence must be given a broad application. Education has only a general relationship to intelligence. . . . It is a curious fact that it is many of the educated who are most refractory to the acceptance of fact. They have learned to believe in things that are not true. It is very obvious that anyone may believe anything he wishes with impunity. But disease brooks no trifling. If you have a ruptured appendix and you choose to believe there is none or that by rubbing the back of the neck the spreading peritonitis will be halted, it is just too bad. The relationship of intelligent people to the laws governing disease is really very complicated. The point is that this is allegedly a free country and if a person sees fit to reject the aid of scientific medicine, no one can say him nay. Perhaps it is Fate's way of eliminating the unfit."

Dr. Hertzler added that scientific medicine "has made advances almost or quite beyond conception. The science becomes an art when applied to the treatment of the sick. Artists differ in capacity. The medical art available to any one person depends on the capacity of the one practicing the art. That is the task now to assure the greater capacity of the individual practitioner. Certainly the ultimate will not be achieved if either the boss of the faculty or a political boss is allowed to select the doctor. Efficiency can be hoped for only if the patient is allowed to select his own doctor. The science of medicine is abstract, the relation of doctor and patient is something else."[8]

These words, written in 1939 by Dr. Hertzler, seem to capture the

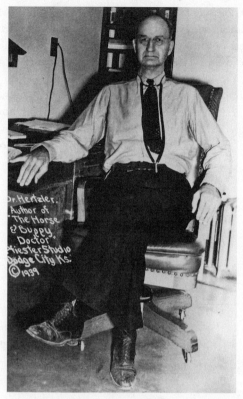

Dr. Arthur E. Hertzler wrote the popular best-selling book The Horse and Buggy Doctor *(1939), plus a two-volume medical work on abdominal surgery and several books of case studies. He spent most of his life in Halstead, Kansas, where he built and operated a hospital. He frequently recommended home remedies in his treatments. (Courtesy Kansas State Historical Society)*

state of medicine in America just before World War II. By 1941, the licensing of physicians was commonplace. Scientific medicine in America was pretty much in place in medical education and the pharmaceutical industry. The high operating standards of modern hospitals were spreading, as were the care and treatment of patients by better-educated physicians. The Food and Drug Administration, and federal and state regulations generally, were providing medical standards unimagined a century earlier. The evidence is strong that 1941 marked the end of medicine's frontier period in America. Since then medicine has pushed ahead with countless new discoveries as it tries to be indifferent to ideas of the supernatural and the spirit, as it concentrates on finding the causes and treatments of illnesses and disease of the human body. It has enabled Americans to live longer. Life expectancy increased from about forty-seven years in 1900 to about sixty years by 1941, and it continues to climb today. Some Americans, however, wonder if its expected benefits have fallen short of what once seemed a realistic goal of conquering all disease and bringing good health to everyone.

A COMPENDIUM OF OLD MEDICAL
TERMS AND SLANG

Ablepsia/Ablepsy: blindness

Abscess: a localized collection of pus buried in tissues, organs, or confined spaces of the body, often accompanied by swelling and inflammation and frequently caused by bacteria

Accoucheur: a man who acts as a midwife

Accoucheuse: a midwife

Accubation: the act or posture of reclining, as in childbirth

Achor: an eruption on the scalp

Acknowledge the Corn: to admit the truth

Acute Indigestion: often listed as a cause of death; probably a heart attack

Acute Mania: severe insanity

Addison's Disease: a destructive disease marked by severe weakness, loss of weight, low blood pressure, gastrointestinal disturbances, and brownish pigmentation of the skin and mucous membranes. Sometimes called *Bronzed Skin Disease*

African Consumption: tuberculosis

Ague: used to define the recurring fever and chills of malarial infection; was sometimes called "chill fever," "the shakes," or "fever and ague," and in Louisiana was often labeled "swamp fever"

Alastrim: a milder form of smallpox

All-Fired: hell-fired

Allopath: a physician practicing conventional or mainstream medicine, as opposed to homeopathy

American Plague: yellow fever

Anasarea: generalized massive swelling

Aphonia: laryngitis

Aphtha: thrush, a disorder caused by infection of the mouth with the fungus (yeast) *Candida albicans*—most common in infants and in the elderly

Apoplexy: synonym for stroke, also used to mean bleeding

Asphyesia: bluish discoloration of the skin and mucous membranes due to lack of oxygen in the blood

Asphyxia: choking due to lack of oxygen

Atrophy: muscles wasting away generally from lack of use

Bad Blood: syphilis

Barber's Itch: infection of the hair follicles of the beard area

Barrel Fever: vomiting or illness due to excessive drinking of alcohol

Baseborn: illegitimate

Bazoo: mouth

Bender: bout of drunkenness

Biggest Toad in the Puddle: the most important person in a group

Biliousness: typhoid, malaria, hepatitis, jaundice, or other conditions or symptoms associated with liver disease, or any upset leading to vomiting bile or just vomiting

Black Death: bubonic plague

Black Fever: typhus or Rocky Mountain spotted fever

Black Jaundice: common term for *Wiel's Disease*, caused by a bacterial infection of the liver carried by rats and secreted in their urine

Black Plague: bubonic plague

Black Pox: black smallpox

Black Vomit: vomiting old black blood due to ulcers or yellow fever

Blackwater Fever: severe form of malaria in which the urine contains so much blood it appears to be black

Bladder in Throat: sometimes used to describe diphtheria

Blood Poisoning: the effects of bacteria in the blood

Bloody Flux: bloody stools

Bloody Sweat: sweating sickness including a discharge of blood

Bone Orchard: cemetery

Bone Shave: sciatica, pain along the large sciatic nerve that runs from the lower back down the back of each leg

Brain Fever: meningitis

Brain Wasting: dementia

Breakbone Fever: dengue fever, a disease caused by one of four viruses transmitted to humans by infected mosquitoes

Brick in One's Hat: to be drunk

Bright's Disease: a catchall label for chronic inflammatory disease or disorders of the kidney

Bronze John: yellow fever

Bronzed Skin Disease: see *Addison's Disease*

Brucellosis: a disease affecting humans who come into contact with animals or animal products contaminated with bacteria; see *Milk Fever/Sickness*

Bubo: inflamed gland in the groin, usually a symptom of bubonic plague

Buck: Irish slang for tuberculosis

Bulimia: an eating disorder where a person engages in recurrent binge eating and purging, following by feelings of guilt, depression, and self-condemnation

Cachexy: malnutrition

Cacigastrue: upset stomach

Cacospysy: irregular pulse

Cadiceis: an individual who is subject to falling sickness or epilepsy

Camp Colic: appendicitis

Camp Fever: typhus or diarrhea in camp

Canine Madness: hydrophobia, rabies

Canker: ulceration of mouth or lips or herpes simplex

Carditis: inflammation of the heart wall

Catalepsy: seizures or trances

Catarrh: inflammation of the mucous membrane

Catarrhal: nose and throat discharge from cold or allergy

Cerebritis: inflammation of the cerebrum or lead poisoning

Chilblain: swelling of extremities caused by exposure to cold

Child Bed Fever: infection following birth of a newborn

Chin Cough: whooping cough

Chlorosis: iron-deficiency anemia

Cholecystitus: inflammation of the gallbladder

Cholelithiasis: gallstones

Cholera: acute, severe contagious disease consisting of diarrhea with sloughing of the intestinal lining with contortions and convulsions

Cholera Morbus: nausea, vomiting, abdominal cramps, and elevated temperature; often an appendicitis

Clap: gonorrhea, a sexually transmitted bacterial disease

Cold as a Wagon Tire: dead

Cold Plague: ague

Colic: abdominal pain and cramping

Commotion: concussion

Congestion: any collection of fluid in an organ such as the lungs

Conniption Fit: a fit of hysteria

Coon's Age: a long time

Consumption: tuberculosis

Corned: drunk

Corruption: infection

Coryza: a cold

Costiveness: constipation

Cramp Colic: appendicitis

Crop Sickness: overextended stomach from overeating

Croup: laryngitis, diphtheria, or strep throat, often in infants, with difficult breathing and cough

Day Fever: sweating sickness fever lasting one day

Death from Teething: tooth infections with inflammation and cellulitis, an acute inflammation of the connective tissue of the skin; such conditions caused death before advances occurred in dentistry

Debility: being weak or feeble due to illness or age

Decrepitude: feebleness due to old age

Deef: deaf

Delirium Tremens: hallucinations caused by alcoholism

Dentition: cutting of teeth

Deplumation: tumor of the eyelids that causes hair loss

Diary Fever: a fever that lasts one day

Diphtheria: contagious disease of the throat

Distemper: usually an animal disease with malaise, discharge from nose and throat, anorexia

Dock Fever: yellow fever

Domestic Illness: polite label for mental breakdown, depression, Alzheimer's, Parkinson's, or the aftereffects of a stroke, or any illness that kept a person housebound and probably in need of regular nursing

Dragged Out: fatigued, worn out

Dropsy: edema or swelling, often caused by kidney or heart disease; today called congestive heart failure

Dropsy of the Brain: encephalitis, brain inflammation caused by a virus

Dry Bellyache: lead poisoning

D.T.'s: delirum tremens caused by withdrawal or abstinence from alcohol following habitual excessive drinking

Dysentery: inflammation of the colon with frequent passage of mucus and blood

Dyspepsia: acid indigestion, heartburn, sometimes heart attack symptoms

Dysury: difficulty in urination

Ecstasy: a form of catalepsy characterized by loss of reason, or unusual postures or facial expressions, as seen in schizophrenia and some diseases of the nervous system

Edema: nephrosis, a disease of the kidney with swelling of tissues

Empirie: an individual who practices medicine without formal training, also called a quack or charlatan

Encephalitis: swelling of the brain, as in sleeping sickness

Eneuresis Nocturna: bedwetting

Enteric Fever: typhoid fever

Enteritis: inflammation of the bowels

Enterocolitis: inflammation of the intestines

Epilepsy: a disorder of the nervous system that can cause loss of attention or sleepiness or severe convulsions with loss of consciousness

Epitaxis: a nosebleed

Euphoria: an exaggerated feeling of elation or well-being not based on reality, often due to mania or fatigue following a battle or fight (e.g., Civil War); post-engagement stress syndrome, sometimes associated with narcotic medication

Exhaustion: sometimes used to describe a lingering death before death certificates required a cause or diagnosis of death

Extravasted Blood: rupture of a blood vessel

Falling Sickness: epilepsy

Felo-de-Se: suicide by one of sound mind

Flux: the drainage or discharge of liquid from a body cavity

Flux of Humour: circulation

French Fever: venereal disease

French Pox: syphilis, so named because of a serious outbreak of it in the French army

Full as a Tick: very drunk

Furuncle: boil

Glandular Fever: mononucleosis

Glister: enema

Go Through the Mill: gain experience

Gout: any inflammation caused by the buildup of uric acid in the body;

often occurs in joints where circulation is poor, and can cause gall- or kidney stones

Great Pox: syphilis

Green Sickness: anemia caused by iron deficiency

Grip/Gripe: influenza

Grocer's Itch: skin disease caused by mites in sugar or flour

Habiliments: clothing

Heart Sickness: condition caused by loss of salt from body

Hip Gout: osteomyelitis, an acute and chronic bone infection, usually caused by bacteria

Homeopath: a physician who treats disease on the principle that "like cures like"; a homeopath believes that a substance that produces a set of symptoms in a well person will, in minute "potentized" doses, cure those same symptoms in a sick individual

Horizontal Refreshments: intercourse

Horn: penis

Horrors: delirium tremens

Impetigo: contagious skin disease characterized by pustules

In Apple Pie Order: in top shape

Incubus: a nightmare where a demon takes on the male form to have sexual intercourse with a sleeping woman

Infantile Paralysis: polio

Intestinal Colic: abdominal pain due to improper diet

Jail Fever: typhus

King's Evil: tubercular infection of the throat lymph glands, called *Scrofula;* term sometimes used to describe syphilis

Kink: coughing or choking fit

Kinkcough: whooping cough

Knocked into a Cocked Hat: fouled up, rendered useless

La Grippe: flu

Lockjaw: tetanus or infectious disease affecting the muscles of the neck and jaw; usually fatal if not treated in eight days

Long Sickness: tuberculosis

Lues: syphilis

Lues Venera: often used to describe syphilis but also other venereal diseases

Lumbago: back pain

Lung Fever: pneumonia

Lung Sickness: tuberculosis

Lunger: slang for someone with tuberculosis

Lying In: time of delivery of a baby

Malaria: a disease caused by a parasite in the blood transmitted by mosquitoes

Mania: insanity

Marasmus: progressive emaciation or wasting away of the body due to malnutrition

Materia medica: that branch of medical science concerning the sources, nature, properties, and preparation of drugs

Membranous Croup: hoarse cough

Milk Fever/Sickness: poisoning resulting from the drinking of milk produced by a cow that has eaten a plant known as white snakeroot

Milk Leg: a painful swelling of the leg beginning at the ankle and ascending the thigh, or from the groin and extending down the thigh; the usual cause is infection after labor; also called *Phlebitis*

Monkey: vagina

Morbus Gallicus: syphilis

Mormal: gangrene

Mortification: infection

Mortis: death

Mountain Bitters: one pint of water with one-fourth gill of buffalo gall

Namby-pamby: sickly, timid, or effeminate

Neurasthenia: neurotic condition

Nostalgia: homesickness

Nostrum Remedium: a Latin phrase meaning "our remedy," commonly used by physicians in the seventeenth and eighteenth centuries to describe the medicines they used; the ingredients of such medications were usually secret and often of questionable efficacy

Old Adam: penile erection

Palsy: paralysis or uncontrolled movement of controlled muscles

Pecker: penis

Phlebitis: see *Milk Leg*

Phthiriasis: lice infestation

Podagra: gout

Pott's Disease: tuberculosis of the spine, with destruction of the bone resulting in curvature of the spine

Prick: penis

Protein Disease: a once relatively common childhood kidney disease that causes the kidney to leak protein—a secondary allergic reaction to certain kinds of strep infections

Puke: to throw up or empty the stomach

Putrid Fever: diphtheria

Quinsy: tonsilitis

Remitting Fever: malaria

Rheumatism: a painful disease affecting muscles and joints, mostly the larger joints

Rickets: disease of skeletal system

Rip: vagina

St. Vitus's Dance: see *Cholera*

Sam Hill: euphemism for the devil

Sanguineous Crust: scab

Scarlet Fever: acute infectious fever caused by infection in the throat

Screws: rheumatism

Scrivener's Palsy: writer's cramp

Scrofula: see *King's Evil*

Scrumpox: impetigo, a pustular disease of the skin

Scurvy: a disease resulting from insufficient intake of vitamin C and characterized by livid spots on the skin, spongy gums, and bleeding from mucous membranes

Septicemia: blood poisoning

Shakes: delirium tremens

Shaking: chills, ague

Ship's Fever: typhus

"Shoot, Luke, or Give Up the Gun": do it or quit talking about it

Smell a Rat: become aware of something suspicious, improper, or out of order

Snatch: vagina

Something in Train: something being considered or planned

Spanish Influenza: epidemic influenza

Stranger's Fever: yellow fever

Strangery: rupture

Summer Complaint: dysentery or baby's diarrhea caused by spoiled milk

Take On: grieve

Tallywhacker: penis

Tetanus: a sometime fatal infection caused by a bacterium that enters the body through wounds

Thrush: childhood disease characterized by spots on the mouth, lips, and throat

Tick Fever: Rocky Mountain spotted fever

Trench Mouth: painful ulcers on the gums caused by poor nutrition and poor hygiene

Undulant Fever: brucellosis

Up the Spout: gone to waste or ruin

Venesection: bleeding

Visitation of God: death from natural causes

Wiel's Disease: see *Black Jaundice*

Winter's Fever: pneumonia

Yellow Fever: an acute, often fatal, infectious disease of warm climates caused by a virus transmitted by mosquitoes

Yellow Jacket: yellow fever

APPENDIX

EPIDEMICS IN NORTH AMERICA
1616–1950

1616 Smallpox outbreak decimated the Indian population in New England
1657 Measles outbreak in Boston
1687 Measles outbreak in Boston
1690 Yellow fever outbreak in New York
1713 Measles outbreak in Boston
1729 Measles outbreak in Boston
1732 Influenza outbreak worldwide, lasting into 1733
1738 Smallpox outbreak in South Carolina
1739 Measles outbreak in Boston, lasting into 1740
1761 Influenza outbreak in North America and West Indies
1772 Measles outbreak in North America
1774 Influenza outbreak worldwide, lasting into 1775
1775 Smallpox outbreak in New England that continued until the early 1780s and spread all the way to the Pacific Northwest
1783 Bilious disorder extremely fatal in and around Dover, Delaware
1788 Measles outbreak in New York and Philadelphia
1793 Influenza and "putrid" fever outbreak in Vermont
1793 Influenza outbreak in Virginia
1793 Yellow fever outbreak in Philadelphia
1793 Outbreak of unknown disease in Harrisburg and Middletown, Pennsylvania
1794 Yellow fever outbreak in Philadelphia
1796 Yellow fever outbreak in Philadelphia, lasting into 1797
1798 Yellow fever outbreak in Philadelphia
1803 Yellow fever outbreak in New York
1820 Fever outbreak that spread across the nation after originating along the Schuylkill River in southeastern Pennsylvania; lasted until 1823
1831 Asiatic cholera outbreak supposedly brought in by English immigrants; lasted into 1832
1832 Cholera outbreak in New York and other large cities
1833 Cholera outbreak in Columbus, Ohio, and Kentucky; lasted into 1834 in Kentucky
1834 Cholera outbreak in New York
1837 Typhus outbreak in Philadelphia

1841 Yellow fever outbreak over much of the nation but especially in the South

1847 Yellow fever outbreak in New Orleans

1847 Influenza outbreak worldwide, lasting into 1848

1848 Cholera outbreak in North America, lasting into 1849; New York especially hard hit

1850 Yellow fever outbreak across the nation

1850 Influenza outbreak in North America, lasting into 1851

1851 Cholera outbreak, beginning in Illinois and spreading westward across the Great Plains

1852 Yellow fever outbreak in New Orleans that spread across much of the nation

1855 Yellow fever outbreak throughout the nation

1857 Influenza outbreak worldwide that lasted into 1859

1860 Smallpox outbreak in Pennsylvania that lasted into 1861

1865 A series of recurring epidemics of smallpox, typhus, cholera, typhoid, scarlet fever, yellow fever, and influenza in Boston, New York, Philadelphia, New Orleans, Baltimore, Memphis, and Washington, D.C.; lasted until 1873

1866 Cholera outbreak in Kansas that lasted into 1867

1873 Influenza outbreak throughout North America

1878 Yellow fever outbreak in New Orleans and Memphis

1885 Typhoid outbreak in Plymouth, Pennsylvania

1886 Yellow fever outbreak in Jacksonville, Florida

1900 Cholera outbreak in Galveston, Texas

1902 Measles outbreak in Alaska

1905 Yellow fever outbreak in New Orleans

1916 Polio outbreak nationwide

1918 Influenza, or "Spanish flu," outbreak worldwide

1949 Polio outbreak nationwide that continued into the early 1950s

NOTES

CHAPTER ONE: INDIAN MEDICINE

1. The federal government established the 50,000-acre Wichita Mountains Wildlife Refuge in 1901 as a habitat for large native grazing animals, including Rocky Mountain elk, white-tailed deer, Texas longhorn cattle, and American buffalo (bison), that were returned to the refuge in 1907. In all, more than 50 species of mammals, about 240 birds, 64 reptiles and amphibians, 36 fish, and 806 plants thrive in the refuge today.

2. Letter to author from Clara Sue Kidwell, director of the Native American Studies Program, University of Oklahoma, April 1, 2004.

3. Eric Stone, M.D., *Medicine Among the American Indians* (New York: Hafner Publishing Co., 1962), pp. 1, 3.

4. Letter to author from Kidwell.

5. Ibid.

6. Thomas Kennard, "Medicine Among the Indians," *St. Louis Medical and Surgical Journal*, vol. 16 (1858), 392–93.

7. Roland B. Dixon, "Some Aspects of the American Shaman," *The Journal of American Folklore*, vol. 21, no. 80 (January–March 1908), 3.

8. Alex D. Krieger, *We Came Naked and Barefoot: The Journey of Cabeza de Vaca Across North America* (Austin: University of Texas Press, 2002), pp. 50, 71, 218.

9. Margarita Artschwager Kay, "The Florilegio Medicinal: Source of Southwest Ethnomedicine," *Ethnohistory*, vol. 24, no. 3 (Summer 1977), 251–59.

10. Marc Simmons, "Francisco Xavier Romero: Too Colorful to Overlook in Local History," *Santa Fe New Mexican*, December 4, 2004, p. B1.

11. Blanton P. Seward, "Pioneer Medicine in Virginia," Part 1, *Annals of Medical History*, vol. 10, no. 1 (January 1930), 62.

12. Henry S. Burrage, ed., *Early English and French Voyages* (New York: Charles Scribner's Sons, 1906), pp. 325–51.

13. Sir William Talbot, *The Discoveries of John Lederer . . .* (London: printed by J. C. for Samuel Heyrick, 1672), pp. 22–23.

14. Albert Cook Myers, *Narratives of Early Pennsylvania, West New Jersey, and Delaware, 1630–1707* (New York: Charles Scribner's Sons, 1912), pp. 227–29, 323.

15. Robert Beverley, *The History and Present State of Virginia* (Chapel Hill: University of North Carolina Press, 1947; orig. pub. in London in 1705), pp. 217–20.

16. Eric Stone, M.D., "Medicine Among the Iroquois," *Annals of Medical History*, vol. 6, no. 6 (November 1934), 351–52.

17. John Lawson, *Lawson's History of North Carolina* (Richmond, Va.: Garrett & Massie, 1937), pp. 235–36. Reprint of the 1714 first edition.

18. John Brickell, *The Natural History of North-Carolina, With an Account of the Trade, Manners, and Customs of the Christian and Indian Inhabitants*, ed. J. Bryan Grimes (Raleigh, N.C.: Trustees of Public Libraries, 1911), p. 394. Reprint of the 1737 first edition.

19. Mark Catesby, *The Natural History of Carolina, Florida, and the Bahama Islands*, vol. 2 (London: C. Marsh, 1743), p. 57.

20. John Wesley, *Primitive Physic; Or, an Easy and Natural Method of Curing Most Diseases* (London: John Mason, 1836), pp. 4–5. First published anonymously in 1747. Not until 1760 did Wesley place his name on it.

21. G. W. Christopher, T. J. Cieslak, J. A. Paylin, and E. M. Eitzen, Jr., "Biological Warfare, a Historical Perspective," *Journal of the American Medical Association*, vol. 278, no. 5 (1997), 278, 412–17.

22. John L. Kessell, *Kiva, Cross, and Crown* (Albuquerque: University of New Mexico Press, 1977), pp. 163, 170.

CHAPTER TWO: EARLY AMERICAN MEDICINE

1. Albert Deutsch, "The Sick Poor in Colonial Times," *American Historical Review*, vol. 46, no. 3 (April 1941), 564.

2. [John Tennent,] *Every Man His Own Doctor; Or, The Poor Planter's Physician* . . . (Williamsburg, Va. and Annapolis, Md.: Wil. Parks, 1736), pp. 10–12. Undated modern facsimile reprint of the third edition, purchased by the author at Williamsburg.

3. Virgil J. Vogel, *American Indian Medicine* (Norman: University of Oklahoma Press, 1970), pp. 392–93. In his appendix, Vogel describes about 170 drugs used by Indians in North America that have been or still are officially listed in either the *Pharmacopoeia of the United States of America* or the *National Formulary*.

4. Benjamin Rush, "An Inquiry into the Natural History of Medicine Among the Indians." Rush presented these remarks on February 4, 1774, before the American Philosophical Society in Philadelphia. They were published as *An Oration* . . . printed by Joseph Cruikshank, Philadelphia, 1774. Rush's negative attitude toward Indian medicine was reinforced by other physicians, and in time would help shape the new U.S. government's health care policy. It also ultimately quashed any effort to scientifically examine Indian medicine.

5. A copy of Rush's list of questions for Meriwether Lewis was obtained from the Thomas Jefferson Foundation, Inc., Monticello, Virginia.

6. Donald Jackson, ed., *Letters of the Lewis and Clark Expedition, with Related Documents, 1783–1854* (Urbana: University of Illinois Press, 1962), vol. 1, pp. 54–55.

7. Joseph Carlisle, a researcher for the Lewis and Clark Bicentennial Exhibition, compiled this information for the Missouri Historical Society from Gary E. Moulton, ed., *The Journals of the Lewis and Clark Expedition* (Lincoln: University of Nebraska Press, 1983–2000), 13 vols. See also Jackson, ed., *Letters of the Lewis and Clark Expedition* (Urbana: University of Illinois Press, 1962).

8. Letter from Benjamin Rush to Meriwether Lewis, June 11, 1803, Thomas Jefferson Papers Series 1, General Correspondence, 1751–1827, Library of Congress.

9. " 'Doctor Lewis' Thunderclappers," *Smithsonian* (June 2004), 22.

10. Bruce C. Paton, M.D., "Olaf Larsell's 'Medical Aspects of the Lewis and Clark Expedition'—a Commentary," *Wilderness and Environmental Medicine*, vol. 14, no. 4 (2003), 263–64.

11. About 1800, Sacagawea, a Shoshone, was kidnapped by a war party of Hidatsa Indians, her tribe's enemies. She was taken from her home in modern Idaho to a Hidatsa-Mandan village near present-day Bismarck, North Dakota. She was later sold as a slave to Toussaint Charbonneau, and became one of his wives. It was at Fort Mandan that she gave birth to Jean-Baptiste Charbonneau. He lived sixty-one years, dying of pneumonia at Danner, Oregon, in 1866.

12. Jim Salter, "Did Sacagawea Have a Miscarriage?," Associated Press report, April 10, 2005. Historians Peter Kastor and Conevery Bolton Valencius were from Washington University, St. Louis, Missouri.

13. Paul Cutright, "The Journal of Private Joseph Whitehouse," *Bulletin of the Missouri Historical Society*, vol. 28, no. 3 (1976), 160.

CHAPTER THREE: OVER THE APPALACHIANS

1. John Anthony Caruso, *The Appalachian Frontier, America's First Surge Westward* (Knoxville: University of Tennessee Press, 2003), p. 13. Reprint of the 1959 first edition.

2. Jo Ann Carrigan, *The Saffron Scourge: A History of Yellow Fever in Louisiana, 1796–1905* (Lafayette, La.: Center for Louisiana Studies at University of Southwestern Louisiana, 1994).

3. *Medicine and Its Development in Kentucky* (Louisville, Ky.: The Standard Printing Co., 1949), p. 31. Compiled and written by the Medical Historical Research Project, Works Project Administration, for the Commonwealth of Kentucky.

4. Dr. Jesse Bennett did not report the operation because no decent physician would operate on his wife. Several of his medical colleagues, however, were aware of the case, which has since been authenticated and recorded. Dr. Bennett owned an English translation of a French book by Dr. Jean-Louis Baudeloque that reviewed thirty-one successful cesarean sections performed during a fifty-year period. Dr. Bennett annotated the margins of his copy after operating on his wife. She lived another twenty-five years. His daughter, delivered during the operation, lived to be seventy-seven. Dr. Bennett performed the operation using laudanum on a platform consisting of two planks set across two barrels. He noted further that he removed both ovaries, because he did not want to be subjected to such an ordeal again. Dr. Bennett died in 1842 at age seventy-three.

5. Biemann Othersen, Jr., "Ephraim McDowell: The Qualities of a Good Surgeon," *Annals of Surgery*, vol. 239, no. 5 (May 2004), 648–50.

6. R. Douglas Hurt, *The Ohio Frontier, Crucible of the Old Northwest, 1720–1830* (Bloomington and Indianapolis: Indiana University Press, 1996), p. 270.

7. Stephen Otto, "Identifying a Family Heirloom: The Indian Doctor's Dispen-

satory," *Canadian Bulletin of Medical History/Bulletin canadien d'histoire de la médecine*, vol. 12 (1995), 443–45.

8. Rachel Engers, "Anatomy of an Insurrection," *Yale Medicine*, vol. 34, no. 2 (Spring 2002).

9. W. D. Snively, Jr., and L. Furbee, "Discoverer of the Cause of Milk Sickness (Anna Pierce Hobbs Bixby)," *Journal of the American Medical Association*, vol. 195 (June 1966), 1055–60. See also Jon Musgrave, "Anna Bixby: In Search of the Real Frontier Medicine Woman," *Daily Register* (Harrisburg, Ill.), May 21, 2005.

10. Daniel Drake, *Daniel Drake, M.D., Frontiersman of the Mind* (Cincinnati: Crossroads Books, History of the Health Sciences Library and Museum, University of Cincinnati, 1985), pp. xvii–xxvi. This work contains a fine brief biography of Drake written by Denise Mobley. See also Mary Louise Marshall, "The Versatile Genius of Daniel Drake," *Bulletin of the Medical Library Association*, vol. 31, no. 4 (October 1943), 291–318.

11. Elizabeth M. Meek, "Two Pioneer Doctors of Southeast Arkansas," *Arkansas Historical Quarterly*, vol. 5 (1946), 121.

12. Willene Hendrick and George Hendrick, *On the Illinois Frontier: Dr. Hiram Rutherford, 1840–1848* (Carbondale and Edwardsville: Southern Illinois University Press, 1981), p. 15.

13. John W. Bright, M.D., *The Mother's Medical Guide: A Plain, Practical Treatise on Midwifery, and the Diseases of Women and Children* (Louisville, Ky.: [printed by A. S. Tilden, Jeffersonville, Ind.], 1844).

14. Carrie Tarleton Goldsborough and Anna Goldsborough Fisher, *William Loftus Sutton, M.D., 1797–1862, Father of Kentucky State Medical Society and of Kentucky's First Vital Statistics Law* (Lexington, Ky.: The Thoroughbred Press, 1948), pp. 101–3.

CHAPTER FOUR: BEYOND THE MISSISSIPPI

1. Biography of Dr. Antoine Saugrain provided by the National Park Service, Jefferson National Expansion Memorial, St. Louis, n.d. See also William Vincent Byars, *The First Scientist of the Mississippi Valley, a Memoir of the Life and Work of Doctor Antoine François Saugrain* (St. Louis: Benjamin von Puhl, [1903]); N. P. Dandridge, M.D., "Antoine François Saugrain (De Vigni.): The First Scientist of the Mississippi Valley," *Ohio History: The Scholarly Journal of the Ohio Historical Society*, vol. 15, no. 2 (April 1906), 192–296; and J. Thomas Scharf, *A History of St. Louis City and County* (Philadelphia: L. H. Everts & Co., 1883), vol. 2, pp. 1517–18.

2. Reimert Thorolf Ravenholt, M.D., M.P.H., "Underlying Cause of Death of Meriwether Lewis," paper presented October 24, 2001, at The Medical History of the American West Conference, Montana State University, Museum of the Rockies, Bozeman, Montana. Earlier, Dr. Ravenholt's "Trail's End for Meriwether Lewis: The Role of Syphilis" appeared in the Cosmos Club journal (1997), Washington, D.C. Ravenholt concludes that had Thomas Jefferson, William Clark, and Lucy Marks not understood that this then unmentionable disease was the underlying cause of Lewis's death, they would likely have actively pursued further investigation into his suicide, as they did not. "No alternative explanation or diagnosis," Ravenhold adds, "fits all of the known facts of his illness and suicide."

3. Thomas B. Hall, "John Sappington," *Missouri Historical Review*, vol. 24, no. 2 (1930), 177–200. See also Thomas B. Hall, Jr., and Thomas B. Hall III, *Dr. John Sappington of Saline County, Missouri, 1776–1856* (Arrow Rock, Mo.: The Friends of Arrow Rock, Inc., 1975). A biographical sketch of Sappington is contained in Scharf's *A History of St. Louis City and County*, vol. 1, pp. 578–79.

4. David Dary, *The Santa Fe Trail: Its History, Legends, and Lore* (New York: Alfred A. Knopf, 2000), pp. 68–73.

5. Zebulon M. Pike, *The Journals of Zebulon Montgomery Pike, with Letters and Related Documents*, ed. Donald Jackson (Norman: University of Oklahoma Press, 1966), vol. 2, pp. 242–43.

6. John Hamilton Robinson's personal and family history is outlined in the Earl Fischer database of the St. Louis Genealogical Society. Before his death in 1999, Fischer spent years compiling the names of nearly 30,000 individuals in nearly 7,500 families. Fischer's research indicates that Robinson was born January 24, 1782, in Augusta County, Virginia. He arrived in St. Louis in the summer of 1805, perhaps at the invitation of Dr. Antoine Saugrain, the first physician in St. Louis. Whether Pike requested that Dr. Robinson accompany his second expedition or Robinson simply volunteered to go for other reasons is not clear. Robinson died in September 1819. One account says he died at Natchez on September 19, while another indicates he died in Washington, Mississippi, on September 29. His widow, Sophie, returned to St. Louis, where she died in 1848. A brief sketch of Dr. Robinson's life is contained in *Dear Brother: Letters of William Clark to Jonathan Clark* (pp. 252–53), edited by James J. Holmberg and published by Yale University Press, New Haven (2002), in association with The Filson Historical Society.

7. The *Western Engineer* could navigate narrow, shallow, and snag-littered channels of inland rivers. Fitted with a strong engine, the boat had a paddlewheel built into the stern to reduce the danger of snags. In case of Indian attack, the boat had a bulletproof pilothouse, mounted cannon on the bow, and howitzers along the side. Perhaps its most unusual feature was its bow, which was shaped like the neck and head of an aquatic monster, possibly intended to impress or frighten potential Indian adversaries. From its mouth rolled clouds of smoke.

8. [Edwin James,] *From Pittsburgh to the Rocky Mountains: Major Stephen Long's Expedition, 1819–1820*, ed. Maxine Benson (Golden, Colo.: Fulcrum, 1988), p. vi.

9. Edwin James, "Remarks on the Sandstone and Floetz Trap Formations of the Western Part of the Valley of the Mississippi," *Transactions of the American Philosophical Society*, New Series, vol. 2 (1825), 193.

10. [Edwin James,] *From Pittsburgh to the Rocky Mountains*, pp. 304, 387.

11. The Topographical Engineers were first authorized for War Department duties in 1813. Reauthorized in 1816, the Topographical Engineers Bureau was assigned to the Engineer Department in 1818. In 1831 the Bureau was separated from the Office of the Chief Engineer and made an independent War Department staff organization under the Chief Engineer. In 1838 they were organized into a separate Corps of Topographical Engineers under the supervision of the Chief of the Topographical Bureau, and one year later (1839) they were transferred to the Corps of Engineers.

12. J. C. Frémont, *Report of the Exploring Expedition to the Rocky Mountains in the Year 1842, and to Oregon and North California in the Years 1843–44* (Washington: Gales and Seaton, Printers, 1845), pp. 174, 240–1.

CHAPTER FIVE: FUR TRADERS AND TRAPPERS

1. Grace Lee Nute, *The Voyageur* (New York and London: D. Appleton and Co., 1931). Reprinted by the Minnesota Historical Society Press, St. Paul, in 1987.

2. Alice M. Johnson, ed., *Saskatchewan Journals and Correspondence: Edmonton House 1796–1800, Chesterfield House 1800–1802* (London: Hudson's Bay Record Society, 1967), p. 25.

3. Alexander Henry, *New Light on the Early History of the Northwest: The Manuscript Journals of Alexander Henry . . .* ed. Elliot Coues (Minneapolis, Minn.: Ross & Haines, 1965), pp. 110–11, 122.

4. Ibid., pp. 96, 679, 836.

5. J. B. Tyrrell, ed., *Journals of Samuel Hearne and Philip Turnor* (New York: Greenwood Press, 1968), p. 139. Reprint of the 1934 first edition.

6. Johnson, ed., *Saskatchewan Journals and Correspondence*, p. 109.

7. Henry, *New Light on Early History of Northwest*, pp. 241, 249, 271, 825.

8. Alexander Mackenzie, *The Journals and Letters of Sir Alexander Mackenzie*, ed. W. Kaye Lamb (London: Cambridge University Press, 1970), p. 248.

9. Gabriel Franchere, *Narrative of a Voyage to the Northwest Coast of America in the Years 1811, 1812, 1813, and 1814*, ed. Milo Milton Quaife (Chicago: The Lakeside Press, 1954), p. 194.

10. Johnson, ed., *Saskatchewan Journals and Correspondence*, p. 25.

11. John McLoughlin, *Letters of Dr. John McLoughlin, Written at Fort Vancouver 1829–1832*, ed. Burt Brown Barker (Portland: Binfords & Mort for the Oregon Historical Society, [1948]), p. 133.

12. James Douglas, "Diary," ed. Herman A. Leader, *Oregon Historical Quarterly*, vol. 32 (March 1931), 8.

13. James Harvey Young. *The Toadstool Millionaires: A Social History of Patent Medicines in America Before Federal Regulation* (Princeton, N.J.: Princeton University Press, 1961), p. 11.

14. Dr. Benjamin Waterhouse of Boston learned of Dr. Edward Jenner's successful inoculation with cowpox matter. Waterhouse obtained specimens of thread impregnated with the vaccine matter from Dr. Jenner, and in 1800 vaccinated his children and household servants. He published his findings and two years later, with the aid of six other Boston physicians, began vaccinating other persons. Thomas Jefferson, then U.S. vice president, vaccinated his family and household at Monticello, and he also promoted smallpox vaccinations in other cities.

15. Aubrey L. Haines, "Hugh Glass," in *The Mountain Men and the Fur Trade of the Far West*, ed. LeRoy R. Hafen (Glendale, Calif.: Arthur H. Clark Co., 1968), vol. 6, pp. 161–71.

16. Charles L. Camp, "James Clyman," in *The Mountain Men and the Fur Trade of the Far West*, ed. LeRoy R. Hafen (1965), vol. 1, pp. 240–41.

17. Alfred Glen Humpherys. "Thomas L. (Peg-leg) Smith," in *The Mountain Men and the Fur Trade of the Far West* (1966), vol. 4, pp. 324–30.

18. Ann W. Hafen, "John Simpson Smith," in *The Mountain Men and the Fur Trade of the Far West* (1968), vol. 5, pp. 326–29.

19. Rev. Samuel Parker, *Journal of the Exploring Tour Beyond the Rocky Mountains . . .* (Ithaca, N.Y.: published by the author, 1838), pp. 76–77.

20. Rev. Louis Pfaller, "Charles Larpenteur," in *The Mountain Men and the Fur Trade of the Far West* (1965), vol. 1, pp. 296–97; 1968, vol. 5, p. 93.

21. Richard J. Fehrman, "The Mountain Men—A Statistical View," in *The Mountain Men and the Fur Trade of the Far West* (1972), vol. 10, pp. 9–15.

CHAPTER SIX: ON THE OREGON TRAIL

1. Dale Morgan, ed., *Overland in 1846: Diaries and Letters of the California-Oregon Trail* (Lincoln: University of Nebraska Press, 1993), vol. 1, pp. 150–58. This two-volume work was first published in 1963.

2. Edwin Bryant, *What I Saw in California* (New York: D. Appleton & Co., 1848), pp. 87–90.

3. Ibid., p. 91.

4. Dr. Benjamin Cory, journal manuscript, Society of California Pioneers, San Francisco.

5. Louise Barry, "Charles Robinson—Yankee '49er: His Journey to California," *Kansas Historical Quarterly*, vol. 34 (1968), 179–88.

6. Boyle's diary was reprinted in the *Columbus* (Ohio) *Dispatch* between October 2 and November 14, 1849. The diary is available on the Web at www .dispatch.com/coincomments/GOLD RUSH/

7. "Diary of Dr. Jonathan Clark: Crossing the Plains," *The Argonaut*, San Francisco, August 1925.

8. A manuscript copy of Dr. Thomas's diary is in the Bancroft Library, University of California, Berkeley.

9. Israel Shipman Pelton Lord, *At the Extremity of Civilization: A Meticulously Descriptive Diary of an Illinois Physician's Journey in 1849 Along the Oregon Trail to the Goldmines and Cholera of California* . . . (Jefferson, N.C.: McFarland Co., 1995).

10. Material on Dr. Augustus B. Caldwell is found in "A Collection of Letters Written by the Scholl Family and Their Kin (1836–1897)," Jackson County Historical Society Research Library and Archives, Independence, Missouri.

11. Charles R. Parke, Jr., "California Log Book," original manuscript, Henry E. Huntington Library, San Marino, California.

12. Lemuel Clarke McKeeby, "Memoirs," *California History*, vol. 3 (1924), p. 59.

13. Albert Watkins, ed., *Publications of the Nebraska State Historical Society* (Lincoln: Nebraska State Historical Society, 1922), vol. 20, pp. 228–29.

14. John D. Unruh, Jr., *The Plains Across* (Urbana: University of Illinois Press, 1979), pp. 139–40.

15. Merrill J. Mattes, *Platte River Road Narratives* (Urbana and Chicago: University of Illinois Press, 1988), p. 3.

16. Ibid., pp. 409–10.

17. Dr. John Hudson Wayman, *A Doctor on the California Trail: The Diary of Dr. John Hudson Wayman from Cambridge City, Indiana, to the Gold Fields in 1852*, ed. Edgeley Woodman Todd (Denver: Old West Publishing Co., 1971), pp. 27–88.

18. Mattes, *Platte River Road Narratives*, pp. 409–10.

19. Ibid., pp. 397–8.

20. Kenneth L. Holmes, comp., *Covered Wagon Women: Diaries & Letters from the Western Trails 1840–1890* (Spokane, Wash.: The Arthur H. Clark Co., 1990), vol. 9, pp. 85–86.

CHAPTER SEVEN: AMONG THE SOLDIERS

1. Richard C. Knopf, ed., "A Surgeon's Mate at Fort Defiance: The Journal of Joseph Gardner Andrews for the Year 1795," *Ohio History: The Scholarly Journal of the Ohio Historical Society*, vol. 66, no. 1 (January 1957), 57–86.
2. Mary C. Gillett, *The Army Medical Department 1775–1818* (Washington, D.C.: GPO, 1990), p. 138.
3. Ibid., p. 151.
4. Ibid., p. 192.
5. For an interesting look at military surgeons who became ornithologists, see Edgar Erskine Hume, *Ornithologists of the United States Army Medical Corps* (Baltimore, Md.: Johns Hopkins Press, 1942).
6. Leonard McPhail, "The Diary of Assistant Surgeon Leonard McPhail, on His Journey to the Southwest in 1835," *Chronicles of Oklahoma*, vol. 18, no. 3 (1940), 281–92.
7. Sgt. Daniel Tyler, *A Concise History of the Mormon Battalion in the Mexican War* (Glorieta, N.M.: The Rio Grande Press, 1969), p. 149. Reprint of the 1881 first edition.
8. Samuel P. Moore, "Sanitary Report from Fort Laramie" (Washington, D.C.: Executive Document No. 96, 34th Congress, 1855).
9. Joseph King Fenno Mansfield, *Mansfield on the Condition of the Western Forts 1853–54* (Norman: University of Oklahoma Press, 1963), p. 176.
10. C. Keith Wilbur, M.D., *Civil War Medicine* (Old Saybrook, Conn.: The Globe Pequot Press, 1998), pp. 9–15.
11. Robert E. Denney, *Civil War Medicine: Care & Comfort of the Wounded* (New York: Sterling Publishing Co., 1994), p. 40.
12. Mary C. Gillett, *The Army Medical Department 1865–1916* (Washington, D.C.: GPO, 1995), p. 4.
13. R. H. McKay, *Little Pills: An Army Story* (Pittsburg, Kans.: Pittsburg Headlight, 1918), pp. 10–11.
14. Joseph H. Bill, "Notes on Arrow Wounds," *American Journal of Medical Science*, vol. 44, 1862. See also *A Report of Surgical Cases Treated in the Army of the United States from 1865 to 1871*, from the U.S. Army Surgeon General's Office (Washington, D.C.: GPO, 1871), and Volney Steele's "Arrow Wounds and the Military Surgeon in the West," *Military History of the West*, vol. 30 (Fall 2000), 155, 170.
15. Francis E. Quebbeman, *Medicine in Territorial Arizona* (Phoenix: Arizona Historical Foundation, 1966), p. 80.

CHAPTER EIGHT: ON HOMESTEAD AND RANCH

1. James Stewart, "The Diary of James R. Stewart, Pioneer of Osage County," *Kansas Historical Quarterly*, vol. 17, nos. 1–4, 1–36, 122–75, 254–95, 360–97.
2. Edith Thompson Hall, "The Biography of a Pioneer Nebraska Doctor, John Wesley Thompson," *Nebraska History*, vol. 44 (1963), 283.
3. Addison E. Sheldon, "The Pioneer Doctor," *Nebraska History*, vol. 7 (1926), 37.
4. Everett Dick, *The Sod-House Frontier 1854–1890* (Lincoln, Neb.: (Johnsen Publishing Co., 1954), p. 439.

5. Thomas N. Bonner, *The Kansas Doctor: A Century of Pioneering* (Lawrence: University of Kansas Press, 1959), pp. 75–78.

6. David Dary, *True Tales of Old-Time Kansas* (Lawrence: University Press of Kansas, 1984), pp. 266–73.

7. Dr. E. E. Morrison, "Pioneer Medicine in Barton County," *Kansas Historical Quarterly*, vol. 6, no. 4 (November 1937), 401–2.

8. Sheldon, "Pioneer Doctor," *Nebraska History*, 37.

9. Etta May Lacey Crowder, "Memoirs," *Journal of History and Politics*, vol. 46, no. 2 (Iowa City: State Historical Society of Iowa, 1948), 34–37. Crowder recorded her memoirs between 1930 and 1932.

10. Doane Robinson, *A History of South Dakota* (Aberdeen, S.D.: B. F. Bower & Co., 1904), vol. 1, p. 479.

11. *New Teller* (York, Neb.), Feb. 5, 1913.

12. Ben Blackstock, "A Special Kind of Man: The Autobiography of Dr. Lindsey L. Long," *The Chronicles of Oklahoma*, vol. 77, no. 4 (1999), 451–58. The passage quoted appears on p. 454.

13. Ibid., pp. 455–56.

14. Henry F. Hoyt, *A Pioneer Doctor* (Boston and New York: Houghton Mifflin Co., 1929), pp. 54–55.

15. Edith L. Crawford, interview in WPA Federal Writers Project, The Library of Congress, 1936–1940. The interview was conducted in Carrizozo, New Mexico and is available on the Library of Congress Web site.

16. *The West Texas Historical Association Year Book*, vol. 7 (June 1931), 35–39.

17. Carl Coke Rister, *Southern Plainsmen* (Norman: University of Oklahoma Press, 1938), pp. 166–8.

18. Ibid.

19. Jack Bailey, *A Texas Cowboy's Journal: Up the Trail to Kansas in 1868*, ed. David Dary (Norman: University of Oklahoma Press, 2006), p. 54.

20. James Emmit McCauley, *A Stove-Up Cowboy's Story* (Austin and Dallas: Texas Folklore Society and University Press, 1943), pp. 73–74.

21. Phil Roberts, "The Fetterman Hospital Association and Health Care Coverage on the Range in the 1880s," *Montana: Magazine of Western History*, vol. 44, no. 3 (1994), 63–69.

CHAPTER NINE: IN WESTERN TOWNS

1. Mrs. A. M. Woodward interview, WPA Federal Writers Project, 1936–40, Library of Congress. The interview was conducted in Bosqueville, Texas, and is available on the Library of Congress Web site.

2. Ibid.

3. J. Roy Jones, *Memories, Men and Medicine: A History of Medicine in Sacramento, California* (Sacramento, Calif.: Society for Medical Improvement, 1950), pp. 389–90.

4. Paul Scholten, M.D., "The Origins of the San Francisco Medical Society: 1868–1998," *San Francisco Medicine*, vol. 71, no. 2 (February 1998), 5–15.

5. Lisa See, *On Gold Mountain: The One-Hundred-Year Odyssey of a Chinese-American Family* (New York: St. Martin's Press, 1995), pp. 4–89.

6. Olga Reifschneider, "Dr. Anderson in Wild & Wooly Carson City, Nevada," in *Nevada Highways and Parks* (Fall 1966), p. 16. See also Olga Reifschneider,

Biographies of Nevada Botanists, 1844–1963 (Reno: University of Nevada Press, 1964), pp. 35–37.

7. H. Miles Moore, *Early History of Leavenworth City and County* (Leavenworth, Kans.: Sam'l Dodsworth Book Co., 1906), pp. 156, 215.

8. P. Peck, "Cornelius Ambrose Logan (1832–1899). A Study of the Kansas Physician, Diplomat and Writer," *The Journal of the Kansas Medical Society* (March 1968), 134–40. See also Gilbert Cuthbertson, "Active Leavenworth Doctors Were Prominent in Early Days," *University Daily Kansan* (Lawrence), June 23, 1959.

9. Material provided by the Dickinson County (Kansas) Historical Society, Abilene, and from the roster of the Forty-fourth Regiment, Iowa Volunteer Infantry.

10. Ibid. A biographical sketch of Dr. C. C. Furley also appears in William G. Cutler, *A History of the State of Kansas* (Chicago: A. T. Andreas, 1883). It appears in the section on Sedgwick County, Kansas.

11. Thelphilus Little, "Early Days in Abilene," unpublished manuscript in the files of the Dickinson County (Kans.) Historical Society, Abilene.

12. Stuart Henry, *Conquering Our Great American Plains* (New York: Dutton, 1930), p. 217.

13. Ida Ellen Rath, *Early Ford County* (North Newton, Kans.: Mennonite Press, 1964), pp. 158–59.

14. Robert M. Wright. *Dodge City: The Cowboy Capital and The Great Southwest* (Wichita, Kans.: published by the author, 1913), pp. 211–14.

15. William E. Connelley, *Kansas and Kansans* (Chicago: Lewis Publishing Co., 1919), vol. 5, p. 253.

16. Karen Holliday Tanner, *Doc Holliday: A Family Portrait* (Norman: University of Oklahoma Press, 1998). Tanner is a distant cousin of Doc Holliday.

17. Numerous works on outhouses have been consulted, including John Pudney, *The Smallest Room: A Discreet Survey Through the Ages* (London: Michael Joseph, 1954), and Ronald S. Barlow, *The Vanishing American Outhouse: A History of Country Plumbing* (El Cajon, Calif.: Windmill Publishing Co., 1992).

CHAPTER TEN: GOING WEST FOR YOUR HEALTH

1. Albert D. Richardson, *Our New States and Territories, Being Notes of a Recent Tour of Observation Through Colorado, Utah, Idaho, Nevada, Oregon, Montana, Washington Territory and California* (New York: Beadle, 1866), p. 10.

2. Harrison Clifford Dale, ed., *The Ashley-Smith Explorations and the Discovery of a Central Route to the Pacific, 1822–1829* (Glendale, Calif.: The Arthur H. Clark Co., 1941), p. 135.

3. Stephen F. Austin, "Descriptions of Texas, 1828," *Southwestern Historical Quarterly*, vol. 28 (1925), 104.

4. Matthew C. Field, *Matt Field on the Santa Fe Trail* (Norman: University of Oklahoma Press, 1960), pp. 118, 205.

5. Josiah Gregg, *Commerce of the Prairies: Or the Journal of a Santa Fe Trader, During Eight Expeditions Across the Great Western Prairies, and A Residence of Nearly Nine Years* (New York: Henry G. Langley, 1844), vol. 1, pp. v, 146–8. In the fall of 1845, following the publication of this two-volume work, Gregg enrolled at the University of Louisville medical school, where he studied for two semes-

ters and became a physician. Following the Mexican War, Gregg practiced medicine with Dr. G. M. Prevost in Saltillo, Mexico.

6. Daniel Drake, *A Systematic Treatise, Historical, Etiological, and Practical, on the Principal Diseases of the Interior Valley of North America, as They Appear in the Caucasion* [sic], *African, Indian, and Esquimaux Varieties of Its Population* (Cincinnati: Winthrop B. Smith & Co.; Philadelphia: Grigg, Elliot & Co.; New York: Mason & Law, 1850), pp. 156, 174–75.

7. Elijah White, *Ten Years in Oregon: Travels and Adventures of Doctor E. White and Lady, West of the Rocky Mountains: With Incidents of Two Sea Voyages via the Sandwich Islands Around Cape Horn* (Ithaca, N.Y.: Mack, Andrus, & Co., 1848), p. 317. Compiled by Miss A. J. Allen

8. Francis Parkman, Jr., *The California and Oregon Trail: Being Sketches of Prairie and Rocky Mountain Life* (New York: George P. Putnam, 1849), p. 299.

9. Joseph Williams, "The Joseph Williams Tour," in *The Far West and Rockies Historical Series, 1820–1875*, ed. LeRoy Hafen (Pasadena, Calif.: The Arthur H. Clark Co., 1966), vol. 3, p. 200.

10. Max Greene, *The Kanzas Region: Forest, Prairie, Desert, Mountain, Vale, and River, Descriptions of Scenery, Climate, Wild Productions, Capabilities of Soil, and Commercial Resources* (New York: Fowler and Wells, 1856), pp. 18–19.

11. Maurice O'Connor Morris, *Rambles in the Rocky Mountains: With a Visit to the Gold Fields of Colorado* (London: Smith, Elder and Co., 1864), pp. 88–89.

12. Samuel Bowles, *Across the Continent* (Springfield, Mass.: S. Bowles & Co., 1869), p. 31.

13. Albert D. Richardson, *Beyond the Mississippi: From the Great River to the Great Ocean* (Hartford, Conn.: American Publishing Co., 1867), p. 218.

14. Augustus A. Hayes, Jr., *New Colorado and the Santa Fe Trail* (New York: Harper and Brothers, 1880), p. 184.

15. On August 4, 1901, Dr. Samuel Edwin Solly, M.D., wrote a letter to the "Physicians of Colorado Springs in the year 2000 A.D." The letter was one of many items placed in 1901 in a metal chest that was a time capsule. The chest was sealed with two hundred rivets to make it airtight. When it was opened in the library of Colorado College in Colorado Springs, January 1, 2001, Dr. Solly's letter was found and read.

16. William W. Hibbard, M.D., "The Climate of Arizona," *New York Medical Record*, vol. 43 (January 28, 1893), 111.

17. "Vacation Aspects of Colorado," *Harper's New Monthly Magazine*, vol. 40 (March 1880), 544–45.

18. Billy M. Jones, *Health-Seekers in the Southwest 1817–1900* (Norman: University of Oklahoma Press, 1967), pp. 145–46.

19. Robert Ward, "Climate and Health, with Special Reference to the United States," *The Scientific Monthly*, vol. 12, no. 4 (April 1921), 355.

CHAPTER ELEVEN: MIDWIVES AND WOMEN DOCTORS

1. Eric Stone, *Medicine Among the American Indians* (New York: Hafner Publishing Co., 1962), pp. 72–75. A reprint of the 1932 first edition.

2. Laurel Thatcher Ulrich, *A Midwife's Tale: The Life of Martha Ballard, Based on Her Diary 1785–1812* (New York: Alfred A. Knopf, 1990). Martha Ballard's descendants preserved the diary until 1930, when a great-great-granddaughter

gave it to the Maine State Library. Half a century later, it was rediscovered there by Ulrich, who realized it was a great source of information on midwifery and early New England life.

3. Amalie Kass, "Walter Channing: Brief Life of a Nineteenth-Century Obstetrician, 1786–1876," *Harvard Magazine*, March–April 2004.

4. Selma Harrison Calmes, "Then and Now: The Women of ASA," *ASA Newsletter*, vol. 69, no. 10 (October 2005).

5. Kenneth L. Holmes, ed., *Covered Wagon Women: Diaries & Letters from Western Trails 1840–1890*, vol. 1 (Glendale, Calif.: The Arthur H. Clark Co., 1983), pp. 13–14, 157–87.

6. John W. Bright, M.D., *The Mother's Medical Guide; A Plain, Practical Treatise on Midwifery and the Diseases of Women and Children . . .* (Louisville, Ky.: privately printed, 1844), p. 169.

7. Biographies of Elizabeth Blackwell, M.D., include Rachel Baker's *"The First Woman Doctor"* (New York: Messner, 1944); and Peggy Chambers's *A Doctor Alone . . .* (London and New York: Abelard-Schuman, 1958). See also a sketch of Dr. Blackwell's life by Ira Peck, published by Millbrook Press, Brookfield, Conn., in 2000.

8. "Susan LaFlesche Picotte (1865–1915)," biographical sketch in the files of the Nebraska State Historical Society, Lincoln.

9. Biographical sketch of Susan Anderson provided by the Colorado Women's Hall of Fame, Denver.

10. Biographical sketch of Justina Laurena Carter Ford located in The African American Registry, Minneapolis, Minnesota.

11. Biographical sketch of Sofie Dalia Herzog may be found in *The Handbook of Texas.*

12. Biographical sketches of Ruth E. Newland, Hattie F. Atwater, and Catherine Nicholas Post may be found in the state archives, Carson City, Nevada.

13. Biographical material on Lucy Hobbs Taylor found in the Watkins Community Museum, Lawrence, Kansas.

14. C. A. Loucks, "Sketch of Amy M. Loucks," in the files of the Finney County Historical Society, Garden City, Kansas.

15. "Memoirs of Etta May Lacey Crowder," *Iowa Journal of History and Politics*, vol. 46, no. 2 (April 1948), 156–98.

CHAPTER TWELVE: PATENT MEDICINES

1. George B. Griffenhagen and James Harvey Young, "Old English Patent Medicines in America," *Contributions from the Museum of History and Technology* (Washington, D.C.: Smithsonian Institution, 1959), paper 10.

2. David B. Haycock, "Medicine within the market: proprietary medicines in seventeenth century England." An undated paper. Haycock was a faculty member, Department of Economic History, London School of Economics.

3. Ibid. See also David B. Haycock and Patrick Wallis, eds., *Quackery and Commerce in Seventeenth-Century London: The Proprietary Medicine Business of Anthony Daffy* (London: The Wellcome Trust, University College London, 2005), supp. 25, pp. 18–25.

4. Jim Cox, "That Quacking Sound in Colonial America," *Colonial Williamsburg Journal* (Spring 2004). Available on the Colonial Williamsburg Web site.

5. Haycock and Wallis, eds., *Quackery and Commerce in Seventeenth-Century London*, pp. 20–21.

6. James Harvey Young, *The Toadstool Millionaires: A Social History of Patent Medicines in America Before Federal Regulation* (Princeton, N.J.: Princeton University Press, 1961), pp. 31, 35–36, 42–43.

7. Bill and Betty Wilson, *19th Century Medicine in Glass* (Eau Gallie, Fla.: 19th Century Hobby & Publishing Co., 1971).

8. William D. Naylor interview, Federal Writers Project, 1936–1940, Library of Congress. The interview was conducted in New York City, November 9, 1938. It is available on the Library of Congress Web site.

9. Young, *The Toadstool Millionaires*, pp. 192–93. The history of William and Donald McKay can be found in Frank T. Gilbert's *Historic Sketches of Walla Walla, Whitman, Columbia, and Garfield Counties, Washington Territory, and Umatilla County, Oregon* (Portland, Ore.: Printing House of A. G. Walling, 1882), p. 25.

10. Grace McCune interview, Federal Writers Project, 1936–1940, Library of Congress. The interview was conducted in Athens, Georgia, in February 1939, and is available on the Library of Congress Web site. Efforts to identify the Indian medicine company and its medicine(s) were unsuccessful.

11. Young, *The Toadstool Millionaires*, pp. 193–94.

12. Clement Flynn interview, Federal Writers Project, 1936–1940, Library of Congress. The interview was conducted in Hastings, Nebraska, during the fall of 1938. It is available on the Library of Congress Web site.

13. Lydia E. Pinkham Medicine Company records, Radcliffe College, Harvard University. See also Sarah Stage's biography and study of Mrs. Pinkham's business, titled *Female Complaints: Lydia Pinkham and the Business of Women's Medicine* (New York: W. W. Norton & Co., 1979).

14. Young, *The Toadstool Millionaires*, pp. 145–49.

15. Glenn Poch, *Bottle Collecting Newsletter #816*, March–April 1997. Information on Soule's Kansas investments may be found in the files of the Kansas State Historical Society. See also Jacqueline Kochak, "The Golden Touch of Asa Soule," *American History Illustrated*, vol. 19 (March 1964).

16. The early history of Dr Pepper is hazy. Standard works consulted include: Harry E. Ellis, *Dr Pepper—King of Beverages* (Dallas: Taylor Co., 1979), and Karen Wright's *The Road to Dr Pepper, Texas: The Story of Dublin Dr Pepper* (Abilene: State House Press/McMurry University, 2006). The first Dr Pepper bottling plant was located in Dublin, Texas. *The Handbook of Texas* also provides a sketch of the soft drink's history, written by Patrick Farl.

17. There are numerous histories of Coca-Cola. The author has relied on a historical sketch of the soft drink provided by the Coca-Cola Company.

CHAPTER THIRTEEN: QUACKS

1. James Harvey Young, "American Medical Quackery in the Age of the Common Man," *The Mississippi Valley Historical Review*, vol. 47, no. 4 (March 1961), 583.

2. *Appleton's Cyclopedia of American Biography* (New York: D. Appleton and Co., 1888). See also Madeleine B. Stern, *Heads and Headlines: The Phrenological Fowler* (Norman: University of Oklahoma Press, 1971).

3. Patrick K. Ober, "The Pre-Flexnerian Reports: Mark Twain's Criticism of

Medicine in the United States," *History of Medicine*, vol. 126, no. 2 (January 15, 1997), 157–63.

4. Fielding H. Garrison, "On Quackery as a Reversion to Primitive Medicine," *Bulletin, New York Academy of Medicine* (November 1933), 601–12.

5. Francis J. Shepherd, "Medical Quacks and Quackeries," *Popular Science Monthly* 23 (June 1883), 162.

6. Bob McCoy, *Quack! Tales of Medical Fraud from the Museum of Questionable Medical Devices* (Santa Monica, Calif.: Santa Monica Press, 2000), pp. 49–69.

7. Austin C. Lescarboura, "Our Abrams Verdict: The Electronic Reactions of Abrams and Electronic Medicine in General Found Utterly Worthless," *Scientific American*, September 1924, pp. 131, 158–59.

8. Indiana Supreme Court decision, *Heil Eugene Crum vs. State Board of Medical Registration and Examination*, November 3, 1941.

9. McCoy, *Quack! Tales of Medical Fraud*, pp. 97–114.

10. Ibid., pp. 169–70.

11. Richard W. Schwarz, *John Harvey Kellogg, M.D.* (Nashville, Tenn.: Southern Publishing Association, 1970).

12. A recent biographical sketch of Dr. John Brinkley may be found in Eric S. Juhnke's *Quarks and Crusaders* . . . (Lawrence: University Press of Kansas, 2002), pp. 1–35. Earlier works about Brinkley include Ralph Titus's "John R. Brinkley, The Radio, and the Promised Gland," in *The Prairie Scout*, vol. 5 (Abilene, Kans.: The Kansas Corral of the Westerners, 1985); and Gerald Carson, *The Roguish World of Doctor Brinkley* (New York: Rinehart & Co., 1960).

13. McCoy, *Quack! Tales of Medical Fraud*, pp. 36–63. For Baker's own story, see Alvin Winston's *Doctors, Dynamiters, and Gunmen: The Life Story of Norman Baker* (Muscatine, Iowa: TNT Press, 1936). Baker paid Winston to write the book.

CHAPTER FOURTEEN: INTO THE TWENTIETH CENTURY

1. Mark Twain, *The Autobiography of Mark Twain*, ed. Charles Neider (New York: Harper & Brothers, 1959), pp. 10–11.

2. Abraham Flexner, *Medical Education in the United States and Canada: A Report to the Carnegie Foundation for the Advancement of Teaching*. Bulletin 4. New York: The Carnegie Foundation, 1910.

3. Sir William Osler, "On Full-time Clinical Teaching in Medical Schools," *Canadian Medical Association Journal*, vol. 87, no. 6 (1962), 762–65.

4. Recollections of Leonard J. Dary provided to the author on May 15, 2004.

5. D. W. Cathell, *Book on the Physician Himself and Things That Concern His Reputation and Success*. Baltimore: Cushing and Bailey, 1882. This first edition contained 194 pages. Later editions were longer.

6. Michael A. Shadid, *Crusading Doctor* (Boston: Meador Publishing Co., 1956).

7. Thomas N. Bonner, *The Kansas Doctors: A Century of Pioneering* (Lawrence: University Press of Kansas, 1959), pp. 120–71. See also the files of the Kansas State Historical Society, Topeka, for detailed material on Samuel J. Crumbine.

8. Arthur E. Hertzler, *The Horse and Buggy Doctor* (New York and London: Harper & Brothers, 1938), pp. 313–22.

BIBLIOGRAPHY

ARTICLES

Austin, Stephen F. "Description of Texas, 1828." *Southwestern Historical Quarterly*, vol. 28, no. 2, October 1924.

Barry, Louise. "Charles Robinson—Yankee '49ers: His Journey to California." *Kansas Historical Quarterly*, vol. 34, 1968.

Bill, Joseph H. "Notes on Arrow Wounds." *American Journal of Medical Science*, vol. 44, October 1862.

Blackstock, Ben. "A Special Kind of Man: The Autobiography of Dr. Lindsey L. Long." *Chronicles of Oklahoma*, vol. 77, no. 4, Autumn 1999.

Christopher, G. W., et al. "Biological Warfare, A Historical Perspective." *Journal of the American Medical Association*, vol. 278, no. 5, August 1997.

Clements, Forrest E. "Primitive Concepts of Disease." In *University of California Publications in American Archaeology and Ethnology*, vol. 32, Berkeley, 1932.

Cox, Jim. "The Quacking Sound in Colonial America." *Colonial Williamsburg Journal*, Spring 2004.

Crowder, Etta May Lacey. "Memoirs." *Journal of History and Politics*. Iowa City: State Historical Society of Iowa, vol. 46, no. 2, 1948.

Cutright, Paul. "The Journal of Private Joseph Whitehouse," *Bulletin of the Missouri Historical Society*, vol. 28, no. 3, 1972.

Dandridge, N. P., M.D. "Antoine François Saugrain (De Vigni): The First Scientist of the Mississippi Valley." *Ohio History: The Scholarly Journal of the Ohio Historical Society*. Columbus: Ohio History Society, vol. 15, no. 2, April 1906.

Deutsch, Albert. "The Sick Poor in Colonial Times." *American Historical Review*, vol. 46, no. 3, April 1941.

Dixon, Roland B. "Some Aspects of the American Shaman." *Journal of American Folklore*, vol. 21, no. 80, January–March 1908.

Engers, Rachel. "Anatomy of an Insurrection." *Yale Medicine*. New Haven: Yale University, Spring 2002.

Garrison, Fielding H. "On Quackery as a Reversion to Primitive Medicine." *Bulletin, New York Academy of Medicine*, November 1933.

Hall, Edith Thompson. "The Biography of a Pioneer Nebraska Doctor, John Wesley Thompson." *Nebraska History*, vol. 7, 1926.

Hall, Thomas B. "John Sappington." *Missouri Historical Review*, vol. 24, no. 2, January 1930.

Hibbard, William W., M.D. "The Climate of Arizona." *New York Medical Record*, vol. 43, January 28, 1893.

Kay, Margarita Artschwager. "The Florilegio Medical Source of Southwest Ethnomedicine." *Ethnohistory*, vol. 24, no. 3, Summer 1977.

Kennard, Thomas. "Medicine Among the Indians." *St. Louis Medical and Surgical Journal*, vol. 16, 1858.

Knopf, Richard C., ed. "A Surgeon's Mate at Fort Defiance: The Journal of Joseph Gardner Andrews for the Year 1795." *Ohio History: The Scholarly Journal of the Ohio Historical Society*, vol. 66, no. 1, January 1957.

Leader, Herman A., ed. "Diary of James Douglas." *Oregon Historical Quarterly*, vol. 32, March 1931.

Marshall, Mary Louise. "The Versatile Genius of Daniel Drake." *Bulletin of the Medical Library Association*, vol. 31, no. 4, October 1945.

McKeeby, Lemuel Clarke. "Memoirs." *California History*, vol. 3, 1924.

McPhail, Leonard. "The Diary of Assistant Surgeon Leonard McPhail, on His Journey to the Southwest in 1835." *Chronicles of Oklahoma*, vol. 18, no. 3, 1940.

Meek, Elizabeth M. "Two Pioneer Doctors of Southeast Arkansas." *Arkansas Historical Quarterly*, vol. 5, 1946.

Morrison, E. E., M.D. "Pioneer Medicine in Barton County." *Kansas Historical Quarterly*, vol. 6, no. 4, November 1937.

Ober, Patrick K. "The Pre-Flexnerian Reports: Mark Twain's Criticism of Medicine in the United States." *History of Medicine*, vol. 126, no. 2, January 15, 1997.

Olch, Peter D., M.D. "Medicine in the Indian-Fighting Army, 1866–1890." *Journal of the West*, vol. 21, no. 3, July 1982.

Osler, Sir William, "On Full-Time Clinical Teaching in Medical Schools." *Canadian Medical Association Journal*, vol. 87, no. 6, October 6, 1962.

Othersen, Biemann, Jr. "Ephraim McDowell: The Qualities of a Good Surgeon." *Annals of Surgery*, May 2004.

Otto, Stephen. "Identifying a Family Heirloom: The Indian Doctor's Dispensatory." *Canadian Bulletin of Medical History/Bulletin canadien d'histoire de la médecine*, vol. 12, no. 2, 1995.

Paton, Bruce C., M.D. "Olaf Larsell's 'Medical Aspects of the Lewis and Clark Expedition'—A Commentary." *Wilderness and Environmental Medicine*, vol. 14, no. 4, December 2003.

Peck, P. "Cornelius Ambrose Logan (1832–1899): A Study of the Kansas Physician, Diplomat and Writer." *Journal of the Kansas Medical Society*, March 1968.

Reifschneider, Olga. "Dr. Anderson in Wild and Wooly Carson City, Nevada." *Nevada Highways and Parks*, Fall 1966.

Roberts, Phil. "The Fetterman Hospital Association and Health Care Coverage on the Range in the 1880s." *Montana: Magazine of Western History*, vol. 44, no. 3, 1994.

Scholten, Paul, M.D. "The Origins of the San Francisco Medical Society, 1868–1998." *San Francisco Medicine*, vol. 71, no. 2, February 1998.

Seward, Blanton P. "Pioneer Medicine in Virginia." *Annals of Medical History*, Part 1, vol. 10, no. 1, January 1930.

Sheldon, Addison E. "The Pioneer Doctor." *Nebraska History*, vol. 7, 1926.

Snively, W. D., Jr., and L. Purbee. "Discoverer of the Cause of Milk Sickness (Ann Pierce Hobbs Bixby)." *Journal of the American Medical Association*, June 20, 1966.

Steele, Volney. "Arrow Wounds and the Military Surgeon in the West." *Military History of the West*, vol. 30, Fall 2000.

Sternberg, George M., M.D. "Medicine for the Military: Dr. George M. Sternberg on the Kansas Plains." *Kansas History*, vol. 17, no. 4, 1994.

Stewart, James. "The Diary of James R. Stewart, Pioneer of Osage County." *Kansas Historical Quarterly*, vol. 17, nos. 1–4, 1949.

Stone, Eric, M.D. "Medicine Among the Iroquois." *Annals of Medical History*, N.S., vol. 6, no. 6, November 1936.

Titus, Ralph. "John R. Brinkley, The Radio and the Promised Gland." in *The Prairie Scout*, vol. 5, Abilene, Kans.: Kansas Corral of the Westerners, 1985.

Ward, Robert. "Climate and Health, with Special Reference to the United States." *Scientific Monthly*, vol. 12, no. 4, April 1921.

Webb, Bernice L. "Lady Doctor on a Homestead." *Journal of the West*, vol. 27, October 1988.

West Texas Historical Association Year Book, vol. 7, June 1931.

Wier, James A. "18th Century Army Doctors on the Frontier and in Nebraska. *Nebraska History*, vol. 61, Summer 1980.

Young, James Harvey. "American Medical Quackery in the Age of the Common Man." *Mississippi Valley Historical Review*, vol. 47, no. 4, March 1961.

BOOKS

Appleton's Cyclopedia of American Biography. New York: D. Appleton and Co., 1883.

Ashburn, Frank D. *The Ranks of Death: A Medical History of the Conquest of America by the Late Colonel P. M. Ashburn, Medical Corps, United States Army*. New York: Coward-McCann Inc., 1947.

Bailey, Jack. *A Texas Cowboy's Journal: Up the Trail to Kansas in 1868*. Ed. David Dary. Norman: University of Oklahoma Press, 2006.

Baker, Rachiel. *The First Woman Doctor*. New York: Messner, 1944.

Barlow, Ronald S. *The Vanishing American Outhouse: A History of Country Plumbing*. El Cajon, Calif.: Windmill Publishing Co., 1992.

Bennett, Henry Hollcom, ed. *The Country of Ross: The History of Ross County, Ohio* . . . Madison, Wis.: Selwyn A. Brant, 1902.

Beverley, Robert. *The History and Present State of Virginia*. Chapel Hill: University of North Carolina Press, 1947.

Bloom, Khaled J. *Mississippi Valley's Great Yellow Fever Epidemic of 1878*. Baton Rouge: Louisiana State University Press, 1993.

Bonner, Thomas N. *The Kansas Doctor: A Century of Pioneering*. Lawrence: University Press of Kansas, 1959.

Bowles, Samuel. *Across the Continent*. Springfield, Mass.: S. Bowles & Co., 1869.

Brickell, John. *The Natural History of North-Carolina*. Raleigh, N.C.: Trustees of Public Libraries, 1911. A reprint of the 1717 first edition.

Bright, John W., M.D. *The Mother's Medical Guide: A Plain, Practical Treatise of Midwifery, and the Diseases of Women and Children*. Louisville, Ky.: [printed by A. S. Tilden Jeffersonville, Ind.], 1844.

Bryant, Edwin. *What I Saw in California*. New York: D. Appleton & Co., 1848.

Buchan, William. *Domestic Medicine, or, the Family Physician*. Philadelphia: J. Dunlap, 1772. First published at Edinburgh in 1769.

Burrage, Henry S., ed. *Early English and French Voyages*. New York: Charles Scribner's Sons, 1906.

Byars, William Vincent. *The First Scientist of the Mississippi Valley: A Memoir of the Life and Work of Doctor Antoine François Saugrain*. St. Louis: Benjamin von Puhl, [1903].

Byrne, Bernard James. *A Frontier Army Surgeon: Life in Colorado in the Eighties*. New York: Exposition Press, 1962.

Carrigan, Jo Ann. *The Saffron Scourge: A History of Yellow Fever in Louisiana, 1796–1905*. Lafayette: Center for Louisiana Studies, University of Southwestern Louisiana, 1994.

Carson, Gerald. *The Roguish World of Doctor Brinkley*. New York: Rinehart & Co., 1960.

Carter, Richard. *Valuable Vegetable Medical Prescriptions, for the Cure of All Nervous and Putrid Disorders*. Frankfort, Ky.: Gerard & Berry, 1815. The book was reprinted in Cincinnati in 1830.

Caruso, John Anthony. *The Appalachian Frontier, America's First Surge Westward*. Knoxville: University of Tennessee Press, 2003. A reprint of the 1859 first edition. New introduction by John C. Inscoe.

Catesby, Mark. *The Natural History of Carolina, Florida, and the Bahama Islands*. 2 vols. London: C. Marsh, 1743.

Cathell, D. W. *Book on the Physician Himself and Things That Concern His Reputation and Success*. Baltimore, Md.: Cushing and Bailey, 1892. Other editions were also consulted.

Chambers, Peggy. *A Doctor Alone: A Biography of Elizabeth Blackwell, the First Woman Doctor, 1821–1910*. London & New York: Abelard-Schuman, 1958.

Clark, William. *Dear Brother: Letters of William Clark to Jonathan Clark*. Ed. James J. Holmberg. New Haven: Yale University Press, 2002.

Connelley, William E. *Kansas and Kansans*. 5 vols. Chicago: Lewis Publishing Co., 1919.

Coolidge, R. H. *Statistical Report on the Sickness and Mortality in the Army of the United States . . . 1839 to 1855*. Washington, D.C.: Surgeon General's Office, 1856.

Curtis, Samuel. *A Valuable Collection of Recipes, Medical and Miscellaneous*. Amherst, N.H.: Elijah Mansur, 1819. Another recipe book for home medical use.

Cutler, William. *History of the State of Kansas*. Chicago: A. T. Andreas, 1883.

Dale, Harrison Clifford, ed. *The Ashley-Smith Exploration and the Discovery of a Central Route to the Pacific, 1822–1829*. Glendale, Calif.: The Arthur H. Clark Co., 1941.

Dary, David. *The Santa Fe Trail: Its History, Legends, and Lore*. New York: Alfred A. Knopf, 2000.

———. *True Tales of Old-Time Kansas*. Lawrence: University Press of Kansas, 1984.

Denney, Robert E. *Civil War Medicine: Care & Comfort of the Wounded*. New York: Sterling Publishing Co., 1994.

Dick, Everett. *The Sod-House Frontier 1854–1890*. Lincoln, Neb.: Johnson Publishing Co., 1954.

Doerksen, Clifford J. *American Babel: Rogue Radio Broadcasters of the Jazz Age*. Philadelphia: University of Pennsylvania Press, 2005.

Drake, Daniel. *A Systematic Treatise, Historical, Etiological, and Practical, on the Principal Diseases of the Interior Valley of North America, as They Appear in the Caucasion [sic], African, Indian, and Esquimaux Varieties of the Population*. Cincinnati:

Winthrop B. Smith & Co.; Philadelphia: Grigg Elliot & Co.; New York: Mason & Law, 1850.

Duffy, John. *The Sanitarians: A History of American Public Health.* Urbana and Chicago: University of Illinois Press, 1992.

———. *Sword of Pestilence, The New Orleans Yellow Fever Epidemic of 1853.* Baton Rouge: Louisiana State University Press, 1966.

Ellis, Harry E. *Dr Pepper—King of Beverages.* Dallas: Taylor Co., 1979.

Erwin, Marie H., comp. *Statistical Reports on the Sickness and Mortality of the Army.* Washington, D.C., GPO, 1943.

Ewell, James. *The Planter's and Mariner's Medical Companion.* Philadelphia: John Bioren, 1807.

Field, Matthew C. *Matt Field on the Santa Fe Trail.* Norman: University of Oklahoma Press, 1960.

Flexner, Abraham. *Medical Education in the United States and Canada: A Report to the Carnegie Foundation for the Advancement of Teaching.* Bulletin 4. New York: The Carnegie Foundation, 1910.

Foster, Robert D. *The North American Indian Doctor: Nature's Method of Curing and Preventing Disease According to the Indians . . .* Canton, Ohio: Smith and Bevin, 1838.

Frachere, Gabriel. *Narrative of a Voyage to the Northwest Coast of America in the Years 1811, 1812, 1813, and 1814.* Ed. Milo Milton Quaife. Chicago: Lakeside Press, 1954.

Frémont, J. C. *Report of the Exploring Expedition to the Rocky Mountains in the Year 1842, and to Oregon and North California in the Years 1843–44.* Washington, D.C.: Gales and Seaton, 1845.

Garner, Pierre. *Voyage médical en Californie.* Paris: Chez l'auteur, 1854. This 43-page pamphlet was translated into English and reprinted in 1967.

Gilbert, Frank T. *Historic Sketches of Walla Walla, Whitman, Columbia, and Garfield Counties, Washington Territory, and Umatilla County.* Portland, Ore.: A. G. Walling, 1882.

Gill, Sam D. *Native American Traditions.* Belmont, Calif.: Belmont Publishing Co., 1983.

Gillett, Mary C. *The Army Medical Department 1775–1818.* Washington, D.C.: GPO, 1990.

———. *The Army Medical Department 1818–1865.* Washington, D.C.: GPO, 1987.

———. *The Army Medical Department 1865–1917.* Washington, D.C.: GPO, 1995.

Goldsborough, Carrie Tarleton, and Anna Goldsborough Fisher. *William Loftus Sutton, M.D. 1797–1862: Father of Kentucky State Medical Society and of Kentucky's First Vital Statistics Law.* Lexington, Ky.: The Thoroughbred Press, 1948.

Goodchild, P. *Survival Skills of the North American Indians.* Chicago: Chicago Review Press, 1984.

Greene, Max. *The Kanzas Region: Forest, Prairie, Desert, Mountain, Vale and River, Descriptions of Scenery, Climate, Wild Productions, Capabilities of Soil and Commercial Resources.* New York: Fowler and Wells, 1856.

Gregg, Josiah. *Commerce of the Prairies; Or, the Journal of a Santa Fe Trader, During Eight Expeditions Across the Great Western Prairies, and A Residence of Nearly Nine Years.* 2 vols. New York: Henry G. Langley, 1844.

Griffenhagen, George B., and James Harvey Young. *Old English Patent Medicines in America: Contributions from the Museum of History and Technology.* Washington, D.C.: Smithsonian Institution, 1959.

Hafen, LeRoy R., ed. *The Far West and Rockies Historical Series, 1820–1873.* 15 vols. Pasadena, Calif.: The Arthur H. Clark Co., 1954–1961.

———. *The Mountain Men and the Fur Trade of the Far West.* 10 vols. Glendale, Calif.: The Arthur H. Clark Co., 1965–1972.

Hall, Thomas B., Jr., and Thomas B. Hall III. *Dr. John Sappington of Saline County, Missouri, 1776–1856.* Arrow Rock, Mo.: The Friends of Arrow Rock, Inc., 1975.

Hastings, Lansford Warren. *The Emigrants' Guide to Oregon and California . . .* Cincinnati: George Conklin, 1845.

Haycock, David B., and Patrick Wallis, eds. *Quackery and Commerce in Seventeenth-Century London: The Proprietary Medicine Business of Anthony Daffy.* London: Welcome Trust, University College London, 2005, supplement 25.

Hayes, Augustus A., Jr. *New Colorado and the Santa Fe Trail.* New York: Harper & Brothers, 1880.

Hendrick, Willene, and George Hendrick. *On the Illinois Frontier: Dr. Hiram Rutherford, 1840–1848.* Carbondale and Edwardsville: Southern Illinois University Press, 1981.

Henry, Alexander. *New Light on the Early History of the Northwest: The Manuscript Journals of Alexander Henry . . .* Ed. Elliott Coues. Minneapolis, Minn.: Ross & Haines, 1965.

Henry, Stuart. *Conquering Our Great American Plains.* New York: Dutton, 1930.

Hertzler, Arthur E., M.D. *The Horse and Buggy Doctor.* New York: Harper & Brothers, 1938.

Hohmann, Johan Georg. *The Long Lost Friend: A Collection of Mysterious and Invaluable Arts and Remedies . . . which appeared in print for the first time in 1820.* Harrisburg, Pa.: T. F. Scheffer, 1856. Originally published in German about 1826. This is the first American edition in English. Contains a collection of folk remedies, and became known as the "Pow-Wow Book."

Holmes, Kenneth L., comp. *Covered Wagon Women: Diaries and Letters from the Western Trails 1840–1890.* 11 vols. Spokane, Wash.: The Arthur H. Clark Co., 1983–1993.

Horsman, Reginald. *William Beaumont: America's First Great Medical Scientist.* Columbia: University of Missouri Press, 1996.

Hoyt, Henry F. *A Pioneer Doctor.* Boston and New York: Houghton Mifflin Co., 1929.

Hume, Edgar Erskine. *Ornithologists of the United States Army Medical Corps.* Baltimore, Md.: Johns Hopkins University Press, 1942.

Hurt, R. Douglas. *The Ohio Frontier: Crucible of the Old Southwest 1720–1830.* Bloomington and Indianapolis: Indiana University Press, 1996.

Jackson, Donald, ed. *Letters of the Lewis and Clark Expedition, with Related Documents 1783–1854.* 2 vols. Urbana: University of Illinois Press, 1978.

[James, Edwin.] *From Pittsburgh to the Rocky Mountains: Major Stephen Long's Expedition 1819–1820.* Ed. Maxine Benson. Golden, Colo.: Fulcrum, 1988.

James, George Wharton. *What the White Race May Learn from the Indians.* Chicago: Forbes & Co., 1908.

Johnson, Alice M., ed. *Saskatchewan Journals and Correspondence: Edmonton House 1796–1800, Chesterfield House 1800–1862.* London: Hudson's Bay Record Society, 1967.

Jones, Billy M. *Health-Seekers in the Southwest 1817–1900.* Norman: University of Oklahoma Press, 1967.

Jones, J. Roy. *Memories, Men and Medicine: A History of Medicine in Sacramento, California.* Sacramento, Calif.: Society for Medical Improvement, 1950.

Juhnke, Eric S. *Quacks and Crusaders: The Fabulous Careers of John Brinkley, Norman Baker, and Harry Hoxsey.* Lawrence: University Press of Kansas, 2002.

Kessell, John L. *Kiva, Cross, and Crown.* Albuquerque: University of New Mexico Press, 1977.

Krieger, Alex D. *We Came Naked and Barefoot: The Journey of Cabeza de Vaca Across North America.* Austin: University of Texas Press, 2002.

Lane, Levi. *The Old Indian Practice, or Botanic Family Physician* . . . Gustavus, Ohio: published by the author, 1849.

Lawson, John. *Lawson's History of North Carolina.* Richmond, Va.: Garrett & Massie, 1937. A reprint of the 1714 first edition.

Lederer, John. *The Discoveries of John Lederer, in three several Marches from Virginia, to the West of Carolina* . . . London: Printed by J.C. for Samuel Heyrick, at Grays-Inne-gate in Holborn, 1672. Lederer's narrative was translated from the Latin by Sir William Talbot, Baronet.

Lee, R. Alton. *The Bizarre Careers of John R. Brinkley.* Lexington: University Press of Kentucky, 2002.

Lord, Israel Shipman Pelton. *At the Extremity of Civilization: A Meticulously Descriptive Diary of an Illinois Physician's Journey in 1849 Along the Oregon Trail to the Goldmines and Cholera of California* . . . Jefferson, N.C.: McFarland Co., 1995.

Mackenzie, Alexander. *The Journals and Letters of Sir Alexander Mackenzie.* Ed. W. Kaye Lamb. London: Cambridge University Press, 1970.

Mahoney, Jas. W. *The Cherokee Physician; or, Indian Guide to Health* . . . New York: James M. Edney, 1857.

Malin, James C. *Doctors, Devils and the Women of Fort Scott, Kansas 1870–1890.* Lawrence, Kans.: Coronado Press, 1975.

Mansfield, Joseph K. F. *Mansfield on the Condition of the Western Forts, 1853–54.* Ed. Robert W. Frazer. Norman: University of Oklahoma Press, 1963.

Mattes, Merrill J. *Platte River Road Narratives.* Urbana: University of Illinois Press, 1988.

McCauley, James. *A Stove-Up Cowboy's Story.* Austin and Dallas: Texas Folklore Society and University Press, 1943.

McCoy, Bob. *Quack! Tales of Medical Fraud from the Museum of Questionable Medical Devices.* Santa Monica, Calif.: Santa Monica Press, 2000.

McKay, R. H. *Little Pills: An Army Story.* Pittsburg, Kans.: Pittsburg Headlight, 1918.

McLoughlin, John. *Letters of Dr. John McLoughlin, Written at Fort Vancouver 1829–1832.* Ed. Burt Brown Barker. Portland: Oregon Historical Society, [1948].

McNamara, Brooks. *Step Right Up.* Garden City, N.Y.: Doubleday, 1976.

Meyers, C. *Narratives of Early Pennsylvania, West New Jersey, and Delaware, 1630–1707.* New York: Charles Scribner's Sons, 1912.

Mobley, Denise. *Daniel Drake, M.D.: Frontiersman of the Mind.* Cincinnati, Ohio: University of Cincinnati, 1985.

Moore, H. Miles. *Early History of Leavenworth City and County.* Leavenworth, Kans.: Sam'l Dodsworth Book Co., 1906.

Morgan, Dale, ed. *Overland in 1846: Diaries and Letters of the California-Oregon Trail.* 2 vols. Lincoln: University of Nebraska Press, 1993.

Morris, Maurice O'Connor. *Rambles in the Rocky Mountains: With a Visit to the Gold Fields of Colorado.* London: Smith, Elder and Co., 1964.

Moulton, Gary E., ed. *The Journals of the Lewis and Clark Expedition.* 13 vols. Lincoln: University of Nebraska Press, 1983–2000.

National Library of Medicine. *Medicine on the Early Western Frontier.* Washington, D.C.: National Library of Medicine, 1978. A 12-page illustrated exhibition program.

Ney, Virgil. *Fort on the Prairie: Fort Atkinson, on the Council Bluff 1819–1827.* Washington, D.C.: Command Publications, 1978.

Nute, Grace Lee. *The Voyageur.* New York and London: D. Appleton and Co., 1931.

Parker, Rev. Samuel. *Journal of the Exploring Tour Beyond the Rocky Mountains . . .* Ithaca, N.Y.: published by the author, 1838.

Parkman, Francis, Jr., *The California and Oregon Trail: Being Sketches of Prairie and Rocky Mountain Life.* New York: George P. Putnam, 1949.

Perrone, Robette, H. Henrietta Stockel, and Victoria Krueger. *Medicine Women, Curanderas, and Women Doctors.* Norman: University of Oklahoma Press, 1989.

Phillips, Paul C. *Medicine in the Making of Montana.* Missoula: Montana State University Press, 1962.

Pike, Zebulon M. *The Journals of Zebulon Montgomery Pike, with Letters and Related Documents.* 2 vols. Ed. Donald Jackson. Norman: University of Oklahoma Press, 1966.

Pudney, John. *The Smallest Room: A Discreet Survey Through the Ages.* London: Michael Joseph, 1954.

Quebbeman, Francis E. *Medicine in Territorial Arizona.* Phoenix: Arizona Historical Foundation, 1966.

Rath, Ida Ellen. *Early Ford County.* North Newton, Kans.: Mennonite Press, 1964.

Reifschneider, Olga. *Biographies of Nevada Botanists 1844–1963.* Reno: University of Nevada Press, 1964.

Richardson, Albert D. *Beyond the Mississippi: From the Great River to the Great Ocean.* Hartford, Conn.: American Publishing Co., 1867.

———. *Our New States and Territories, Being Notes of a Recent Tour of Observation Through Colorado, Utah, Idaho, Nevada, Oregon, Montana, Washington Territory and California.* New York: Beadle, 1866.

Rister, Carl Coke. *Southern Plainsmen.* Norman: University of Oklahoma Press, 1938.

Rivers, W. H. R. *Medicine, Magic, and Religion: The Fitzpatrick Lectures Delivered Before the Royal College of Physicians of London in 1915 and 1916.* London: Kegan Paul, Trench, Trubner & Co., Ltd., 1927.

Robinson, Doane. *History of South Dakota.* 2 vols. Aberdeen: B. F. Bower & Co., 1904.

Rothstein, William G. *American Physicians in the Nineteenth Century from Sects to Science.* Baltimore and London: The Johns Hopkins University Press, 1972.

Rouse, Parke, Jr. *The Great Wagon Road from Philadelphia to the South.* Richmond, Va.: The Dietz Press, 2004. A reprint of the 1973 first edition published in the Great American Trails Series by McGraw-Hill.

Rush, Benjamin. *An Inquiry into the Natural History of Medicine Among the Indians,*

An Oration. Philadelphia: Joseph Cruikshank, 1774. A lecture delivered by Dr. Rush before the American Philosophical Society in Philadelphia, February 4, 1774.

St. Clair County History. Philadelphia: Brink, McDonough and Co., 1881.

Scharf, J. Thomas. *A History of St. Louis City and County.* 2 vols. Philadelphia: L. H. Everts & Co., 1883.

Schwarz, Richard W. *John Henry Kellogg, M.D.* Nashville, Tenn.: Southern Publishing Association, 1970.

See, Lisa. *On Gold Mountain: The One-Hundred-Year Odyssey of a Chinese-American Family.* New York: St. Martin's Press, 1995.

Shadid, Michael A., M.D. *Crusading Doctor.* Boston: Meador Publishing Co., 1956.

Shikes, R. H. *Rocky Mountain Medicine: Doctors, Drugs, and Disease in Early Colorado.* Boulder, Colo.: Johnson Books, 1986.

Smith, Peter. *The Indian Doctor's Dispensatory, Being Father Smith's Advice Respecting Diseases and Their Cure* . . . Cincinnati: printed by Browne and Looker, for the author, 1913. This work was reprinted several times under slightly different titles.

Sohn, Anton Paul. *A Saw, Pocket Instruments, and Two Ounces of Whiskey: Frontier Military Medicine in the Great Basin.* Spokane, Wash.: The Arthur H. Clark Co., 1998.

Stage, Sarah. *Female Complaints: Lydia Pinkham and the Business of Women's Medicine.* New York: W. W. Norton & Co., 1979.

Stern, Madeleine B. *Heads and Headlines: The Phrenological Fowler.* Norman: University of Oklahoma Press, 1971.

Stone, Eric, M.D. *Medicine Among the American Indians.* New York: Hafner Publishing Co., 1962. A reprint of the 1932 first edition.

Stratton, Owen Tully. *Medicine Man.* Ed. Owen S. Stratton. Norman: University of Oklahoma Press, 1989.

Tanner, Karen Holliday. *Doc Holliday: A Family Portrait.* Norman: University of Oklahoma Press, 1998.

[Tennent, John.] *Every Man His Own Doctor; Or, The Poor Planter's Physician* . . . Williamsburg and Annapolis: Wil. Parks, 1736.

Tyler, Sgt. Daniel. *A Concise History of the Mormon Battalion in the Mexican War.* Glorieta, N.M.: Rio Grande Press, 1969. The work was first published in 1881.

Tyrrell, J. B., ed. *Journals of Samuel Hearne and Philip Turnor.* New York: Greenwood Press, 1968.

Ulrich, Laurel Thatcher. *A Midwife's Tale: The Life of Martha Ballard Based on Her Diary 1785–1812.* New York: Alfred A. Knopf, 1990.

Unruh, John D., Jr. *The Plains Across.* Urbana: University of Illinois Press, 1979.

Vogel, Virgil J. *American Indian Medicine.* Norman: University of Oklahoma Press, 1970.

Wallace, Anthony F. C. *Jefferson and the Indians: The Tragic Fate of the First Americans.* Cambridge, Mass.: The Belknap Press of Harvard University Press, 1999.

Walsh, James J. *The Story of the Cures That Fail.* New York: Appleton, 1923.

Watkins, Albert, ed. *Publications of the Nebraska State Historical Society.* Lincoln: Nebraska State Historical Society, 1922.

Wayman, Dr. John Hudson. *A Doctor on the California Trail: The Diary of Dr. John Hudson Wayman from Cambridge City, Indiana, to the Gold Fields in 1852.* Ed. Edgeley Woodman Todd. Denver: Old West Publishing Co., 1971.

Weiss, G., and S. Weiss. *The Healing Herbs.* New York: Wings Books, 1985.

Wesley, John. *Primitive Physic; Or, an Easy and Natural Method of Curing Most Diseases.* London: John Mason, 1836.

White, Elijah. *Ten Years in Oregon: Travels and Adventures of Doctor E. White and Lady, West of the Rocky Mountains: With Incidents of Two Sea Voyages via Sandwich Islands Around Cape Horn.* Ithaca, N.Y.: Andrus & Co., 1848.

Wilbur, C. Keith, M.D. *Civil War Medicine.* Old Saybrook, Conn.: Globe Pequot Press, 1994.

Wilson, Bill and Betty. *19th Century Medicine in Glass.* Eau Gallie, Fla.: 19th Century Hobby and Publishing Co., 1971.

Winston, Alvin. *Doctors, Dynamiters, and Gunmen: The Life Story of Norman Baker.* Muscatine, Iowa: TNT Press, 1936.

WPA Medical Historical Research Project. *Medicine and Its Development in Kentucky.* Louisville, Ky.: The Standard Printing Co., 1949.

Wright, Karen. *The Road to Dr Pepper, Texas: The Story of Dublin Dr Pepper.* Abilene, Tex.: State House Press & McMurry University, 2006.

Wright, Robert M. *Dodge City: The Cowboy Capital and the Great Southwest.* Wichita, Kans.: published by the author, 1913.

Young, James Harvey. *The Medical Messiahs: A Social History of Health Quackery in Twentieth-Century America.* Princeton, N.J.: Princeton University Press, 1967.

———. *The Toadstool Millionaires: A Social History of Patent Medicines in America Before Federal Regulation.* Princeton, N.J.: Princeton University Press, 1961.

COURT DOCUMENT

Indiana Supreme Court decision, *Heil Eugene Crum vs. State Board of Medical Registration and Examination,* November 3, 1941.

GOVERNMENT DOCUMENTS

Moore, Samuel P. "Sanitary Report from Fort Laramie." *Executive Document No. 96, 34th Congress,* Washington, D.C., 1855.

[Robinson, John Hamilton.] Diplomatic Records: A Select Catalog of the National Archives. Microfilm Publications Part 2: General Records of The Department of State, Record Group 59, Records Relating to Special Agents.

WPA FEDERAL WRITERS PROJECT INTERVIEWS, 1936–1940, LIBRARY OF CONGRESS

William D. Baylor in New York City.

Edith L. Crawford in Carrizozo, New Mexico.

Clement Flynn in Hastings, Nebraska.

Grace McCune in Athens, Georgia.

Mrs. A. M. Woodward in Bosqueville, Texas.

OTHER DOCUMENTS, RECORDS, AND PAPERS

"A Collection of Letters Written by the Scholl Family and Their Kin (1836–1897)," Jackson County Historical Society Research Library and Archives, Independence, Missouri.

Anderson, Dr. Susan, biographical sketch provided by the Colorado Women's Hall of Fame, Denver.

A Report of Surgical Cases Treated in the Army of the United States from 1865 to 1871. Washington, D.C.: Government Printing Office, 1871. Issued by the U.S. Army Surgeon General's Office.

Atwater, Dr. Hattie F., biographical sketch in the state archives, Carson City, Nevada.

Billington, Ray Allen. *Words That Won the West 1830–1850.* A published address before the Conference of the Public Relations Society of America, Fairmont Hotel, San Francisco, November 18, 1963.

Caldwell, Dr. Augustus B. His material is found in "A Collection of Letters Written by the Scholl Family and Their Kin (1836–1837)," Jackson County Historical Society Research Library and Archives, Independence, Missouri.

Dickinson County (Kansas) Historical Society. Materials on early Abilene physicians.

Ford, Dr. Justina Laurena Carter, biographical sketch in The African American Registry, Minneapolis, Minnesota.

Herzog, Sofie Dalia, biographical sketch in *The Handbook of Texas.*

Lydia E. Pinkham Medicine Co. records, Radcliffe College, Harvard University.

Newland, Dr. Ruth E., biographical sketch in the state archives, Carson City, Nevada.

Post, Catherine Nicholas, biographical sketch in the state archives, Carson City, Nevada.

Ravenholt, Reimert Thorolf, M.D., M.P.H. "Underlying Cause of Death of Meriwether Lewis." Paper presented to "The Medical History of the American West Conference," Montana State University, Museum of the Rockies, Bozeman, Montana, October 24, 2001.

Rush, Dr. Benjamin. "Questions for Meriwether Lewis." Thomas Jefferson Foundation, Inc., Monticello, Virginia.

St. Louis (Missouri) Genealogical Society, Earl Fischer database containing information on nearly 30,000 early residents of St. Louis.

Taylor, Dr. Lucy Hobbs, biographical material provided by the Watkins Community Museum, Lawrence, Kansas.

MANUSCRIPTS

Cory, Dr. Benjamin. Journal manuscript, Society of California Pioneers, San Francisco.

Flint, Dr. Thomas, Diary, Bancroft Library, University of California, Berkeley.

Haycock, David B. "Medicine within the market proprietary, Medicines in Seventeenth Century England." Undated paper in the files of the Dept. of Economic History, London School of Economics.

"History of Coca-Cola," Coca-Cola Co., Atlanta, Georgia.

Little, Thelphilus. "Early Days in Abilene." Unpublished manuscript in the files of the Dickinson County (Kansas) Historical Society, Abilene.

Loucks, Amy M. "Sketch of Amy M. Loucks" by C. A. Loucks, in the files of the Finney County Historical Society, Garden City, Kansas.

National Park Service. "Biography of Dr. Antoine Saugrain," St. Louis: NPS, Jefferson National Expansion Memorial, n.d.

Parke, Charles R., Jr. "California Log Book," original manuscript, Henry E. Huntington Library, San Marino, California.

Picotte, Susan LaFlesche (1865–1915), biographical sketch in the files of the Nebraska State Historical Society, Lincoln.

"Sketch of Amy M. Loucks" by C. A. Loucks is in the files of the Finney County Historical Society, Garden City, Kansas.

LETTERS

Ayres, Dr. Samuel Matthias. Manuscript collection. University of Missouri and Missouri State Historical Society, Columbia, 1850.

Dary, Leonard J., to author, May 15, 2004.

Dr. George W. Beinecke Davis Library, Yale University, 1850.

Kidwell, Clara Sue, Ph.D., director, Native American Studies Program, University of Oklahoma, to author, April 1, 2004.

Rush, Dr. Benjamin, to Meriwether Lewis, June 11, 1803. Thomas Jefferson Papers Series 1, General Correspondence, 1751–1827, Library of Congress, image 570.

Solly, Samuel Edwin, M.D., letter written in 1901 and addressed to the "Physicians of Colorado Springs in the year 2000 A.D." Removed from a time capsule in Colorado Springs, January 1, 2001.

MAGAZINES

"Diary of Dr. Jonathan Clark: Crossing the Plains." *The Argonaut*, San Francisco, August 1925.

" 'Doctor' Lewis' Thunderclappers." *Smithsonian*, June 2004.

Kass, Amalie. "Walter Channing: Brief Life of a Nineteenth-Century Obstetrician, 1786–1878." *Harvard Magazine*, March–April 2004.

Kochak, Jacqueline. "The Golden Touch of Asa Soule." *American History Illustrated*, vol. 19, March 1964.

Lescarboura, Austin C. "Our Abrams Verdict: The Electronic Reactions of Abrams and Electronic Medicine in General Found Utterly Worthless." *Scientific American*, September 1924.

Olch, Peter D., M.D. "Western Americana: Tracking Frontier Medicine." *AB Bookman's Weekly*, October 9, 1989.

Shepherd, Francis J. "Medical Quacks and Quackeries." *Popular Science Monthly*, June 1883.

"Vacation Aspects of Colorado." *Harper's New Monthly Magazine*, vol. 40, March 1880.

NEWSPAPERS

Columbus (Ohio) *Dispatch*, October 2 through November 14, 1849.

Cuthbertson, Gilbert. "Active Leavenworth Doctors Were Prominent in Early Days," *University Daily Kansan*, Lawrence, June 23, 1959.

Musgrave, Jon. "Anna Bixby: In Search of the Real Frontier Medicine Woman," *The Daily Register* (Harrisburg, Ill.), May 21, 2005.

New Teller (York, Neb.), February 5, 1913.

Salter, Jim. "Did Sacagawea Have a Miscarriage?," The Associated Press, April 10, 2005. Report on findings by historians Peter Kastor and Conevery Bolton Valencius of Washington University, St. Louis.

Simmons, Marc. "Francisco Xavier Romero: Too Colorful to Overlook in Local History, *The Santa Fe New Mexican*, September 4, 2004.

NEWSLETTERS

Calmes, Selma Harrison. "Then and Now: The Women of ASA," *ASA Newsletter*, vol. 69, no. 10, October 2005.
Poch, Glenn. *Bottle Collecting Newsletter #816*, March–April 1997.

ACKNOWLEDGMENTS

Many people have helped in researching and writing this work. Special thanks go to writer and physician Don Coldsmith, M.D.; writer Robert Conley, a Cherokee Indian whose research and writing have dealt with Indian medicine; Clara Sue Kidwell, Ph.D., of the University of Oklahoma; historian and writer Mark Gardner; the late Sam Arnold of Colorado; Mary Olch, widow of Peter D. Olch, M.D., an authority on the medical history of the American West; and Steve Hanley, who first suggested I tackle a book on frontier medicine.

Thanks also to those institutions whose files contained the illustrations used, including the Kansas State Historical Society, the Missouri Historical Society, the Western History Collections in the University of Oklahoma Libraries, the Illinois Historical Society, the Utah State Historical Society, the State Historical Society of North Dakota, the Texas State Historical Association and the Texas State Library and Archives in Austin, the University of North Carolina Libraries, the John Wesley House and Museum of Methodism and the Florence Nightingale Museum in London, in the West Midlands of England the University of Birmingham Special Collections, the National Library of Medicine at Bethesda, Maryland, and in nearby Washington, D.C., the Library of Congress, National Archives, National Portrait Gallery of the Smithsonian Institution, the White House Historical Association, and the National Park Service. In Pennsylvania there are the University of Pennsylvania Archives, Carpenters' Hall, the Pennsylvania Historical Society, and the Independence National Historic Park in Philadelphia.

On the West Coast: Lane Medical Library at Stanford, Oregon State Archives, Jedediah Strong Smith Collection at the University of the Pacific, California State Library, Bancroft Library at Berkeley, the San Diego Historical Society, and the Kelton Foundation of San Monica. Thanks also to McDowell House Museum in Danville, Kentucky, the Dykes Library at the University of Kansas Medical Center, Wood Library Museum of Anesthesiology at Park Ridge, Illinois, University of Missouri at Columbia, University of Denver Press, Canadian Ministry of Natural Resources and the National Archives of Canada in Ottawa, Pikes Peak Library District, Mark L. Gardner of Cascade, Colorado, Marcus Kaar of Vienna, Austria, the Schlesinger Library–Radcliffe Institute at Harvard University, the Colorado Women's Hall of Fame, American Institute of the History of Pharmacy at Madison, Wisconsin, and the Lewis Walpole Library at Yale University.

I would be remiss if I did not acknowledge the many physicians and others connected with medicine who through the years put down their recollections in books and papers as medicine in America evolved. Without their contributions this work would not have been possible. Appreciation also goes to the authors of other works listed in the bibliography.

INDEX

PATRIOT PIRATES
The Privateer War for Freedom and Fortune in
the American Revolution
by Robert H. Patton

American privateering—essentially legalized piracy—began with a ragtag squadron of New England schooners in 1775. It quickly erupted into a massive seaborne insurgency of money-mad patriots plundering Britain's maritime trade throughout the Atlantic. Patton's extensive research brings to life the extraordinary adventures of privateers as they hammered the British economy, infuriated the Royal Navy, and humiliated the crown.

History/978-0-307-39055-4

BLOOD AND THUNDER
The Epic Story of Kit Carson and
the Conquest of the American West
by Hampton Sides

At the center of this sweeping tale is Kit Carson, the trapper, scout, and soldier whose adventures made him a legend. Sides shows us how this illiterate mountain man understood and respected the Western tribes better than any other American, yet willingly followed orders that would ultimately devastate the Navajo nation. Rich in detail and spanning more than three decades, this is an essential addition to our understanding of how the West was won.

History/Biography/978-1-4000-3110-8

BUFFALO BILL'S AMERICA
William Cody and the Wild West Show
by Louis S. Warren

William F. "Buffalo Bill" Cody was the most famous American of his age. He claimed to have worked for the Pony Express when only a boy and to have scouted for General George Custer. But what was his real story? And how did a frontiersman become a worldwide celebrity? This definitive biography reveals the genius of America's greatest showman, and the startling history of the American West that drove him to the world stage.

Biography/978-0-375-72658-3

LEWIS AND CLARK THROUGH INDIAN EYES
Nine Indian Writers on the Legacy of the Expedition
by Alvin M. Josephy, Jr.

At the heart of this landmark collection of essays rests a single question: What impact, good or bad, did Lewis and Clark's journey have on the Indians whose homelands they traversed? The nine writers in this volume each provide their own unique answers; from Pulitzer Prize–winner N. Scott Momaday, who offers a haunting essay evoking the voices of the past; to Roberta Conner's comparisons of the explorer's journals with the accounts of the expedition passed down to her. Incisive and compelling, these essays shed new light on our understanding of this landmark journey into the American West.

History/978-1-4000-7749-6

FAITH AND BETRAYAL
A Pioneer Woman's Passage in the American West
by Sally Denton

In the 1850s, Jean Rio, a deeply spiritual widow, was moved by the promises of Mormon missionaries and set out from England for Utah. Traveling across the Atlantic by steamer, up the Mississippi by riverboat, and westward by wagon, Rio kept a detailed diary of her extraordinary journey. In *Faith and Betrayal*, Sally Denton, an award-winning journalist and Rio's great-great-granddaughter, uses the long-lost diary to re-create Rio's experience. Unusually intimate and full of vivid detail, this is an absorbing story of a quintessential American pioneer.

Biography/History/978-1-4000-3473-4

VINTAGE BOOKS / ANCHOR BOOKS
Available at your local bookstore, or visit
www.randomhouse.com